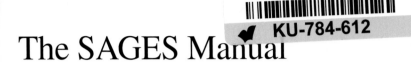

# The SAGES Manual

## Volume 1 Basic Laparoscopy and Endoscopy

Third Edition

Nathaniel J. Soper, MD
Northwestern University Feinberg School of Medicine, Chicago, IL, USA

and

Carol E.H. Scott-Conner, MD, PhD
University of Iowa Hospitals and Clinics, Iowa City, IA, USA

Editors

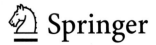 Springer

*Editors*
Nathaniel J. Soper
Department of Surgery
Northwestern University Feinberg
School of Medicine
Chicago, IL, USA

Carol E.H. Scott-Conner
Department of Surgery
University of Iowa Hospitals
and Clinics
Iowa City, IA, USA

ISBN 978-1-4614-2343-0      e-ISBN 978-1-4614-2344-7
DOI 10.1007/978-1-4614-2344-7
Springer New York Dordrecht Heidelberg London

Library of Congress Control Number: 2012932411

Printed on acid-free paper

Springer is part of Springer Science+Business Media (www.springer.com)

# Foreword

As the Society of American Gastrointestinal and Endoscopic Surgeons completes its 30th year, our commitment to education burns as brightly as ever. The first SAGES manual was published in 1998. Since then, it has continued to be a well-organized, clear, and to the point reference in minimally invasive surgery written by experts in the field and aimed at the surgical resident. That said, it will also be useful to students and attending surgeons alike. This third addition of the SAGES manual reflects the best of what has been a leading reference in minimally invasive surgery yet at the same time incorporating many new concepts that have evolved since the second addition. This is mirrored by the tireless efforts of Carol E.H. Scott Connor, MD who has overseen this project since its inception and the addition of Ninh T. Nguyen, MD and Nathanial (Nat) Soper, MD as editors of the third edition. Together, this team has organized this brilliant reference in the field of minimally invasive surgery.

Surgical residents and practicing surgeons will find this addition completely reorganized as the field of minimally invasive surgery continues to grow. Dividing the manual into two volumes allows for a convenient method of keeping it handy as well as reorganizing this book into basic (volume 1) and advanced procedures (volume 2). Students of history, who recall that SAGES' roots grew out of flexible endoscopy, will also no doubt notice the increasing prominence of flexible endoscopy in this manual. This reflects the rise in interest of *surgeon* performed endoscopy as a therapeutic tool complementing other MIS techniques. Surgical residents interested in a career in gastrointestinal surgery should pay close attention to the increasing role that the endoscope will play in their future. While the first two chapters of this edition of the SAGES manual highlight the roles of the Fundamentals of Laparoscopic Surgery (FLS) and Maintenance of Certification (MOC) in the educational process, future editions will clearly also include information on the Fundamentals of Endoscopic Surgery (FES) and other key offerings as well.

Even as this book comes to press, controversies concerning optimal treatment strategies continue to swirl as issues of endoluminal therapies, surgical robotics, and natural orifice translumenal endoscopic surgery (NOTES) are debated around the world. Even the issue concerning the optimal number and size(s) of trocars in our bread and butter commodity procedure such as laparoscopic cholecystectomy remains unsettled. Clearly we should get working on the fourth edition.

I have recently been asked if medical texts are destined for the same desolate fate as ice boxes, typewriters, and mimeographs in the annals of history, all supplanted by newer technologies. Clearly, the organization of medical information is evolving rapidly with so much information now available at our fingertips in digital form. The available "infostream" is coming at us like water spouting wildly from a fire hose, but amidst all that data, where do we find truly useful information concisely organized? I suspect it will be in places such as the SAGES Manual, and yes, this reference too will be available in a digital format for those who wish to abandon paper altogether.

Whether on paper or in a digital format, I am sure that you will enjoy using this reference (at least until the next edition comes out).

*Steven D. Schwaitzberg, MD*
SAGES President 2011–2012
Cambridge, MA, USA

# Preface

In creating this third edition of *The SAGES Manual*, we have completely restructured, reorganized, and revised the entire manual. Rather than put the manual on a diet, we have separated it into two volumes for better portability. Volume 1 covers the fundamentals and procedures performed during surgical residency. We anticipate that Volume 1 will be the first volume used by students, residents, and allied health-care professional trainees, do not be deceived, however; we have added material to these fundamentals and procedures that should also be of interest to experienced surgeons. Volume 2 covers more advanced procedures, generally taught during fellowship. If you own an old, dog-eared copy of the second edition, you will find much that is new in both volumes.

All of the sections have been reorganized with a critical eye to the needs of the modern minimal access surgeon. Two new editors have been added. Although many chapters have new authors, many stalwart authors have continued to contribute. We have also added color photographs.

As before, the manual strives to strike a balance between completeness and conciseness. Significant additional information, including videos, is available from the SAGES Web site (see Appendix, at the end of Volume 1). But, as always, we want you to think of this manual as a way to take SAGES experts along with you throughout your surgical journey.

*Nathaniel J. Soper*
Saint Louis, MO, USA
*Ninh T. Nguyen*
Orange, CA, USA
*Carol E.H. Scott-Conner*
Iowa City, IA, USA

# Contents

**Part I  Basic Laparoscopy and Endoscopy:
General Principles**

## Part II    Diagnostic Laparoscopy and Biopsy

## Part III    Laparoscopic Cholecystectomy and Common
##             Duct Exploration

## Part IV    Basic Laparoscopic Gastric Surgery

## Part V    Basic Laparoscopic Procedures
## of the Small Intestine, Appendix, Colon

## Part VI    Hernia Repair

## Part X    Flexible Endoscopy: Basic Lower
             Gastrointestinal Endoscopy

# Contributors

*Sajida Ahad, MD*
Department of Surgery, Southern Illinois University
School of Medicine, Springfield, IL, USA

*Mohan C. Airan, MD, FACS*
Advocate Good Samaritan Hospital, Lombard, IL, USA

*Richard A. Alexander Jr., MD*
Department of General Surgery, South East Baptist Hospital,
San Antonio, TX, USA

*Maurice E. Arregui, MD*
Department of General Surgery, St. Vincent's Hospital and Healthcare
Center, Indianapolis, IN, USA

*Michael M. Awad, MD, PhD, FACS*
Section of Minimally Invasive Surgery, Division of General Surgery,
Department of Surgery, Washington University in St. Louis
School of Medicine, St. Louis, MO, USA

*Aman Banerjee, MD*
Department of Surgery, University Hospitals Case Medical Center,
Cleveland, OH, USA

*William C. Beck, MD*
Department of Surgery, Vanderbilt University Medical Center,
Nashville, TN, USA

*James G. Bittner IV, MD*
Department of Surgery, Medical College of Georgia
School of Medicine, Augusta, GA, USA

*David M. Brams, MD*
Department of Surgery, Lahey Clinic, Burlington, MA, USA

*L. Michael Brunt, MD*
Department of Surgery, Washington University School of Medicine, St. Louis, MO, USA

*Jo Buyske, MD*
American Board of Surgery, Philadelphia, PA, USA

*John Byrn, MD*
Department of Surgery, University of Iowa Carver College of Medicine, Iowa City, IA, USA

*Mark P. Callery, MD*
Department of Surgery, Division of General Surgery, Beth Israel Deaconess Medical Center, Boston, MA, USA

*I. Bulent Cetindag, MD*
Department of Surgery, Southern Illinois University School of Medicine, Springfield, IL, USA

*Bipan Chand, MD, FACS*
Department of Bariatric and Metabolic Surgery, Cleveland Clinic Foundation, Cleveland, OH, USA

*John A. Coller, MD*
Department of Colon & Rectal Surgery, Lahey Clinic, Burlington, MA, USA

*Joseph J. Cullen, MD, FACS*
Department of Surgery, University of Iowa Carver College of Medicine, Iowa City, IA, USA

*Brian R. Davis, MD*
Department of Surgery, Paul L. Foster School of Medicine, Texas Tech University, El Paso, TX, USA

*Daniel J. Deziel, MD*
Department of General Surgery, Rush University Medical Center, Chicago, IL, USA

*James A. Dickerson II, MD*
Department of Surgery, Duke University Medical Center, San Antonio, TX, USA

*Kevin El-Hayek, MD*
Department of General Surgery, Cleveland Clinic, Cleveland, OH, USA

*Aaron S. Fink, MD*
VA Medical Center Atlanta, Emory University School of Medicine, Decatur, GA, USA

*Morris E. Franklin Jr., MD, FACS*
Texas Endosurgery Institute, San Antonio, TX, USA

*Frederick L. Greene, MD, FACS*
Department of Surgery, Carolinas Medical Center, Charlotte, NC, USA

*Rahul Gupta, MBBS, MS, DNB*
Division of General Surgery, Department of Surgery,
Beth Israel Deaconess Medical Center, Boston, MA, USA

*Michael D. Holzman, MD, MPH*
Department of Surgery, Vanderbilt University Medical Center, Nashville, TN, USA

*Michael D. Honaker, MD*
Department of General Surgery, Carolinas Medical Center, Charlotte, NC, USA

*Jennifer Hrabe, MD*
Department of Surgery, University of Iowa Carver College of Medicine, Iowa City, IA, USA

*Eric S. Hungness, MD, FACS*
Department of Surgery, Northwestern University Feinberg School of Medicine, Northwestern Memorial Hospital, Chicago, IL, USA

*Amila Husic, MD*
Department of General Surgery, Lahey Clinic, Burlington, MA, USA

*Daniel B. Jones, MD, MS*
Department of Surgery, Division of General Surgery, Beth Israel Deaconess Medical Center, Boston, MA, USA

*Andreas Kirakopolous, MD*
Department of Minimally Invasive Surgery, The Ohio State University, Columbus, OH, USA

*Michael Lalla, MD*
Department of Surgery, St. Vincent's Hospital, Indianapolis, IN, USA

*Minh B. Luu, MD*
Department of General Surgery, Rush University Medical Center, Chicago, IL, USA

*Bruce V. MacFadyen Jr., MD, FACS*
Department of Surgery, Medical College of Georgia,
Augusta, GA, USA

*Jeffrey M. Marks, MD, FACS*
Department of General Surgery, Case Western Reserve Medical Center,
University Hospitals of Cleveland, Cleveland, OH, USA

*Timothy Mayfield, MD*
Surgix Minimally Invasive Surgery Institute, Shawnee Mission
Medical Center, Shawnee Mission, KS, USA

*John J. Meehan, MD*
Robotic Surgery Center, Seattle Children's Hospital, Seattle, WA, USA

*John D. Mellinger, MD, FACS*
Department of Surgery, Southern Illinois University School
of Medicine, Springfield, IL, USA

*W. Scott Melvin, MD, FACS*
Department of Surgery, The Ohio State University,
Columbus, OH, USA

*Carmen L. Mueller, BSc, MD*
Division of General Surgery, University of Toronto, Toronto,
ON, Canada

*Allan Okrainec, MD, MHPE, FRCSC, FACS*
Department of Surgery, University of Toronto, Toronto, ON, Canada

*Dmitry Oleynikov, MD*
Department of Surgery, University of Nebraska Medical Center,
Omaha, NE, USA

*Pradeep Pallati, MBBS*
Department of Surgery, University of Nebraska Medical Center,
Omaha, NE, USA

*Adrian Park, MD, FRCSE, FACS, FCS (ECSA)*
Department of Surgery, Anne Arundel Health System,
Annapolis, MD, USA

*Chan W. Park, MD*
Department of Surgery, Duke University Medical Center,
Durham, NC, USA

*Joseph B. Petelin, MD, FACS*
Department of Surgery, University of Kansas School of Medicine,
Shawnee Mission, KS, USA

*Melissa S. Phillips, MD*
Department of Surgery, University of Tennessee Graduate
School of Medicine, Knoxville, TN, USA

*Jeffrey L. Ponsky, MD, FACS*
Department of Surgery, University Hospitals Case Medical Center,
Cleveland, OH, USA

*Aurora D. Pryor, MD*
Department of Surgery, Duke University Medical Center,
Durham, NC, USA

*John Rodriguez, MD*
Department of General Surgery, Cleveland Clinic Foundation,
Cleveland, OH, USA

*Michael J. Rosen, MD*
Department of Surgery, University Hospitals Case Medical Center,
Cleveland, OH, USA

*Karla Russek, MD*
Texas Endosurgery Institute, San Antonio, TX, USA

*Byron F. Santos, MD*
Department of Surgery, Northwestern University Feinberg School
of Medicine, Northwestern Memorial Hospital, Chicago, IL, USA

*Bruce David Schirmer, MD, FACS*
Department of Surgery, University of Virginia,
Charlottesville, VA, USA

*Carol E.H. Scott-Conner, MD, PhD*
Department of Surgery, University of Iowa Hospitals and Clinics,
Iowa City, IA, USA

*Jessica K. Smith, MD*
Department of Surgery, Iowa City VA Medical Center,
University of Iowa Hospitals and Clinics, Iowa City, IA, USA

*Nathaniel J. Soper, MD*
Department of Surgery, Northwestern University Feinberg School
of Medicine, Chicago, IL, USA

*Steven C. Stain, MD*
Department of Surgery, Albany Medical School, Albany, NY, USA

*Nathaniel Stoikes, MD*
Department of Surgery, Washington University School of Medicine,
St. Louis, MO, USA

*Raphael Sun, MD*
Department of Surgery, University of Iowa Carver College
of Medicine, Iowa City, IA, USA

*Erica R.H. Sutton, MD*
University of Louisville School of Medicine, Louisville, KY, USA

*Lee L. Swanstrom, MD, FACS*
Department of Surgery, Oregon Health Sciences University, Portland,
OR, USA

*Thadeus L. Trus, MD*
Department of Surgery, Dartmouth-Hitchcock Medical Center,
Lebanon, NH, USA

*Brian T. Valerian, MD*
Department of Surgery, Albany Medical School, Albany, NY, USA

*J. Esteban Varela, MD, MPH, FACS*
Division of General Surgery, Section of Minimally Invasive Surgery,
Department of Surgery, Washington University in St. Louis School
of Medicine, St. Louis, MO, USA

*Gary C. Vitale, MD*
Department of Surgery, University of Louisville, Louisville, KY, USA

*Jarrod Wall, MB, BCh, PhD*
Department of Surgery, Southern Illinois University School
of Medicine, Springfield, IL, USA

*Jeremy A. Warren, MD*
Department of Surgery, Georgia Health Sciences University,
Augusta, GA, USA

*Jessemae Welsh, MD*
Department of Surgery, University of Iowa Carver College
of Medicine, Iowa City, IA, USA

Part I

# Basic Laparoscopy and Endoscopy: General Principles

# 1. Fundamentals of Laparoscopic Surgery (FLS) and of Endoscopic Surgery (FES)

*Jeffrey M. Marks, M.D., F.A.C.S.*

The Fundamentals of Laparoscopic surgery (FLS) is a validated program for the teaching and evaluation of the basic knowledge and skills required to perform laparoscopic surgery. The educational component includes didactic, Web-based material and a simple, affordable physical simulator with specific tasks and a recommended curriculum. FLS certification requires passing both a written multiple-choice examination and a proctored manual skills examination in the FLS simulator. The metrics for the FLS program has been rigorously validated to meet the highest educational standards and certification is now a requirement for the American Board of Surgery. This chapter summarizes the validation process and the FLS related research that has been done to date.

The FLS program was developed by surgeons, educators, and administrators, under the leadership of the Society of American Gastrointestinal and Endoscopic Surgeons (SAGES). The impetus to create this curriculum was born out of the need to safely introduce laparoscopic techniques into clinical practice and by the demand to demonstrate basic competence in the application of this new technology. In the early years of laparoscopy, some surgeons integrated these techniques into their practices after cursory weekend courses or animal labs. Unfortunately, an increase in bile duct injuries and other complications occurred during the early experience with laparoscopic cholecystectomies. This critical issue of patient safety was the initial driver for the FLS effort. Around the same time, the concept of simulation in medicine was also starting to gain popularity, especially in light of restricted resident work hours and limited operating room resources.

N.J. Soper and C.E.H. Scott-Conner (eds.), *The SAGES Manual: Volume 1 Basic Laparoscopy and Endoscopy*, DOI 10.1007/978-1-4614-2344-7_1,
© Springer Science+Business Media, LLC 2012

# A. Program Description and Components

The FLS Program is not procedure or discipline-specific. It includes both teaching and assessment components.

## 1. Web-Based Study Guide

    a.   Didactic modules (Fig. 1.1)
        i.   Preoperative considerations
        ii.   Intraoperative considerations
        iii.   Basic laparoscopic procedures
        iv.   Postoperative care and complications
        v.   Manual skills practice
    b.   Patient scenarios
    c.   Technical skills explanations

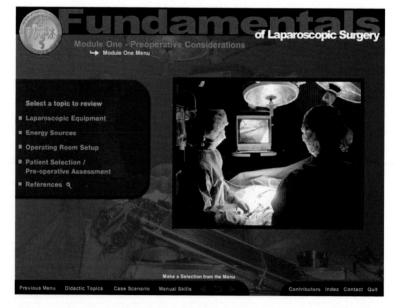

Fig. 1.1. Web-based study guide for FLS.

## 2. Assessment Tool

The assessment of this didactic material is done in the form of a 90-min multiple-choice examination of 75 questions. The computer-based test must be taken in a proctored setting at designated testing centers. It includes standard multiple-choice questions as well as case-based scenarios, and sometimes asks the examinee to interpret digital images.

## 3. Manual Skills (Fig. 1.2)

a.  Five tasks performed in a box trainer with a built-in camera that is connected to a monitor (not included).
b.  The kit also contains a set of instruments and disposable supplies. FLS is modeled after the original program developed by Fried et al., and previously referred to as the McGill Inanimate System for the Training and Evaluation of Laparoscopic Skills (MISTELS).

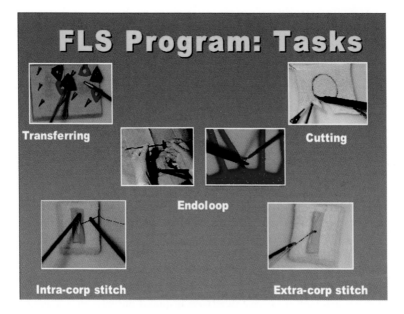

Fig. 1.2. Manual skills tests for FLS.

   c.   The tasks are scored for efficiency and precision, and each task has a predetermined cutoff time. The scores have been normalized and are equally weighted. A higher score indicates superior performance.

      i.   Peg transfer
     ii.   Precision cutting
   iii.   Placement of a ligating loop
   iv.   Suturing using extracorporeal knot tying
    v.   Suturing using intracorporeal knot tying

## 4. Global Operative Assessment of Laparoscopic Skills (GOALS)

The Global Operative Assessment of Laparoscopic Skills (GOALS) is a validated measure of intraoperative laparoscopic skill, and a high positive correlation exists between FLS manual skill performance and GOALS scores in the operating room during dissection of the gallbladder from the liver bed.

# B. FLS Simulator Practice Improves Operating Room Performance

The true test regarding the effectiveness of the FLS manual skills program as a training program is whether or not the skills acquired and measured in the simulator transfer to the operating room. Sroka et al. recently conducted a randomized controlled trial examining the effects of training using the FLS proficiency based curriculum described by Ritter and Scott on operating room performance as measured by GOALS. The FLS-trained group achieved the proficiency goals and improved significantly (increased by $6.1 \pm 1.3$, $p < 0.01$) in the operating room compared to the control group whose GOALS scores remained unchanged (increased by $1.8 \pm 2.1$, $p = 0.47$). After 2.5 h of supervised practice, and 5 h of individual deliberate practice, the simulator group, composed of first and second year residents performed at the level of third and fourth year residents in a previous study. They acquired skills in the simulator in 7.5 h that they may have otherwise acquired during 1 or 2 years of residency training!

# C. Fundamentals of Endoscopic Surgery (GOALS)

Many of the same issues that prompted the development of FLS are apparent in the training of competent flexible endoscopists both in the fields of gastroenterology and gastrointestinal surgery. The importance of these skills for surgeons is rapidly increasing as we work toward the development of increasingly less invasive methods to treat gastrointestinal disease. In response to the need for an objective way to teach and assess the knowledge and skills required to perform basic flexible endoscopy, members of SAGES began to discuss the possibility of developing a flexible gastrointestinal endoscopy teaching and evaluation program, similar to FLS, that could serve as a benchmark for physicians of all specialties. Through this discussion, Fundamentals of Endoscopic Surgery (FES) was born. At the time of preparation of this chapter, the program is still being developed and validated, with the intention to launch the program by Fall 2011.

Similar to FLS, the FES Program is not procedure or discipline-specific and includes teaching and assessment components.

## 1. Web-Based Study Guide

    a.   Didactic modules (Figs. 1.3 and 1.4)
- i. Technology
- ii. Patient preparation
- iii. Sedation and analgesia
- iv. Upper gastrointestinal endoscopy
- v. Lower gastrointestinal endoscopy
- vi. Performing lower GI procedures
- vii. Lower GI anatomy, pathology, and complications
- viii. Didactic Endoscopic Retrograde Cholangiopancreatography (ERCP)
- ix. Hemostasis
- x. Tissue removal
- xi. Enteral access
- xii. Endoscopic therapies

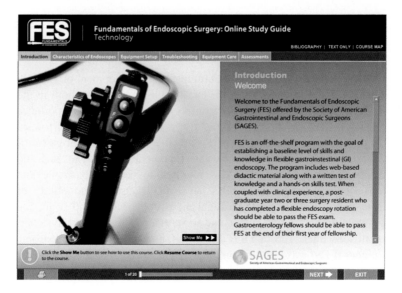

Fig. 1.3.   Web-based study guide pages for FES.

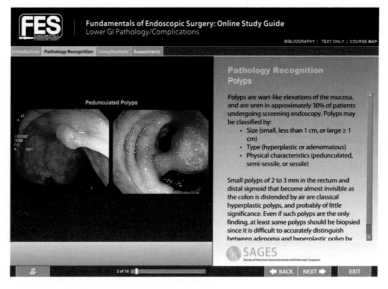

Fig. 1.4.   Web-based study guide pages for FES.

## 2. Assessment Tool

The assessment of this didactic material is done in the form of a 90-min multiple-choice examination of 75 questions. The computer-based test must be taken in a proctored setting at designated testing centers. It includes standard multiple-choice questions as well as case-based scenarios, and sometimes asks the examinee to interpret digital images.

## 3. Manual Skills

a. It consists of five separate modules administered on the Simbionix GI Mentor II platform (Fig. 1.5).
b. Because of the cost of this platform, it is envisioned that the test will initially be given at regional testing centers around the world. Eventually, the goal is to develop a desktop testing

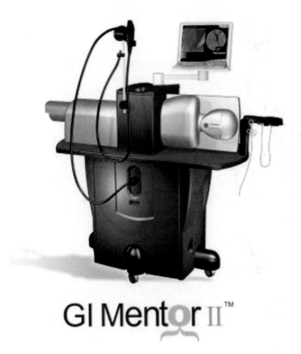

Fig. 1.5. Simbionix GI Mentor II for FES hands on skills (GI Mentor, Simbionix, USA).

platform, which could be more easily distributed to individual training programs.

   i.   Module 1—Navigation (traversal, tip deflection, and torque) (Fig. 1.6a)

  ii.   Module 2—Loop reduction

 iii.   Module 3—Retroflexion (Fig. 1.6b)

 iv.   Module 4—Mucosal evaluation (Fig. 1.6c)

  v.   Module 5—Targeting (Fig. 1.6d)

## 4. Global Assessment of Gastrointestinal Endoscopic Skills (GAGES)

The Global Assessment of Gastrointestinal Endoscopic Skills (GAGES) was developed by expert endoscopists and educators. The fundamental skills required for flexible endoscopy were identified and

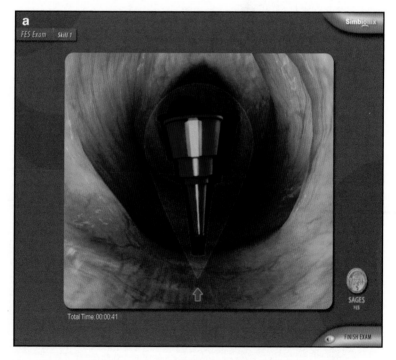

Fig. 1.6. Manual skills tests for FES. (**a**) Navigation (traversal, tip deflection, and torque); (**b**) Retroflexion; (**c**) Mucosal evaluation; (**d**) Targeting (GI Mentor, Simbionix, USA).

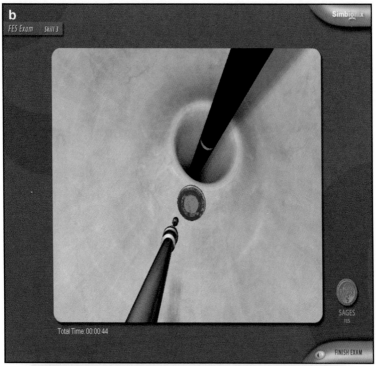

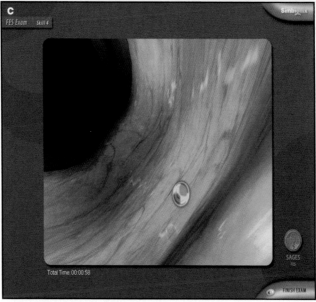

Fig. 1.6. (continued)

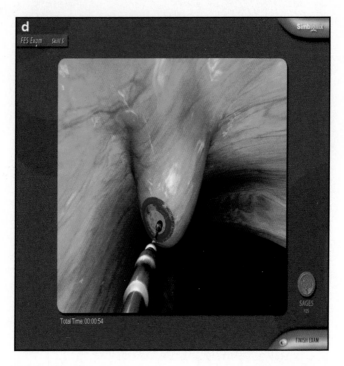

Fig. 1.6. (continued)

then distilled into two global assessments: GAGES Upper Endoscopy (GAGES-UE) and GAGES Colonoscopy (GAGES-C). The assessments were modeled after the Objective Structured Assessment of Technical Skills (OSATS) for open surgery and the GOALS for laparoscopic surgery and consist of itemized skills rated on a 5-point Likert scale with anchors at 1, 3, and 5.

## D. Conclusion

The concept that merits reiteration is the notion that passing FLS, and eventually FES, does not indicate that an individual is a competent surgeon or endoscopist, but that they have demonstrated competence in the basic knowledge and technical skills required to safely perform these procedures. Just as one would expect that a trainee learn the differences between needle drivers and suture materials and how to suture and tie knots outside of the operating room, these programs attempt to assure a basic level of knowledge and skill before entering the clinical arena. Overall, the goal is to optimize patient safety and the utilization of operating room resources while improving the efficiency and quality of surgical education.

## Selected References

Clarke JR. Making surgery safer. J Am Coll Surg. 2005;200:229.

Derossis AM, Antoniuk M, Fried GM. Evaluation of laparoscopic skills: a 2-year follow-up during residency training. Can J Surg. 1999;42:293.

Fried GM, Feldman LS, Vassiliou MC, et al. Proving the value of simulation in laparoscopic surgery. Ann Surg. 2004;240:518–25. discussion 525–8.

McCluney AL, Vassiliou MC, Kaneva PA, et al. FLS simulator performance predicts intraoperative laparoscopic skill. Surg Endosc. 2007;21:1991–5.

Sroka G, Feldman LS, Vassiliou MC, et al. Fundamentals of Laparoscopic Surgery simulator training to proficiency improves laparoscopic performance in the operating room—a randomized controlled trial. Am J Surg. 2010;199(1):115–20.

Strasberg SM, Hertl M, Soper NJ. An analysis of the problem of biliary injury during laparoscopic cholecystectomy. J Am Coll Surg. 1995;180:101.

# 2. Maintenance of Certification

*Jo Buyske, M.D.*

## A. Introduction

### 1. Definition of Maintenance of Certification

Maintenance of Certification (MOC) is the documentation of a personal program of continuous learning and improvement. MOC is required for ongoing certification by the American Board of Surgery and starts immediately upon initial certification or recertification. MOC crosses all specialties. It was established in 2002 by the American Board of Medical Specialties, a federation of 24 member boards. It is the logical continued growth of the process of board certification and also answers the public demand for demonstration of quality and ongoing acquisition of knowledge.

### 2. History of Board Certification

Board certification in the USA has evolved since its inception in 1917. The American Board of Ophthalmology was the first board formed, inspired by a 1908 speech to the American Academy of Ophthalmology and Otolaryngology by Derrick Vail, an ophthalmologist. He stated:

> I hope to see the time when ophthalmology will be taught in this country as it should be taught. That day will come when we demand… that a certain amount of preliminary education and training be enforced before a man may be licensed to practice ophthalmology. After a sufficiently long term of service in an ophthalmic institution … he should be permitted to appear before a proper examining board for examination… and if he is found competent let him then be permitted and licensed to practice ophthalmology.

N.J. Soper and C.E.H. Scott-Conner (eds.), *The SAGES Manual: Volume 1 Basic Laparoscopy and Endoscopy*, DOI 10.1007/978-1-4614-2344-7_2,
© Springer Science+Business Media, LLC 2012

That speech inspired the formation of the American Board of Ophthalmology in 1917, and in 1937 the American Board of Surgery was formed. The original mission statement of the ABS notes that the Board is formed to **"protect the public and improve the specialty"** which was to be accomplished by the establishment of a comprehensive, standardized certification process, including periodic assessment of individual hospitals as appropriate places of training, the requirement of 5 years of training beyond internship, and the development of an examination process designed to assess both knowledge and judgment.

## 3. Background of MOC

From 1937 until 1976 certification was lifelong: once certified, nothing further was required for the duration of one's surgical career. In 1976, the American Board of Surgery formally recognized that surgery is a field that requires ongoing active engagement in learning and that this should be supported by requiring recertification. Recertification requirements included: submission of a case log, assessment of knowledge by a broad-based multiple choice exam with a passing score, proof of active license and hospital privileges, and testimonials from hospital officials including the chief of surgery. The decision to implement intermittent reassessment for recertification was supported by the outcome. The results of those first recertification exams confirmed that the body of knowledge of surgeons 20 or 30 years out of training was not the same as that of surgeons within 10 years of their training; the former group failed the exam in high numbers.

A confluence of events at the turn of the century caused the specialty boards to revisit the duration of certification yet again. Increased public scrutiny of patient safety, the issuance of the IOM report "To Err is Human" in 1999, and the highly successful safety campaign by the airline industry all drove focus towards more oversight of knowledge and training. In addition, surgery underwent a series of rapid changes, including the widespread adoption of laparoscopy, the development of endovascular surgery, the introduction of sentinel node technology, the discovery of *Helicobacter pylori*, the penetration of interventional endoscopy, and the increased use of noninvasive management of blunt trauma. All these things combined to make it clear that surgical training and practice were dynamic arenas that required ongoing attention and self-education.

# B. Defining MOC

MOC is a result of that reassessment. MOC changes the emphasis from a burst of studying every 10 years to that of an ongoing process of learning and assessment. It is broken into four categories, based upon the ABMS/ACGME Six Competencies, adopted in 1999. The Six Competencies are a rubric for resident education and assessment across all specialties. Programs are required to demonstrate that their curriculum addresses these arenas.

The competencies are as follows:

- **Patient Care and Procedural Skills**: Provide care that is compassionate, appropriate and effective treatment for health problems and to promote health.
- **Medical Knowledge**: Demonstrate knowledge about established and evolving biomedical, clinical, and cognate sciences and their application in patient care.
- **Interpersonal and Communication Skills**: Demonstrate skills that result in effective information exchange and teaming with patients, their families, and professional associates (e.g., fostering a therapeutic relationship that is ethically sound, uses effective listening skills with nonverbal and verbal communication; working as both a team member and at times as a leader).
- **Professionalism**: Demonstrate a commitment to carrying out professional responsibilities, adherence to ethical principles and sensitivity to diverse patient populations.
- **Systems-Based Practice**: Demonstrate awareness of and responsibility to larger context and systems of health care. Be able to call on system resources to provide optimal care (e.g., coordinating care across sites or serving as the primary case manager when care involves multiple specialties, professions or sites).
- **Practice-Based Learning and Improvement**: Able to investigate and evaluate their patient care practices, appraise and assimilate scientific evidence, and improve their practice of medicine.

# C. Components of MOC

## 1. Categories/Components of MOC for Surgeons

MOC combines the Six Competencies and condenses them into four categories. The components of MOC are as follows:

- **Part 1—Professional standing** through maintenance of an unrestricted medical license, hospital privileges and satisfactory references.
- **Part 2—Lifelong learning and self-assessment** through continuing education and periodic self-assessment.
- **Part 3—Cognitive expertise** based on performance on a secure examination.
- **Part 4—Evaluation of performance in practice** through tools such as outcome measures and quality improvement programs, and the evaluation of behaviors such as communication and professionalism.

## 2. Fulfilling the MOC Requirements for Surgery

As is true of the field of surgery, MOC is an evolving field. Parts I and 3 are straightforward. Part 1 includes submission of documentation of an unrestricted license, and hospital privileges, as well as a testimonial form filled out by the chief of surgery and chair of the credentials committee. This is to be submitted once every 3 years.

Part 3 is the familiar "recertification" examination, which still must be taken once every 10 years. Admissibility to that exam will include timely fulfillment of all other MOC requirements, as well as a case log.

Parts 2 and 4 have a lot of promise, and are both more complicated and more interesting. Part 2 is self-assessment. In surgery, this will be fulfilled by CME I credits, especially those that require self-assessment. 30 credits will be required each year, 20 of which must be self-assessment. Standards for satisfactory self-assessment are under development by the ABS. Standards currently include CME 1 products that include a self test, which must be passed with a minimum 75% correct. Live activities, enduring materials, journal-based reading, and skills training are all offerings eligible for self-assessment. SAGES offers vehicles for self-assessment, both at the annual meeting and via the online SAGES University (http://www.sages.org/education/university.php).

SAGES University is available free to SAGES members and includes SAGES Journal Club, Online Self-Assessment Program (OSAP), and my CME/MY MOC Web page. A partial list of other self-assessment vehicles are listed on the ABS Web page (http://home.absurgery.org/ default.jsp?exam-moccme). Part II MOC reporting to the ABS will be required each 3-year cycle, along with Parts 1 and 4. Future plans for Part 2 MOC include linking the CME subject areas to case logs and practice, as well as using this venue for continuing education in ethics, professionalism, and perhaps systems-based practice. Ideally, Part 2 requirements will eventually link to requirements of other certifying and licensing groups, such as state licensing boards, hospital credential committees, the Joint Commission, and others. Professional societies including SAGES are providing multiple pathways to achieve those self-assessments credits that are meaningful to an individual's learning and pertinent to his or her practice.

Part 4 is the evaluation of performance in practice. To fulfill Part IV, the ABS currently requires participation in an outcomes database. At present a wide variety of databases fulfills this requirement, including the American College of Surgeons National Surgical Quality Improvement Program (ACS NSQIP), the American College of Surgeons Case Log, Mastery of Breast Surgery (The American Society of Breast Surgeons), participation in the United Network for Organ Sharing (UNOS), participation in bariatric surgery databases offered either by the American College of Surgeons or the American Society of Metabolic and Bariatric Surgery, and many others (for a partial list see http://home.absurgery.org/ default.jsp?exam-mocpa). Currently, participation alone is adequate to fulfill requirements; practice data does not need to be provided. Although the ABS recognizes that actual analysis of one's own practice and outcomes compared those of one's peers is ideal, at present no one perfect database exists that allows for such a requirement. Therefore, for now, participation alone is adequate, on the theory that the process of recording one's own practices is valuable in and of itself. Future plans for Part 4 MOC include a single, unified database for ABS use that is currently under development by the American College of Surgeons. In addition, a requirement of assessment of communication skills based upon patient surveys will likely be included in Part IV as well (Table 2.1).

MOC, when mature, will provide both a vehicle and a requirement for surgeons to structure their learning and measure their practices and outcomes. In practice, the ABS Web site will guide practitioners through the existing requirements, as well as updates as high-quality vehicles for Parts 2 and 4 continue to emerge.

Table 2.1. ABS MOC requirements timeline.

| MOC year | MOC requirement |
|----------|-----------------|
| 0 | Year of certification or recertification |
| 1 | Yearly CME (30 h Category I, 50 overall) |
| 2 | Yearly CME |
| 3 | Yearly CME |
|   | → Diplomate submits information through the ABS Web site regarding medical license, hospital privileges, references, CME and practice assessment participation |
| 4 | Same as Year 1 |
| 5 | Same as Year 2 |
| 6 | Same as Year 3 |
| 7 | Same as Year 1 |
| 8 | Same as Year 2 |
| 9 | Same as Year 3 |
| 8–10 | Secure examination (application and 12-month operative log required) |

*MOC Year* July 1 to June 30, starting July 1 following certification or recertification
Used with permission of the American Board of Surgery

## Selected References

ACGME Outcomes Project. http://www.acgme.org/outcome/comp/GeneralCompetencies Standards21307.pdf. Accessed 6 July 2011.

Maintenance of Certification. http://home.absurgery.org/default.jsp?exam-moc. Accessed 6 July 2011.

SAGES ACCME Compliance. http://www.sages.org/education/university.php. Accessed 6 July 2011.

To Err is Human: 1999 Reports Brief. http://www.iom.edu/~/media/Files/Report%20 Files/1999/To-Err-is-Human/To%20Err%20is%20Human%201999%20%20 report%20brief.pdf. Accessed 6 July 2011.

# 3. Equipment Setup and Troubleshooting

*Mohan C. Airan, M.D., F.A.C.S.*

## A. Room Layout and Equipment Position

1. **General considerations** include the size of the operating room, location of doors, outlets for electrical and anesthetic equipment, and the procedure to be performed. The time required to position the equipment and operating table is well spent. Arrive at the operating room sufficiently early to assure proper setup and to ascertain that all instruments are available and in good working order. This is particularly important when a procedure is being done in an operating room not normally used for laparoscopic operations, or when the operating room personnel are unfamiliar with the equipment (e.g., an operation performed after hours).

2. **Determine the optimum position and orientation for the operating table**. If the room is large, the normal position for the operating table will work well for laparoscopy.

3. **Small operating rooms** will require diagonal placement of the operating table and proper positioning of the laparoscopic accessory instruments around the operating table.

4. **Robotic systems and their effect on operating room space**. If used, the **da Vinci® robot** requires significant space for surgeon console, slave CRT screens for operating room team viewing, as well as the surgical arm cart.

5. **An equipment checklist** helps to ensure that all items are available and minimizes delays once the patient has arrived in the operating room. The following is an example of such a checklist. Most of the equipment and instruments listed here will be needed for operative laparoscopy. Additional equipment

may be needed for advanced procedures. This is discussed in subsequent sections.

a. Anesthesia equipment
b. Electric operating table with remote control if available
c. Two video monitors
d. Suction irrigator
e. Electrosurgical unit, with grounding pad equipped with current monitoring system
f. Ultrasonically activated scissors, scalpel, or other specialized unit if needed
g. Laparoscopic equipment, generally housed in a cart on wheels:
    i. Light source
    ii. Insufflator
    iii. Videocassette recorder (VCR), other recording system, tapes
    iv. Color printer (optional)
    v. Monitor on articulating arm
    vi. Camera-processor unit
h. C-arm X-ray unit (if cholangiography is planned) with remote monitor
i. Mayo stand or table with the following instruments:
    i. #11, #15 scalpel blades and handles
    ii. Towel clips
    iii. Veress needle or Hasson cannula
    iv. Gas insufflation tubes with micropore filter
    v. Fiber-optic cable to connect laparoscope with light source
    vi. Video camera with cord
    vii. Cords to connect laparoscopic instruments to the electrosurgical unit and other energy sources
    viii. 6-in. curved hemostatic forceps
    ix. Small retractors (Army-Navy or S-retractors)
    x. Trocar cannulae (size and numbers depend on the planned operation, with extras available in case of accidental contamination)
    xi. Laparoscopic instruments
    Atraumatic graspers
    Locking toothed jawed graspers
    Needle holders

Dissectors: curved, straight, right angled
Bowel grasping forceps
Babcock clamp
Scissors: Metzenbaum, hook, microtip
Fan retractors: 10 mm, 5 mm
Specialized retractors, such as endoscopic curved retractors
Biopsy forceps
Tru-Cut biopsy-core needle
   xii.   Port site closure devices
   xiii.   Monopolar electrocautery dissection tools
L-shaped hook
Spatula tip dissector/coagulator
   xiv.   Ultrasonically activated scalpel (optional)
Scalpel
Ball coagulator
Hook dissector
Scissors dissector/coagulator/transector
   xv.   Endocoagulator probe (optional)
   xvi.   Basket containing:
Clip appliers
Endoscopic stapling devices
Pretied suture ligatures—endoloops, etc.
Endoscopic suture materials
Extra trocars
  j.  Robot holder if available

# B. Room and Equipment Setup

1. **With the** operating **table positioned**, and all equipment in the room, reassess the configuration. Once the patient is anesthetized and draped, it is difficult to reposition equipment. Consider the room size (as previously discussed), location of doors (particularly if a C-arm is to be used), and the quadrant of the abdomen in which the procedure will be performed. Figure 3.1 shows a typical setup for a laparoscopic cholecystectomy or other procedure in the upper abdomen. Figure 3.2 illustrates a typical setup in a small operating room.

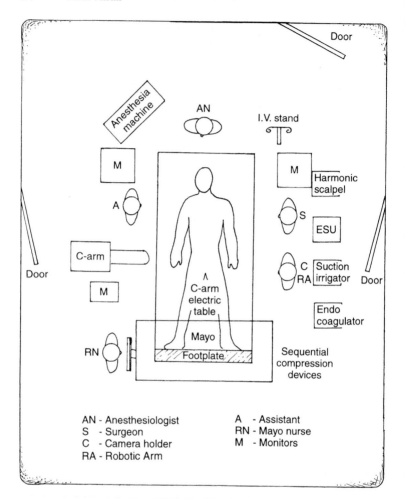

Fig. 3.1. **Basic room setup**. This is the typical setup for laparoscopic cholecystectomy. The room must be sufficiently large to accommodate all of the equipment (see Fig. 3.2 for setup for smaller room). A similar setup can be used for hiatus hernia repair or other upper abdominal surgery. In these cases, one 21-in. or larger monitor can be used in the center where the anesthesiologist usually sits, with the anesthesiologist positioned to the side. The position of the surgeon (S), camera holder (C), and the assistant (A) depends on the procedure that is planned. The best position for the monitor is opposite the surgeon in his line of sight. A C-arm, if used, should be placed perpendicular to the operating table. A clear pathway to the door facilitates placement of the C-arm, and should be planned when the room is set up.

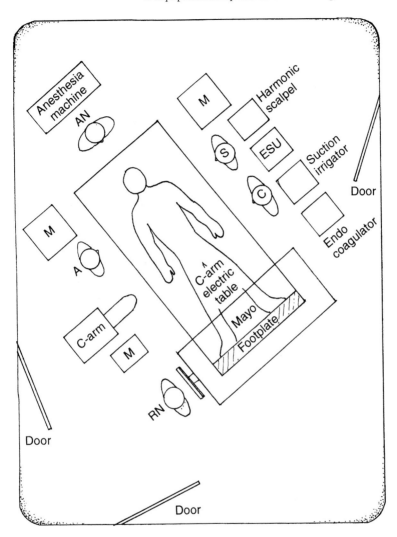

Fig. 3.2. **Laparoscopic cholecystectomy, small operating room**. The monitors, anesthesia machine, and relative position of surgeon and first assistant have been adapted to the diagonal operating table placement.

2. **Set up the equipment** before bringing the patient into the operating room. A systematic approach, starting at the head of the table, is useful.

   a. There should be sufficient space to allow the anesthesiologist to position the anesthesia equipment and work safely.

   b. Next, consider the position of the monitors and the paths that connecting cables will take. Try to avoid "fencing in" the surgeon and assistants. This is particularly important if surgeon and assistant need to change places or move (for example, during cholangiography).

   c. The precise setup must be appropriate to the planned procedure. The setup shown is for laparoscopic cholecystectomy or other upper abdominal procedures. Room and equipment setups for other laparoscopic operations are discussed with each individual procedure in the chapters that follow. A useful principle to remember is that the laparoscope must point toward the quadrant of the abdomen with the pathology, and the surgeon generally stands opposite the pathology and looks directly at the main monitor.

   d. If a C-arm or other equipment will need to be brought in during the procedure, plan the path from the door to the operating table in such a manner that the equipment can be positioned with minimal disruption. This will generally require that the cabinet containing the light source, VCR, insufflator, and other electronics be placed at the side of the patient farthest from the door. Consider bringing the C-arm into the room before the procedure begins.

   e. Additional tables should be available so that water, irrigating solutions, and other items are not placed on any electrical units where spillage could cause short circuits, electrical burns, or fires.

3. **Check the equipment** and ascertain the following:

   a. If no piped-in lines are available, there should be two full carbon dioxide cylinders in the room. One is used for the procedure, and the second is a spare in case the pressure in the first cylinder becomes low. The cylinder should be hooked up to the insufflator and the valve turned on. The pressure gauge should indicate that there is adequate gas in the cylinder. If the cylinder does not appear to fit properly, **do not force it**. Each type of gas cylinder has a unique kind of fitting, and failure to fit properly may indicate that the cylinder contains a different kind of gas (e.g., oxygen). The piped-in lines should be color coded and connected to appropriate intake valves.

b. If the carbon dioxide cylinder needs to be changed during a procedure:

    i. Close the valve body with the proper handle to shut off the gas (old cylinder).

    ii. Unscrew the head fitting.

    iii. Replace the gasket in the head fitting with a new gasket, which is always provided with a new tank of gas.

    iv. Reattach the head fitting so that the two prongs of the fitting are seated in the two holes in the carbon dioxide gas tank valve body.

    v. Firmly align and tighten the head fitting with the integral pointed screw fixture.

    vi. Open the carbon dioxide gas tank valve body, and pressure should be restored to the insufflator.

c. Look inside the back of the cabinet housing the laparoscopic equipment. Check to be certain that the connections on the back of the units are tightly plugged in (Fig. 3.3).

4. **Attention to detail** is important. The following additional items need careful consideration, and can be checked as the patient is brought into the room and prepared for surgery:

a. Assure table tilt mechanism is functional, and that the table and joints are level and the kidney rest down.

b. Consider using a footboard and extra safety strap for large patients.

c. Position patient and cassette properly on operating table for cholangiography.

d. Notify the radiology technologist with time estimate.

e. Assure proper mixing and dilution of cholangiogram contrast solution for adequate image.

f. Assure availability of Foley catheter and nasogastric tube, if desired.

g. Assure all power sources are connected and appropriate units are switched on. Avoid using multiple sockets or extension cords plugged into a single source, as circuits may overload.

h. Check the insufflator. Assure that insufflator alarm is set appropriately.

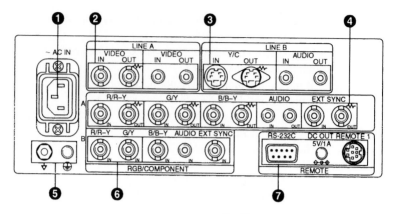

(The ⌁ mark indicates automatic termination.)

Fig. 3.3. **Connections on rear panel**. The actual configuration of connections on the rear panels varies, but there are some general principles that will help when tracing the connections. The video signal is generated by the camera box. A cable plugs into the "video out" port of the camera box and takes the video signal to the VCR or monitor by plugging into a "video in" port. A common arrangement takes the signal first to the VCR, and then from the "video out" port of the VCR to the "video in" port of the monitor. (see Chap. 9, Documentation). Some cameras have split connectors that must be connected to the proper ports. Once connected, these should not be disturbed. The surgeon should be familiar with the instrumentation, as connections frequently are loose or disconnected. The last monitor plugged in should have an automatic termination of signal port to avoid deterioration of the picture quality.

    i.    Assure full volume in the irrigation fluid container (recheck during case).

    j.    Assure adequate printer film and video tape if documentation is desired.

    k.    Check the electrosurgical unit; make sure the auditory alarm of the machine is functioning properly and the grounding pad is appropriate for the patient, properly placed, and functioning.

    l.    The surgeon should specify the electrosurgical unit that he uses.

    m.    Apply S.C.D.'s

5. **Once you are gowned and gloved**, connect the light cable and camera to the laparoscope. Focus the laparoscope and white balance it. Place the laparoscope in warmed saline or electrical warmer. Verify the following:
   a. Check Veress needle for proper plunger/spring action and assure easy flushing through stopcock and/or needle channel.
   b. Assure closed stopcocks on all ports.
   c. Check sealing caps for cracked rubber and stretched openings.
   d. Check to assure instrument cleaning channel screw caps are in place.
   e. Assure free movements of instrument handles and jaws.
   f. If Hasson cannula to be used, assure availability of stay sutures and retractors.

# C. Types of Equipment Available

## 1. Electrosurgical Units

   a. Simple E.S.U.—coagulation and cut features—use AEM technology overlay machine.
   b. Complex E.S.U.—ForceTriad™ energy platform comprises monopolar, bipolar, and proprietary functions utilizing LigaSure™ tissue fusion technology, the Force Triverse™ electrosurgical device, and Valleylab™ mode (Figs. 3.4–3.6).
   c. Ultrasonic machines.

# D. Troubleshooting

1. **Laparoscopic procedures** are inherently complex. Many things can go wrong. The surgeon must be sufficiently familiar with the equipment to troubleshoot and solve problems. Table 3.1 gives an outline of the common problems, their cause, and suggested solutions.

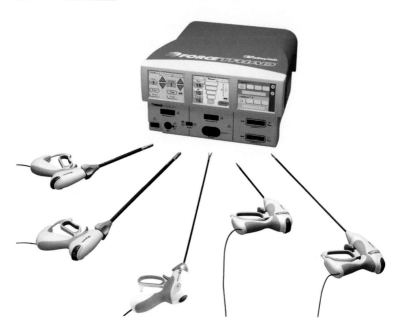

Fig. 3.4. **ForceTriad™ energy platform front panel**. ©2010 Covidien. All rights reserved. Image reprinted with permission from the Energy-based Devices division of Covidien. The ForceTriad™ is an electrosurgical all in one unit. The bipolar device allows surgeons, urologists, gynecologists to perform in a saline environment. Tissue fusion technology permanently fuses vessels up to 7 mm, lymphatic and tissue bundles. The devices can divide the structures as soon as fusion is accomplished. Valleylab™ mode provides equal or superior hemostasis than standard valley lab E.S.U. The touch screens' screen displays change based on instrument recognition technology. Each instrument has its own electronic signature recognized by the unit.

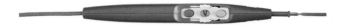

Fig. 3.5. **Force TriVerse™ electrosurgical device**. ©2010 Covidien. All rights reserved. Image reprinted with permission from the Energy-based Devices division of Covidien. The surgeon can change the settings from the sterile field freeing up the circulating RN for other duties.

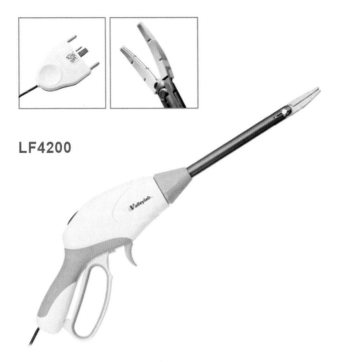

LF4200

Fig. 3.6. **LigaSure™ Impact instrument**. ©2010 Covidien. All rights reserved. Image reprinted with permission from the Energy-based Devices division of Covidien. Used for open surgery to fuse and divide. The function is more economical than using vascular staplers for small vessels.

2. **General Troubleshooting Guidelines—ForceTriad™ energy platform**. If the Force Triad™ energy platform malfunctions, check for obvious conditions that may have caused the problem:

   a. Check the system for visible signs of physical damage.
   b. Make sure the fuse drawer is tightly closed.
   c. Verify that all cords are connected and attached properly.
   d. If an error code is displayed on the touch screens, note the code along with all information on the error screen, then turn the system off and turn it back on.

Table 3.1. Common problems, causes, and solutions.

| Problem | Cause | Solution |
|---|---|---|
| 1. Poor insufflation/loss of pneumoperitoneum | $CO_2$ tank empty or volume low | Change tank |
| | Accessory port stopcock(s) open | Inspect all accessory ports. Open/close stopcock(s) as needed |
| | Leak in sealing cap, reducer | Change cap or stopcock cannula |
| | Excessive suctioning pressure | Allow time to reinsufflate, lower suction |
| | Loose, disconnected, or kinked insufflation tubing | Tighten connections or reconnect at source or at port, unkink tubing |
| | Hasson stay sutures loose | Replace or secure sutures |
| | $CO_2$ flow rate set too low | Adjust flow rate |
| | Valve on $CO_2$ tank not fully open | Use valve wrench to open fully |
| | Leak at skin where port enters cavity | Apply penetrating towel clip or suture around port |
| | Veress needle or cannula tip not in peritoneal space | Reposition needle or cannula under visualization if possible |
| 2. Excessive pressure required for insufflation (initial or subsequent) | Occlusion of tubing (kinking, table joints, etc.) | Inspect full length of tubing |
| | $CO_2$ port stopcock turned off | Fully open stopcock |
| | Patient is "light" | Communicate to anesthesia |
| | Morbidly obese patient | Use longer Veress needle |
| 3. Inadequate lighting (partial/complete loss) | Light is dim | Increase gain. Check scope for adequate fiber-optics |
| | | Replace light cable and/or camera |
| | Light is on standby | Take light off standby |
| | Loose connection at source or at scope | Adjust connection |
| | Light is on "manual-minimum" | Go to "automatic" |
| | Fiber-optics is damaged | Replace light cable |

| Problem | Cause | Solution |
| --- | --- | --- |
| | Automatic iris adjusting to bright reflection from instruments | Reposition instruments, or switch to "manual" |
| | Monitor brightness turned down | Readjust brightness setting, adjust gain |
| | Room brightness floods monitors | Dim room lights |
| | Bulb is burned out | Replace bulb |
| | Scope dark | Check white balance |
| 4. Lighting too bright | Light is on "manual-maximum" | "Boost" on light source activated |
| | Monitor brightness turned up | Go to "automatic," deactivate "boost," readjust setting |
| 5. No picture on monitor(s) | Camera control or other components (VCR, printer, light source, monitor) "not on" | Make sure all power sources are plugged in and turned on |
| | Cable connector between camera control unit and/or monitors not attached properly | Cable should run from "video out" on camera control unit to "video in" on primary monitor. Use compatible cables for camera unit and light source |
| | Cable between monitors not connected | Cable should run from "video out" on primary monitor to "video in" on secondary monitor |
| | Input selection button on monitor doesn't match "video in" choice | Assure matching selection |
| | Input selection button on monitor or video peripherals (e.g., VCR, digital capture, printer) not selected | Adjust input selection |
| 6. Poor-quality picture | Flickering electrical interference, poor cable shielding | Replace cautery cables, switch camera head, make sure cables don't cross, use different plug points |
| | Color problems | White balance camera, monitor chrome on monitor, check printer, VCR, digital capture cables |
| | Glare not caused by lighting | Check for loose cables not plugged in |

(continued)

Table 3.1. (continued)

| Problem | Cause | Solution |
|---|---|---|
| a. Fogging, haze | Condensation on lens from cold scope entering warm abdomen | Use antifog solution or warm water, wipe lens externally |
| | Condensation on scope eyepiece, camera lens | Detach camera from scope (or camera from coupler); inspect, and clean lens as needed |
| b. Flickering, electrical interference | Moisture in camera cable connecting plug | Use suction or compressed air to dry out moisture (don't use cotton-tip applicators on multipronged plug) |
| | Poor cable shielding | Move electrosurgical unit to different circuit or away from video equipment, make sure cables don't cross, switch camera head; replace cables as necessary |
| | Insecure connection of video cable between monitors | Reattach video cable at each monitor |
| c. Blurring, distortion | Incorrect focus | Adjust camera focus ring |
| | Cracked lens, internal moisture | Inspect scope/camera, replace if needed |
| | Too grainy | Adjust enhancement and/or grain setting for units with this option |

| 7. Inadequate suction/ irrigation | Occlusion of tubing (kinking, blood clot, etc.) | Inspect full length of tubing. If necessary, detach from instrument and flush tubing with sterile saline |
| | Occlusion of valves in suction/irrigator device | Detach tubing, flush device with sterile saline |
| | Not attached to wall suction | Inspect and secure suction and wall source connector |
| | Irrigation fluid container not pressurized | Inspect pressure bag or compressed gas source, connector, pressure dial setting |
| 8. Absent or "weak" cauterization | Patient not grounded properly | Assure adequate grounding pad contact |
| | Connection between electrosurgical unit and instrument loose | Inspect both connecting points |
| | Foot pedal or hand-switch not connected to electrosurgical unit | Make connection |
| | Wrong output selected | Correct output choice |
| | Connected to the wrong socket on the electrosurgical unit | Check that cable is attached to endoscopic socket |
| | Instrument insulations failure outside of the surgeon's view | Use new instrument and inspect insulation |

Reprinted with permission from the Society of American Gastrointestinal and Endoscopic Surgeons (SAGES)

    e.   If a solution is not readily apparent, refer to Table 3.2, Correcting Malfunctions, to help identify and correct specific malfunctions. After the malfunction is corrected, verify that the system completes a prescribed self-test. If the malfunction persists, the system may require service. Contact the institution's biomedical engineering department.

3.  **REM Alarms**. If the ForceTriad™ energy platform does not sense the correct impedance for the connected REM patient return electrode, monopolar energy will be disabled, the REM symbol will illuminate red and enlarge on both the center and left touchscreen displays, and an alarm tone will sound twice. The REM symbol will return to its smaller size but will remain red, and RF energy will remain disabled until the REM alarm is corrected. When the REM alarm is corrected, the system is enabled and the REM alarm indication illuminates green. Valleylab recommends the use of Valleylab REM patient return electrodes. Return electrodes from other manufacturers may not provide proper impedance to work correctly with the ForceTriad™ energy platform. To correct a REM alarm condition, follow these steps:

    a.   Inspect the return electrode plug and cord. If there is evidence of cracks, breaks, or other visible damage, replace the return electrode and/or the cord.

    b.   Verify that the patient return electrode cord is correctly connected to the energy platform.

    c.   Verify that the return electrode is in good contact with the patient. Follow the instructions for use provided with the Valleylab REM patient return electrode.

    d.   If the REM alarm persists it may be necessary to use more than one patient return electrode. Refer to the troubleshooting flow chart in the Valleylab REM patient return electrode instructions for use.

# E. Patient Safety Issues—Thermal Injury

1.  **The surgeon must be aware** of the possibility of thermal injury when utilizing any of these devices.

2.  **Unintended radiofrequency burns**—Visceral burns may occur by inadvertent direct coupling, capacitive coupling, and/or insulation failures. This can happen during da Vinci® robotic surgery, single port surgery, or NOTES surgery.

Table 3.2. Correcting malfunctions.

| Situation | Possible causes | Solution |
|---|---|---|
| Abnormal neuromuscular stimulation (stop surgery Immediately) | Metal-to-metal sparking | Check all connections to the energy platform, patient return electrode, and active electrodes |
| | Can occur during coagulation | Use a lower power setting for the Fulgurate and Spray modes |
| | Abnormal 50–60 Hz leakage currents | Contact your biomedical engineering department or a Valleylab technical service representative for assistance |
| Energy platform does not respond when turned on | Disconnected power cord or faulty wall outlet | Check power cord connections (energy platform and wall outlet). Connect the power cord to a functional outlet |
| | Faulty power cord | Replace the power cord |
| | Fuse drawer is open or fuses are blown | Replace the blown fuses(s). Close the fuse drawer Refer to the ForceTriadEnergy Platform Manual |
| | Internal component malfunction | Use a backup energy platform. Contact your biomedical Engineering department or a Valleylab technical service representative for assistance |
| System is on, but did not complete the self-test | Software malfunction | Turn off, then turn on the system |
| | Internal component malfunction | Note the code along with all information on the error screen |
| | | Note the number and refer to System Alarms in the User's manual |
| | | Use a backup energy platform. Contact your biomedical Engineering department or a Valleylab technical service representative for assistance |

(continued)

Table 3.2. (continued)

| Situation | Possible causes | Solution |
| --- | --- | --- |
| Energy platform is on and instrument is activated but system does not deliver output | Malfunctioning footswitch or handswitching instrument | Turn off the energy platform. Check and correct all instrument connections<br>Turn on the energy platform. Replace the instrument if it continues to malfunction |
| | Power is set too low | Increase the power setting |
| | An alarm conditions exists | Note the code along with all information on the error screen. Note the number and refer to System Alarms in the User's manual<br>In case of a REM alarm, refer to Correcting a REM Alarm Condition in the User's manual |
| | Internal component malfunction | Contact your biomedical engineering department or a Valleylab technical service representative for assistance |
| | System does not detect tissue fusion instrument | Firmly insert the LigaSmart connector into the appropriate receptacle on the energy platform front panel. Ensure the vessel fusion touch screen indicates that it has detected the instrument |
| | System does not detect monopolar instrument | Firmly insert the Smart connector into the appropriate receptacle on the energy platform front panel. Ensure the monopolar touch screen indicates that it has detected the instrument |

| Status/Screen | Cause | Action |
|---|---|---|
| CHECK INSTRUMENT screen appears, a six-pulsed tone sounds, and RF output is disabled | System does not detect bipolar instrument | Firmly insert the connector into the appropriate receptacle on the energy platform front panel. Ensure the bipolar touch screen indicates that it has detected the instrument |
| | Excessive tissue/eschar on electrode tips or jaws | Clean electrode tips and jaws with a wet gauze pad |
| | Electrodes have come loose from the instrument jaws | Reinsert the electrode into the instrument jaws making sure that all the electrode pins are firmly seated |
| | Electrode pins may have been compromised or bent during assembly to the instrument and may need to be replaced | |
| | Metal or other foreign object is grasped within jaws | Avoid grasping objects, such as staples, clips, or encapsulated sutures in the jaws of the instrument |
| | Tissue grasped within jaws is too thin | Open the jaws and confirm that a sufficient amount of tissue is inside the jaws. If necessary, increase the amount of tissue and repeat the procedure |
| REACTIVATE screen appears, a four-pulsed tone sounds, and RF output is disabled | Pooled fluids around instrument tip | Minimize or remove excess fluids |
| | The seal cycle was interrupted before completion. The handswitch or footswitch was released before the end tone activated | Reactivate the seal cycle without removing or repositioning the instrument |
| | Additional time and energy are needed to complete the fusion cycle | |
| Continuous monitor | Malfunctioning monitor | Replace the monitor |

(continued)

Table 3.2. (continued)

| Situation | Possible causes | Solution |
| --- | --- | --- |
| Interference | Faulty chassis-to-ground connections | Check and correct the chassis ground connections for the monitor and for the energy platform |
| | | Check other electrical equipment in the room for defective grounds |
| | Electrical equipment is grounded to different objects rather than a common ground. The energy platform may respond to the resulting voltage differences between grounded objects | Plug all electrical equipment into line power at the same location. Contact your biomedical engineering department or a Valleylab representative for assistance |
| Interference with other devices only when the energy platform is activated | Metal-to-metal sparking | Check all connections to the energy platform, patient return electrode, and instruments instrument |
| | High settings used for fulguration | Use lower power settings for fulguration |
| | Electrically inconsistent ground wires in the operating room | Verify that all ground wires are as short as possible and go to the same grounded metal |
| | If interference continues when the energy platform is activated, the monitor is responding to radiated frequencies | Some manufacturers offer RF choke filters for use in monitor leads. The filters reduce interference when the energy platform is activated and minimize the potential for an electrosurgical burn at the site of the monitor electrode |

| Pacemaker interference | Intermittent connections or metal-to-metal sparking | Check the active and patient return electrode cord connections |
| | | It may be necessary to reprogram the pacemaker |
| | Current traveling from active to return electrode during monopolar electrosurgery is passing too close to pacemaker | Consult the pacemaker manufacturer or hospital cardiology department for further information when use of electrosurgical appliances is planned in patients with cardiac pacemakers |
| | | Use bipolar instruments, if possible |
| | | If you must use a monopolar instrument, place the patient return electrode as close as possible to the surgical site. Make sure the current path from the surgical site to the patient return electrode does not pass through the vicinity of the heart or the site where the pacemaker is implanted |
| | | Always monitor patients with pacemakers during surgery and keep a defibrillator available |
| Internal Cardiac Defibrillator (ICD) activation | ICD is activated by energy platform | Stop the procedure and contact the ICD manufacturer for instructions |

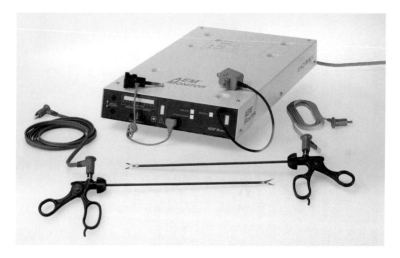

Fig. 3.7. **Encision® active electrode monitoring unit**. ©2010 Encision. All rights reserved. Image reprinted with permission from Encision, Inc.

3. **These injuries can be avoided** by use of bipolar RF, harmonics, or laser or use of active electrode monitoring system such as Encision® (Fig. 3.7).

   a. Monopolar devices—Thermal injuries can occur at the tip of monopolar instruments.

   b. Bipolar devices—Bipolar instruments usually do not have an extensive spread around the operating tip if the current used is brief.

   c. Valleylab ForceTriad™ energy platform—LigaSure™ platform also limits the thermal spread at the operating tip.

   d. Ultrasonic scalpels can also have thermal spread at the operating tip.

4. **Operating room fires**.

   a. Be aware that the light cord tip can become very hot, i.e., the end that goes into the light generator. Do not disconnect hot light cord from light generator if it is close to an oxygen source, i.e., nasal cannula, masks, oropharyngeal tube, endotracheal tubes. This hazard is deadly during extubation. Many patients have been burned.

   b. Chlora-Prep has alcohol base. The vapors from the preparation can be ignited by Bovie tips, hot ultrasonic tips, etc.

# Acknowledgments

Berdelle, Susan. Office Manager, Mohan C Airan, MD SC. Riechert, John Brian. Energy Based Sales Representative. Covidien.

## Selected References

Podnos Y, Williams R. Fires in the operating room. American College of Surgeons, Committee on Perioperative Care. http://www.facs.org/about/committees/cpc/oper0897.html. Accessed 28 Mar 2011.

Encision Inc. Developer and manufacturer of the patented AEM technology. http://www.encision.com. Accessed 19 Jan 2011.

Energy Based Division, Covidien. User's Guide ForceTriad™ energy platform. Boulder, CO; 2008.

ForceTriad Web site. http://www.forcetriad.com. Accessed 19 Jan 2011.

SAGES Continuing Education Committee. Laparoscopy Troubleshooting Guide. SAGES, Santa Monica, CA; 2006. http://www.sages.org/publications/troubleshooting/. Accessed 4 Mar 2011.

Sony Corporation. Rear panel diagram for Trinitron color video monitor. 1995.

# 4. Ergonomics in Operating Room Design

*Erica R.H. Sutton, M.D.*
*Adrian Park, M.D., F.R.C.S.E., F.A.C.S., F.C.S. (ECSA)*

## A. The Human–Machine Interface

The operating room (OR) is a complex working environment reliant on high-stakes decision-making that increasingly must take into account interfaces between humans and machines. With the opportunities for error frequent and the consequences potentially grave, the gathering of full, accurate, applicable knowledge regarding these interfaces must be considered of utmost importance. As nearly three decades of minimally invasive surgical advancements have indicated, the cost of conditions ergonomically unfavorable to the surgeon cannot safely be disregarded, for the resulting consequences are surely borne by doctor and patient alike. Achievement of optimal human–machine interfaces in the OR depends on the systematic discovery and implementation of ergonomically sound principles in this challenging workspace.

## B. Ergonomics Defined

The objective of the applied science of ergonomics is ensuring that efficient and safe interaction is possible between things and persons. Ergonomics seeks—as suggested by its Greek roots translatable as "the natural laws of work"—to establish and define people's relationship to work, which may at once be both physical and cognitive.

Ergonomics as applied to OR design is still taking shape as an informative, evidence-based field of research. A good number of mechanical ergonomics studies have appeared that take as their focus the optimal

N.J. Soper and C.E.H. Scott-Conner (eds.), *The SAGES Manual: Volume 1 Basic Laparoscopy and Endoscopy*, DOI 10.1007/978-1-4614-2344-7_4, © Springer Science+Business Media, LLC 2012

physical and technological working conditions of the OR—monitor placement and display characteristics, table height, instrument design and capability, surgical workflow. Standard ergonomic research into OR design and equipment has elucidated many shortcomings of the working environment, thus far with particular regard to open surgery performance. The research to date, however, primarily offers only suggestions as to what a prototype might do or how it and its end user should interface. Ergonomics, theoretical and applied, has not yet determined what constitutes an ideal OR suite or even the most advantageous prototypes needed for efficacious research.

Similarly, while staples of our evidence-based literature, the metrics by which we assess cognitive ergonomics—subjective reports of well-being or psychological stress, gaze and attention disruptions, heart-rate variability, or complex indices of mental workload—are not well or often defined in relation to one another and even more rarely in terms of consequence to surgeon or surgical outcome. Correlations to professional longevity and patient safety are often suggested but infrequently measured. While the definitions of mechanical ergonomics and cognitive ergonomics have gained consensus, their component metrics are at present subjective and substantially lacking validation in the field of medicine.

## C. Influence of Nonsurgical Ergonomics

Given the reality of the significant consideration that must be accorded to the human–machine interface, the introduction of ergonomics as a primary consideration in the design of the OR suite has been in many ways as unsystematic as was the introduction of MIS itself. Prior to its recent acceptance of the potentials to be gained by obtaining and applying ergonomic data gathered in its environments and from its staffs, the medical field when initially grappling with the need to implement differently conceived operative environments looked elsewhere. Work environments that recapitulate the complexities of the OR are rare, and those that mimic the demands of the minimally invasive work environment even more. Thus, only in components has surgical ergonomics been able to borrow lessons from other disciplines. Where similarities such as dependence on visual displays and similar high levels of mental workload have existed, the ergonomic lessons of related fields have been co-opted.

## 1. Visual Display Technology

Similarities have been profitably drawn in regard to surgical visual display technology and that used in the work of video display terminal (VDT) workers, pilots, and professional drivers. Areas for concern include eye and neck strain symptoms as experienced by surgeons, who in their practice of minimally invasive techniques now view video monitors several hours per day, multiple days per week.

    a.   Ocular discomfort

        i.   The **cumulative nature of eye strain** such as that experienced by workers performing VDT work an average of 6.5 h daily compared with those performing work not done at VDTs workers has been studied.

        ii.   Significantly **higher levels of eye strain** are experienced as a day progresses.

        iii.   **Increased eye strain** has been demonstrated to impact the accommodative response of the pupil and subject reaction time.

    b.   Visual awareness

        i.   The brain's capacity to attend to visual stimuli dictates **situational awareness**.

        ii.   **Perceptual misjudgments of speed and distance**—factors that have been investigated in regard to drivers and pilots—must be deemed pertinent to the performance of surgeons as well. Examples of such instances termed "look, but fail to see" being motor vehicle collisions with parked cars or missed aircraft landings. The central failings implicated in such accidents are perceptual misjudgments of speed and distance. The minimally invasive surgical setting is such that perception difficulties may be encountered by surgeons with respect to depth of dissection and object size.

## 2. Mental Workload

The mental workload associated with military pilots and civil aviators is that of high-stakes decision-making occurring in an environment considered safety critical much as is the case with surgeons. Pilot mental workload and performance during both real and simulated combat missions have been well researched.

a. Information handling
   i.   Effective pilot performance has been positively correlated with capabilities in terms of information handling.
   ii.  Such findings were rightly determined to be of interest to laparoendoscopic surgeons transitioning from open to more technically demanding MIS techniques with impacting changes such as altered perception effected by use of a two-dimensional video monitor, tactile feedback loss, a variable array of hand-held instruments, foot-controlled diathermy, and an influx of varied technical information.
   iii. The **dramatically more complex stream of information** has substantially increased the mental workload of minimally invasive surgeons.
b. Information complexity
   i.   Even **moderate levels of information complexity interfere** with task performance.
   ii.  Increases in levels of flight complexity have been shown to cause escalations in eye movements, heart rate, and pilot-reported mental workload.

# D. Surgical Workflow

The value of defining a workspace in terms of series of both predictable and quantifiable repetitive movements that take place within it is clear. This section addresses the knowledge acquired and the strengths and limitations in the quantification of cognitive and physical surgical OR workflow.

## 1. Workflow Patterns

a. Individual physical/repetitive movement
   An **individual pattern to physical and repetitive movement** exists for each member of the surgical team—the surgeon, scrub technician, circulating nurse, and anesthesiologist (Fig. 4.1). The surgeon maintains a relatively static posture throughout MIS procedures. The circulating nurse must acquire equipment and supplies inside and outside of the room, connect wires and tubing, and adjust the lighting and laparoscopic

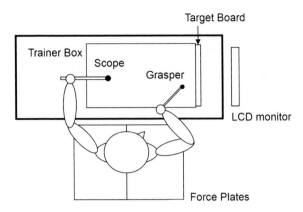

Fig. 4.1. Experimental setup in which kinematic data is being acquired through force plates for the purpose of determining ergonomic physical risk (Adapted with permission from Lee G, Lee T, Dexter D, et al. Ergonomic risk associated with assisting in minimally invasive surgery. Surg Endosc. 2009;23(1): 182–188).

equipment throughout the procedure. That one pattern of movement—for example connecting the light cable to the laparoscope when the next surgical task is insufflation via the Veress needle—can interfere with the task performance of other team members an individual pattern to physical and repetitive movement is being under investigation.

b.  Instrument flow

Of equal importance with the identification of the patterns demonstrated by personnel is the characterization of the **flow of instruments within the surgical procedure** (Fig. 4.2). Contrast the MIS surgeon's relatively static body posture with the constant and complex choreography of instruments that contributes significantly to task efficiency and optimized ergonomics in the operating room. Instrument flow during surgical procedures—either as they take place in the OR or as they have been captured in video recordings—have been traditionally characterized by direct observation, resulting in manually tabulated accounts detailing instrument position and movement. Automated methods resulting from medical imaging aimed at the creation of contextually sensitive OR systems now provide equally useful delineations of surgical workflow. Research focused on the robotic surgical system as a provider of data rich signals contributory to knowledge of instrument flow in the context aware

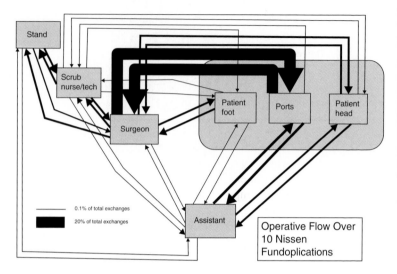

Fig. 4.2. A schematic of the different locations where instruments can be during a procedure. Each line between locations has a weight that is proportional to the frequency of exchanges between those locations during a case averaged over the ten cases. This method does not show where specific instruments are, but rather gives a general view of where the majority of the action is during a case.

integrated OR system is underway and proving of value. Visual data and surgical timing have recently allowed creation of a prototype automated scrub nurse capable of "understanding" a surgical sequence and automatically handing the surgeon the correct instrument as needed.

c. Cognitive workflow

Individually and also interconnected, error, stress, and teamwork first significantly investigated in aviation have now been recognized as critical in surgery and medicine. One survey of 30,000 cockpit crew members and 1,033 doctors, nurses, and surgical trainees that examined perceptions of error, stress, and teamwork found surgeons and anesthesiologists more likely than pilots to deny the effect of fatigue on performance and more likely to abstain from using steep hierarchies of command (indicating that input from junior members of the team is more acceptable in aviation than in medicine). Fatigue, communication issues, and error potential (awareness) are three components of the OR environment that have been implicated in increasing the cognitive workload and stressing the capabilities of team members. Communication intervals—roughly one third of which have been classified as communication failures—have been demonstrated to visibly alter workflow and to place OR staff responsible for patient safety responsible in harm's way. These intervals were shown to increase what the surgeon and team had to cognitively process, disturb routine, and exacerbate tension. The use of surgical checklists and preprocedural briefings are among the solutions now in use to mitigate fatigue and error and their ramifications. Use of a preprocedural briefing structured by a surgical checklist was found to reduce communication failures by one third and to significantly improve core surgical improvement measures such as antibiotic administration.

## 2.  Adaptation

As evidenced within both individual and team performance as well as demonstrable in workflow sequences, adaptability constitutes a crucial yet largely unstudied area contributory to surgical workflow knowledge acquired by applied ergonomics research. Surgical staff may make any number of ergonomically influenced adaptations in order to achieve efficient, error-minimized performance. A study of cognitive distraction in relation to simulated laparoscopic tasks concluded that experienced surgeons have achieved "automation" in the performance of laparoscopic skill sequences such that they are less affected by cognitive distraction than novice surgeons who merely have achieved task proficiency. The adaptive behavior that is employed, strategically or reflexively, by experienced surgeons in response to distraction is described. Adaptation is also common in the physical realm. A case study of adaptive behavior used by a highly skilled laparoscopic surgeon developing bilateral carpal tunnel syndrome demonstrated that what otherwise might be viewed as poor joint kinematics and postural instability (Fig. 4.3) actually functioned as strategic and compensatory movements evoked to preserve surgical performance of laparoscopic skills tasks.

## 3.  Quantification

Creation of suitable models for detailing surgical workflow patterns has too rarely been undertaken. The challenge in regard to the surgical

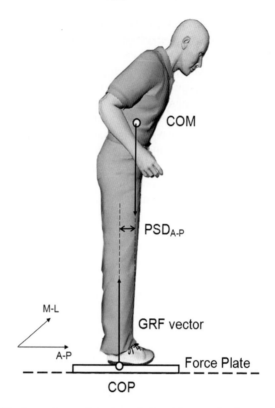

Fig. 4.3. The importance of surgeons being able to maintain a stable posture while performing laparoscopic tasks is accepted wisdom. Ergonomic research investigating postural balance control from data acquired through force plates that record ground reaction force direction and amplitude and where the center of pressure (COP) is located can tell us exactly what the demand is on the body in terms of stable or adaptable posture maintenance (Adapted with permission from Lee G, Park A. Development of a more robust tool for postural stability analysis of laparoscopic surgeons. Surg Endosc. 2007;22:1087–1092.).

workspace is that its quantification is not easily obtainable. Constructing workflow patterns has often been laborious, relying on manual creation dependent on direct observation and hand tabulation. New modeling technology, while not without prohibitive limitations, is promising. Motion analysis, available in a variety of forms including radio frequency ID (RFID) tags, has permitted the generation of diagrams descriptive of clinical and personnel workflow—despite minimally invasive OR barriers such as the number of personnel with unique and, at times, conflicting tasks.

The impact of distractions and interruptions to surgical workflow has also been evaluated. A mean rate of 0.29 distracting events per min (range 1–39 events per case) was demonstrated in a study of 50 surgical procedures—both open and laparoscopic. The study defined an event as a visible pause either in the workflow of the surgeon or another surgical team member. In related research seeking to quantify cognitive workflow interruption, disruptions of the surgeon's gaze during laparoscopic cholecystectomy were recorded and demonstrated that on average—40 breaks—most frequently occasioned by instrument exchange and downward gaze for extracorporeal work occurred in the operating surgeon's attention per 15 min of operating time. Another investigation examining surgical flow disruptions in 31 cardiac procedures found surgical errors escalated significantly with increases in flow disruptions. Disruptions categorized by the study as either teamwork or communication failures were the strongest predictors of surgical errors.

# E. OR Environmental Demands

Specific elements affect the cognitive and physical demands of the OR environment and many may be positively remedied through ergonomic research and application.

## 1. Lighting

a. **Situation**: Dim to no OR lighting is required to adequately expose the operative field for the MIS surgeon.

b. **Risk**: The darkened work environment makes the OR high risk for slips, trips, and falls, especially as regards safety for other OR personnel.

c. **Resolve**: In future ORs, floor lighting is needed to provide a clear view of the OR floor.

Overhead OR lights that are capable of being repositioned with one hand as well as controlled remotely from the nurses' centralized position within the room can also bring resolution.

## 2. Monitors

a. **Situation**: The MIS surgeon is reliant on monitor-displayed images to perform procedures in the same fashion as traditional, open surgery but with smaller, multiple incisions.

b. **Risk**: Placement, adjustability, and image resolution have been identified as issues that would continue to benefit from ergonomic research.

c. **Resolve**: Monitors should be ceiling-mounted and adjustable in height and inclination. These features better allow for realignment of the motor and visual axes, thus avoiding axial rotation of the spine, contributory to ergonomically unsound body posture for the surgeon. The optimal position allowing for gaze-down viewing is ideally 15° downward in that its use has been shown to almost completely minimize neck extension. A viewing distance—though it will be variable based on the visual acuity of the surgeon—should be established so as to avoid the problem of convergence and resultant eye strain.

## 3. Table height

a. **Situation**: The height issue arises as the result of interaction among three factors: surgeon height, instrument handle design, and patient body habitus after pneumoperitoneum.

b. **Risk**: The standard OR table has been proven to be too high for 95% of surgeons performing MIS procedures, a risk contributory among other issues to ergonomically poor body posture for the surgeon.

c. **Resolve**: MIS suite operating tables need to be adjustable to heights from 30 to 60.5 cm, a range allowing for elbow flexion between 90 and 120°. Surgeons and equipment falling off of the standing platforms that now often serve as accommodations to ameliorate the limited range of table height continues to be a safety hazard in the MIS OR suite.

## 4. Instrument handles

a. **Situation**: Overall, the level of satisfaction in regard to instrument handle size is reported to be high.

b.   **Risk**: In some few instances—the laparoscopic stapler being one—reported as being considered "too big" or as necessitating two-handed operation.

c.   **Resolve**: The challenge is to design for the full range of hand sizes. Women account for an increasing percentage of the surgical workforce and the range of hand and body sizes accordingly has become more varied. Going forward, a consideration in the manufacture of surgical instruments should be design that—through altered or adjusted placement of activation buttons or firing mechanisms—addresses the smaller handspan.

## 5.   Cables and tubes

a.   **Situation**: Cables, tubes, wiring, cords increased in the MIS OR environment.

b.   **Risk**: Over 50% of surgeons in one study reported that cables and tubes hindered their work. Cords, cables, wiring, and tubes remain a main source of tripping hazards even in ergonomically improved operating rooms.

c.   **Resolve**: Operating rooms of the future must provide a means by which to reduce the numbers of cables and tubes that cross the OR floor and surgical workspace. Enough floor space must be provided as well as so that remaining cables and tubes can be kept visible even when safely secured.

## 6.   Foot pedals

a.   **Situation**: During laparoscopic procedures, the surgeon operates diathermic and ultrasonic equipment by means of floor-stationed foot pedals.

b.   **Risk**: Postural instability for the surgeon is one ergonomic issue. Foot pedals additionally account for yet one more cord—often presenting a task disruption when its position shifts and it must be visually relocated—within the operative field.

c.   **Resolve**: Future ORs would benefit from hand-activated controls.

# F. Integrated OR Suites

When the twenty-first century began, MIS surgery was being accorded widespread acceptance by both surgeons and patients, and hospitals worldwide were discovering that the then current OR design did not allow for safe and comfortable workflow during performance of procedures. Many hospitals rose to the challenges of renovating and redesigning their operating rooms to accommodate the requirements, technological and otherwise, imposed by MIS surgical techniques, specialized equipment, and spatial demands. Based on the institutional renovation experiences undertaken by many hospitals, a number of formulated principles, many addressing the ergonomic factors as outlined, arose to guide the design of the minimally invasive workspace with a result being integrated OR suites.

## 1. General concepts in OR integrated suite design

   a.  **Centralization of control with optimal economy of workflow**—interoperative, comprehensive workflow efficiency sought that took into consideration the entire surgical team, including the circulating RN, surgical scrub technician, surgeon, and anesthesiologist

   b.  **Control of information flow**—necessitated in part by increased needs for communicating, broadcasting, and receiving video and audio information from points outside of the operating room

   c.  **Patient safety**

   d.  **Protection of the OR staff**

   e.  **Flexibility, expandability, and modular design**

## 2. Integrated computer-controlled ORs

Computer control is now a standard factor in the operating suite and a design element that must be regarded in relation to the situation awareness it promotes for all surgical team members. There are now, for instance, monitors for the scrub technician, the circulating RN, and the anesthesiologist as well as in areas devoted to centralized checklist use and surgical briefing. Design elements such as computer control that promote situation awareness also merit consideration as they have been found to promote patient safety.

# G. Ergonomic Knowledge: Surgical Staff and OR Application

1. **Need for guidelines**: Two recent surveys—each of over 230 surgeons—indicated large numbers of surgeons—American and European—to be experiencing somatic complaints they attributed to operating and all of the European surgeons indicating ergonomics to be important.

2. **Awareness of guidelines**—A general lack of ergonomic guideline awareness among surgeons was reported in both surveys—with 58% of American surgeons and 80% of European surgeons reporting being unaware of ergonomic guidelines. Another recent study confirmed the discrepancy between accurate ergonomics and surgeons' awareness, demonstrating that a third of surgeons indicating the video monitor as being in a proper position actually did not have it situated straight ahead between eye and hand level.

3. **Resolve**—The importance of educating surgeons in regard to both needed and proven ergonomic principles cannot be overstated. Participation and input of surgeons and surgical staff are critical to producing safe and efficient operating rooms in the future.

## Selected References

Ahmadi SA, Sielhorst T, Stauder R. Recovery of surgical workflow without explicit models. Med Image Comput Comput Assist Interv. 2006;9(Pt 1):420–8.

Albayrak A, Kazemier G, Meijer DW, Bonjer HJ. Current state of ergonomics of operating rooms of Dutch hospitals in the endoscopic era. Mini Invas Ther Allied Technol. 2004;13:156–60.

Berguer R. Ergonomics in the operating room. Am J Surg. 1996;171:385–6.

Brogmus G, Leone W, Butler L, Hernandez E. Best practices in OR suite layout and equipment choices to reduce slips, trips, and falls. AORN J. 2007;86:384–98.

Buzink S, van Lier L, de Hingh IHJT, Jakimowicz JJ. Risk-sensitive events during laparoscopic cholecystectomy: the influence of the integrated operating room and a preoperative checklist tool. Surg Endosc. 2010;24:1990–5.

Catchpole K, Mishra A, Handa A, McCulloch P. Teamwork and error in the operating room: analysis of skills and roles. Ann Surg. 2008;247:699–706.

Chou CD, Funk K. Management of multiple tasks: cockpit task management errors. IEEE International Conference on Systems, Man, and Cybernetics. 1990. p. 1154–6.

Davis G. Characteristics of attention and visual short-term memory: implications for visual interface design. Philos Transact A Math Phys Eng Sci. 2004;362:2741–59.

Einav Y, Gopher D, Kara I, et al. Preoperative briefing in the operating room: shared cognition, teamwork, and patient safety. Chest. 2010;137:443–9.

Gallagher A, Smith C. From the operating room of the present to the operating room of the future. Human-factors lessons learned from the minimally invasive surgery revolution. Semin Laparosc Surg. 2003;10:127–39.

Gilbreth FB. Motion study in surgery. Can J Med Surg. 1916;40:22–31.

Healey A, Sevdalis N, Vincent CA. Measuring intra-operative interference from distraction and interruption observed in the operating theatre. Ergonomics. 2006;49:589–604.

Herron DM, Gagner M, Kenyon TL, Swanström LL. The minimally invasive surgical suite enters the 21st century. A discussion of critical design elements. Surg Endosc. 2001;15: 415–22.

Hsu KE, Man FY, Gizicki RA, Feldman LS, Fried GM. Experienced surgeons can do more than one thing at a time: effect of distraction on performance of a simple laparoscopic and cognitive task by experienced and novice surgeons. Surg Endosc. 2008;22: 196–201.

Lee G, Kavic SM, George IM, Park AE. Postural instability does not necessarily correlate to poor performance: case in point. Surg Endosc. 2007;21:471–4.

Lingard L, Regehr G, Cartmill C. Evaluation of a preoperative team briefing: a new communication routine results in improved clinical practice. BMJ Qual Saf. 2011; 20(6):475–82.

Matern U, Koneczny S. Safety, hazards and ergonomics in the operating room. Surg Endosc. 2007;21:1965–9.

Matern U, Waller P, Giebmeyer C, Rückauer KD, Farthmann EH. Ergonomics: requirements for adjusting the height of laparoscopic operating tables. JSLS. 2001;5:7–12.

Miyawaki F, Masamune K, Suzuki S, Yoshimitsu K, Vain J. Scrub nurse robot system – intraoperative motion analysis of a scrub nurse and timed- automata-based model for surgery. IEEE Trans Ind Electron. 2005;52:1227–35.

Murata K, Araki S, Yokoyama K, Yamashita K, Okumatsut T, Sakou S. Accumulation of VDT work-related visual fatigue assessed by visual evoked potential, near point distance and critical flicker fusion. Ind Health. 1996;34:61–9.

Ossenblok P, Spekreijse H. Visual evoked potentials as indicators of the workload at visual display terminals. Ergonomics. 1988;31:1437–48.

Park A, Lee G, Seagull FJ, Meenaghan N, Dexter D. Patients benefit while surgeons suffer: an impending epidemic. J Am Coll Surg. 2010;210:306–13.

Padoy N, Blum T, Ahmadi SA, Feussner H, Berger MO, Navab N. Statistical modeling and recognition of surgical workflow. Med Image Anal. 2010 Dec 8.

Seagull FJ, Sutton E, Lee T, Godinez C, Lee G, Park A. A validated subjective rating of display quality: the Maryland Visual Comfort Scale. Surg Endosc. 2011;25:567–71.

Sexton JB, Thomas EJ, Helmreich RL. Error, stress, and teamwork in medicine and aviation: cross sectional surveys. Br Med J. 2000;320:745–9.

Sutton E, Youssef Y, Meenaghan N, et al. Gaze disruptions experienced by the laparoscopic operating surgeon. Surg Endosc. 2010;24:1240–4.

Svensson E, Angelborg-Thanderz M, Sjöberg L, Olsson S. Information complexity – mental workload and performance in combat aircraft. Ergonomics. 1997;40:362–80.

Thuemmler C, Buchanan W, Fekri AH. Radio frequency identification (RFID) in pervasive healthcare. Int J Healthc Technol Manag. 2009;10:119–31.

van Det M, Meijerink W, Hoff C, Pierie JPEN. Interoperative efficiency in minimally invasive surgery suites. Surg Endosc. 2009;23:2332–7.

Van Det M, Meijerink W, Hoff C, van Veelen MA, Pierie JPEN. Ergonomic assessment of neck posture in the minimally invasive surgery suite during laparoscopic cholecystectomy. Surg Endosc. 2008;22:2421–7.

Vereczkei A, Feussner H, Negele T, et al. Ergonomic assessment of the static stress confronted by surgeons during laparoscopic cholecystectomy. Surg Endosc. 2004;18:1118–22.

Vincent C, Moorthy K, Sarker SK, Chang A, Darzi AW. Systems approaches to surgical quality and safety: from concept to measurement. Ann Surg. 2004;239:475–82.

Wauben LS, van Veelen MA, Gossot D, Gossot D, Goossens RHM. Application of ergonomic guidelines during minimally invasive surgery: a questionnaire survey of 284 surgeons. Surg Endosc. 2006;20:1268–74.

Wiegmann DA, ElBardissi AW, Dearani JA, Daly RC, Sundt TM. Disruptions in surgical flow and their relationship to surgical errors: an exploratory investigation. Surgery. 2007;142:658–65.

# 5. Access to Abdomen

*Nathaniel J. Soper, M.D.*

## A. Equipment

Two pieces of equipment are needed to gain access to the abdomen and create a pneumoperitoneum: an insufflator and a Veress needle (or Hasson cannula, see Sect. C).

## 1. Insufflator

Turn the insufflator on and check the carbon dioxide ($CO_2$) cylinder to ascertain that it contains sufficient gas to complete the procedure. If there is any doubt, bring an extra $CO_2$ container into the operating room. In any event, always keep a spare tank of $CO_2$ immediately available.

Check the insufflator to assure that it is functioning properly. Connect the sterile insufflation tubing (with in-line filter) to the insufflator. Turn the insufflator to high flow (>6 L/min); with the insufflator tubing not yet connected to a Veress needle, the intra-abdominal pressure indicator should register 0 (Fig. 5.1).

Lower the insufflator flow rate to 1 L/min. Kink the tubing to shut off the flow of gas. The pressure indicator should rapidly rise to 30 mmHg and flow indicator should go to zero (Fig. 5.2). The pressure/flow shutoff mechanism is essential to the performance of safe laparoscopy. These simple checks verify that it is operating properly.

Next, test the flow regulator at low and high inflow. With the insufflator tubing connected to the insufflator and the Veress needle (before abdominal insertion), low flow should register 1 L/min and at high flow should register 2–2.5 L/min; measured pressure at both settings should be less than 3 mmHg. A pressure reading 3 mmHg or higher indicates a blockage in the insufflator tubing or the hub or shaft of the Veress needle;

N.J. Soper and C.E.H. Scott-Conner (eds.), *The SAGES Manual: Volume 1 Basic Laparoscopy and Endoscopy*, DOI 10.1007/978-1-4614-2344-7_5,
© Springer Science+Business Media, LLC 2012

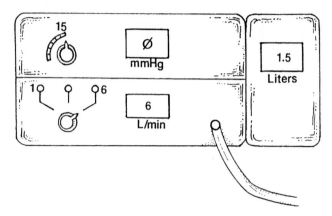

Fig. 5.1. **Insufflator testing**. With insufflator tubing open (i.e., not connected to Veress needle) and flow rate set at 6 L/min, the intra-abdominal pressure reading obtained through the open insufflation line should be 0 mmHg.

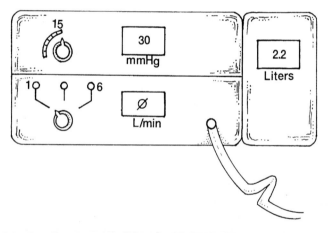

Fig. 5.2. **Insufflator testing**. With the insufflation tubing kinked, the intra-abdominal pressure should rapidly rise (e.g., 30 mmHg), thereby exceeding the preset 15 mmHg pressure set point. The flow of $CO_2$ should immediately cease (0 L/min) and an alarm should sound.

if this occurs, replace the needle. Maximal flow through a Veress needle is only about 2.5 L/min, regardless of the insufflator setting, because it is only 14 gauge. A Hasson cannula has a much larger internal diameter and can immediately accommodate the maximum flow rate of most insufflators (i.e., >6 L/min).

During most laparoscopic procedures, the pressure limit should be set at 12–15 mmHg; intra-abdominal pressures higher than this limit can diminish visceral perfusion and vena caval return, but may be required in obese individuals to achieve adequate visualization.

## 2. Veress Needle

Both disposable and reusable (nondisposable) Veress needles are available. The former is a one-piece plastic design (external diameter, 2 mm; 14 gauge; length, 70 or 120 mm), whereas the latter is made of metal and can be disassembled. Check the Veress needle for patency by flushing saline through it. Then occlude the tip of the needle and push fluid into the needle under moderate pressure to check for leaks. Replace a disposable Veress needle if it leaks; check the screws and connections on a reusable Veress needle.

Next, push the blunt tip of the Veress needle against the handle of a knife or a solid, flat surface to be certain that the blunt tip will retract easily and will spring forward rapidly and smoothly (Fig. 5.3). A red indicator in the hub of the disposable needle can be seen to move upward as the tip retracts.

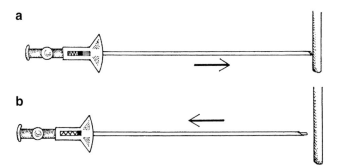

Fig. 5.3. **Testing retractable tip of disposable Veress needle**. (**a**) Blunt tip as it contacts resistance (e.g., a knife handle). (**b**) When the needle is pulled away from the point of resistance, the blunt tip springs forward and protrudes in front of the sharp edge of the needle.

# B. "Closed" Technique with Veress Needle

## 1. Umbilical Puncture

Place the supine patient in a 10–20° head-down position. If there are no scars on the abdomen, choose a site of entry at the superior or inferior border of the umbilical ring (Fig. 5.4). There are several ways to immobilize the umbilicus and provide resistance to the needle. The inferior margin of the umbilicus can be immobilized by pinching the superior border of the umbilicus between the thumb and forefinger of the nondominant hand and rolling the superior margin of the umbilicus in a cephalad direction. Alternatively, in the anesthetized patient, a small towel clip can be placed on either side of the upper margin of the umbilicus; this makes it a bit easier to stabilize the umbilicus and lift it upward.

Next, make a stab incision in the midline of the superior or inferior margin of the umbilicus. With the dominant hand, grasp the shaft (not the hub) of the Veress needle like a dart and gently pass the needle into the incision—either at a 45° caudal angle to the abdominal wall (in the asthenic or minimally obese patient) or perpendicular to the abdominal wall in the markedly obese patient. There will be a sensation of initial resistance, followed by a give, at two points. The first point occurs as the needle meets and traverses the fascia and the second as it touches and traverses the peritoneum (Fig. 5.5). As the needle enters the peritoneal cavity, a distinct click can often be heard as the blunt tip portion of the Veress needle springs forward into the peritoneal cavity.

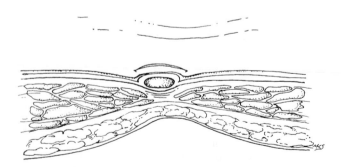

Fig. 5.4. Site of Veress needle insertion at superior crease of umbilicus; stab incision has been made. Transverse oblique section at superior crease of umbilicus; the peritoneum is closer to the skin at the umbilicus and is more densely adherent to the umbilicus than at any other site along the abdominal wall.

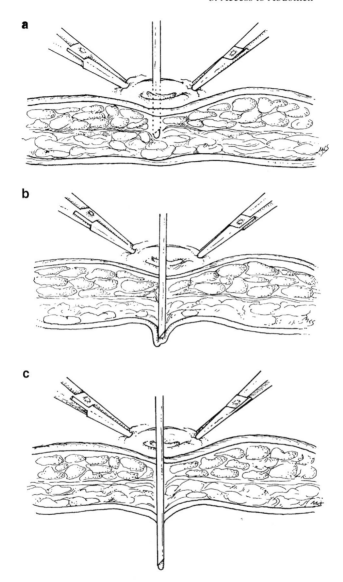

Fig. 5.5. (**a**) Veress needle inserted at umbilicus (sagittal view; the blunt tip retracts as it encounters the fascia of the linea alba). (**b**) As the sharp edge of the needle traverses the fascia, the blunt tip springs forward into the preperitoneal space and then retracts a second time as it encounters the peritoneum. (**c**) Blunt tip springs forward as Veress needle passes across the peritoneum to enter the abdominal cavity.

Connect a 10-mL syringe containing 5 mL of saline to the Veress needle. There are five tests that should be performed in sequence to confirm proper placement of the needle.

a.  Aspirate to assess whether any blood, bowel contents, or urine enter the barrel of the syringe.

b.  Instill 5 mL of saline, which should flow into the abdominal cavity without resistance.

c.  Aspirate again. If the peritoneal cavity has truly been reached, no saline should return.

d.  Close the stopcock and disconnect the syringe from the Veress needle, then open the stopcock and observe as any fluid left in the hub of the syringe falls rapidly into the abdominal cavity (especially if the abdominal wall is elevated slightly manually). This is the so-called drop test. If free flow is not present, the needle either is not in the abdominal cavity, or it is adjacent to a structure.

e.  Finally, if the needle truly lies in the peritoneal cavity, it should be possible to advance it 1–2 cm deeper into the peritoneal cavity without encountering any resistance. Specifically, the tip indicator or the hub of the needle should show no sign that the blunt tip of the needle is retracting, thereby indicating the absence of fascial or peritoneal resistance. Similarly, resistance to the needle tip may be caused by impingement on intra-abdominal viscera or adhesions.

Always be cognizant of anatomic landmarks when placing the needle, and carefully stabilize the needle during insufflation. Minimize side-to-side and back-and-forth movements of the needle to avoid inadvertent injuries.

After ascertaining that the tip of the Veress needle lies freely in the peritoneal cavity, connect the insufflation line to the Veress needle. Turn the flow of $CO_2$ to 1 L/min, and reset the indicator on the machine for total $CO_2$ infused to 0. The pressure in the abdomen during initial insufflation should always register less than 10 mmHg (after subtracting any pressure noted when the needle was tested by itself and with the insufflator) (Fig. 5.6).

If high pressures are noted or if there is no flow because the 15 mmHg limit has been reached, gently rotate the needle to assess whether the opening in the shaft of the needle is resting against the abdominal wall, the omentum, or the bowel. The opening is on the same side of the needle as the stopcock. If the abdominal pressure remains high (i.e., needle in adhesion, omentum, or preperitoneal space), withdraw the needle and

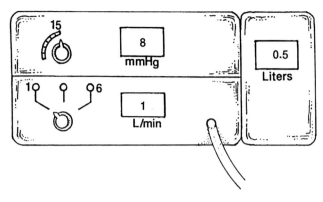

Fig. 5.6. Initial insufflation readings: proper inflow at beginning of $CO_2$-Veress needle insufflation.

make another pass of the Veress needle. If necessary, repeat this process several times until you are certain that the needle resides within the peritoneal cavity. Do not continue insufflation if you are uncertain about the appropriate intraperitoneal location of the tip of the Veress needle. Multiple passes with the Veress needle are not problematic, provided the error is not compounded by insufflating the "wrong" space.

One of the first signs that the Veress needle lies freely in the abdomen is loss of the dullness to percussion over the liver during early insufflation. When the needle is correctly placed, the peritoneum should effectively seal off the needle around the puncture site; if $CO_2$ bubbles out along the needle's shaft during insufflation, suspect a preperitoneal location of the needle tip. During insufflation, a previously unoperated abdomen should appear to expand symmetrically, and there should be loss of the normal sharp contour of the costal margin.

Monitor the patient's pulse and blood pressure closely for a vagal reaction during the early phase of insufflation. If the pulse falls precipitously, allow the $CO_2$ to escape, administer atropine, and reinstitute insufflation slowly after a normal heart rate has returned.

After 1 L of $CO_2$ has been insufflated uneventfully, increase the flow rate on the insufflator to 36 L/min (Fig. 5.7). When the 15 mmHg limit is reached, the flow of $CO_2$ will be cut off. At this point, approximately 3–6 L of $CO_2$ should have been instilled into the abdomen (Fig. 5.8). When percussed, the abdomen should sound as though you are thumping a ripe watermelon.

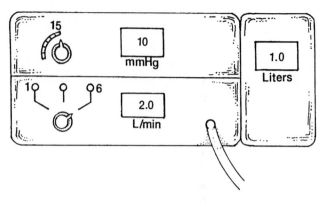

Fig. 5.7.  After 1 L has been insufflated, the set flow is increased to the highest rate.

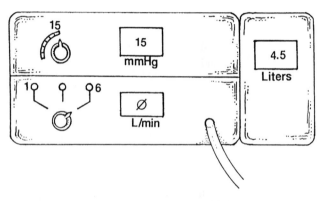

Fig. 5.8.  At 15 mmHg intra-abdominal pressure, 3–6 L of $CO_2$ will usually have been insufflated; the registered flow should then fall to 0.

## 2. Alternate Puncture Sites

Prior abdominal surgery mandates care in selection of the initial trocar site, and may prompt consideration of use of the open technique (see Sect. C). If the previous incisions are well away from the umbilicus, the umbilical site may still be used, with either a closed or open technique.

A midline scar in the vicinity of the umbilicus increases the risk that adhesions will be tethering intra-abdominal viscera to the peritoneum at that level. In this situation, the closed technique may still be used, but it is safer to use an alternate insertion site. This site should be well away from the previous scar and lateral to the rectus muscles, to minimize the thickness of abdominal wall traversed and avoid the inferior epigastric vessels.

In general, patients with prior low vertical midline scars should be approached through a trocar placed at the lateral border of the rectus muscle in either the left or right upper quadrant (Fig. 5.9). With previous upper vertical midline incision or multiple incisions near the midline, the right lower quadrant site may be appropriate. Alternatively, it is possible to perform an open technique with the Hasson cannula.

> **Upper abdomen**. In the upper abdomen, the subcostal regions are good choices. Carefully percuss the positions of the liver and spleen to avoid inadvertent injury to these organs, and decompress the stomach with a nasogastric or orogastric tube.

> **Lower abdomen**. The right lower quadrant, near McBurney's point, is preferable to the left because many individuals have congenital adhesions between the sigmoid colon and anterior abdominal wall. Decompress the bladder when using a closed insertion technique at, or caudad to, the umbilicus.

## 3. Placement of Trocar

A wide variety of trocars are available in both disposable and reusable forms. Most have sharp tips of either a tapered conical or pyramidally faceted configuration. Several new disposable trocar designs incorporate unique design features such as direct serial incision of the tissue under visual control (optical trocars—see below), or radial dilatation of the Veress needle tract. This section describes blind entry with the basic sharp trocar, with or without a "safety shield."

Always inspect the trocar to ensure that all valves move smoothly, that the insufflation valve is closed (to avoid losing pneumoperitoneum), and that any safety shields work properly. Make sure that you are familiar with the trocar; with the variety of designs available, it is not uncommon to be handed a different device (especially if it is less costly!).

Once you have attained a full pneumoperitoneum, remove the Veress needle. Most surgeons augment the pneumoperitoneum by lifting up on the fascia or abdominal wall to provide additional resistance against which to push the trocar. In a slender individual, the distance to the viscera and retroperitoneal structures is slight, and it is prudent to aim the trocar down into the pelvis. In an obese patient, this is less a problem and

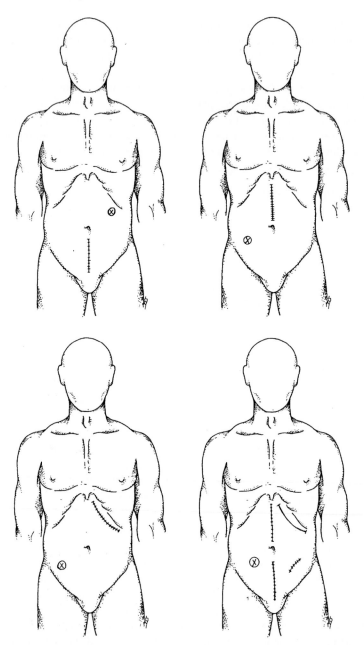

Fig. 5.9. Optional trocar sites in previously operated abdomen. Consider the open cannula technique.

the trocar may be passed in a more direct path. There should be moderate resistance as the trocar is inserted. Excessive resistance may indicate that the trocar is dull or the safety shield (if one is present) has not released, or that the skin incision is too small. The resistance suddenly decreases when the peritoneum is entered. Open the stopcock briefly to confirm intraperitoneal placement by egress of $CO_2$. Insert the laparoscope and visually confirm entry. Connect the insufflator tubing and open the valve to restore full pneumoperitoneum. Subsequent trocars should be placed under direct vision.

If the trocar has been placed preperitoneally, it is rarely possible to redirect it. Time is often saved in this situation by converting to an open technique for placement of the initial trocar.

Optical trocars are generally blunt-tipped. Place an end-viewing (0°) laparoscope in the trocar and use a blunt twisting motion (or activate the built-in knife) to advance the trocar through fascia and preperitoneal fat. The peritoneal cavity will appear as a black layer through the last translucent remnants of preperitoneal fat. These trocars are most commonly used for initial entry after production of pneumoperitoneum; subsequent trocars are placed under direct laparoscopic vision.

## C. "Open" Technique with Hasson Cannula

The open (e.g., Hasson) cannula provides the surgeon with an alternative, extremely safe method to enter the abdomen, especially in a patient who has previously undergone intra-abdominal procedures. In these patients in particular, the blind insertion of a trocar would be fraught with the potential for injury to the abdominal viscera. Some surgeons use the open cannula routinely in all patients for placement of the initial umbilical trocar.

The open cannula consists of three pieces: a cone-shaped sleeve, a metal or plastic sheath with a trumpet or flap valve, and a blunt-tipped obturator (Fig. 5.10). On the sheath or on the cone-shaped sleeve, there are two struts for affixing two fascial sutures. The cone-shaped sleeve can be moved up and down the sheath until it is properly positioned; it can then be tightly affixed to the sheath. The two fascial sutures are then wrapped tightly around the struts, thereby firmly seating the cone-shaped sleeve into the fasciotomy and peritoneotomy. This creates an effective seal so the pneumoperitoneum will be maintained.

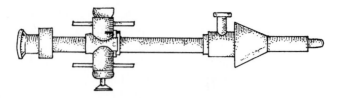

Fig. 5.10.   Open (Hasson) cannula, reusable type.

Make a 2–3-cm transverse incision at the selected entry site (in the quadrant of the abdomen farthest away from any of the preexisting abdominal scars or in the periumbilical skin crease if there has been no prior midline surgery). Dissect the subcutaneous tissue with scissors, and identify and incise the underlying fascia (Fig. 5.11). Exposure is usually facilitated by the use of small L- or S-shaped retractors. Gently sweep the preperitoneal fat off the peritoneum in a very limited area. Grasp the peritoneum between hemostats and open sharply. This incision should be just long enough to admit the surgeon's index finger. Confirm entry into the abdominal cavity visually and by digital palpation, to ensure the absence of adhesions in the vicinity of the incision. Place a #0 absorbable suture on either side of the fascial incision. Some surgeons place the fascial sutures first, use these to elevate the fascia, and then incise the fascia and peritoneum under direct vision.

Insert the completely assembled open cannula through the peritoneotomy with the blunt tip of the obturator protruding. When the obturator is well within the abdominal cavity, advance the conical collar of the open cannula down the sheath until it is firmly seated in the peritoneal cavity. Secure the collar to the sheath with the setscrew. Next, twist or tie the two separate fascial sutures around the struts on the sheath or collar of the open cannula, thereby fixing the cannula in place. Connect the $CO_2$ line to the sidearm port of the cannula and withdraw the blunt-tipped obturator. Establish pneumoperitoneum with the insufflator set at high flow. Increase intra-abdominal pressure to 12–15 mmHg.

With facility, it is possible to establish pneumoperitoneum just as fast (or faster) with the open technique as can be done with Veress needle and "closed" trocar passage. Indeed, many surgeons consider this to be the safest way to establish pneumoperitoneum.

If a Hasson cannula is not available, a standard laparoscopic cannula can be placed by an open technique. For this maneuver, place two concentric purse-string monofilament sutures in the midline fascia and make an incision into the free peritoneal cavity through the center of the purse

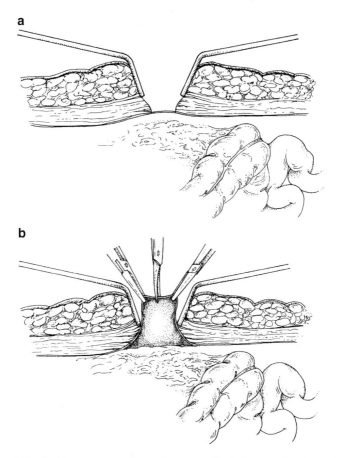

Fig. 5.11. (**a**) Retractors expose peritoneum. (**b**) Peritoneum is elevated and sharply incised. Two fascial sutures are secured to the struts on the sheath of the open cannula. The cone-shaped sleeve is then pushed firmly into the incision and the setscrew is tightened, thereby fixing the sleeve to the sheath of the open cannula. The sutures are wound tightly around the struts on the sheath, thereby securing it in place and sealing the incision.

strings. Keep both sutures long, and pass the tails of each suture through a 3-cm segment of a red rubber catheter, thereby creating two modified Rummel tourniquets. Place a standard laparoscopic sheath (with the sharp-tipped trocar removed), cinch the purse-string sutures against the sheath, and secure by placing a clamp on the red rubber catheter. At the conclusion of the operation, close the fascia by simply tying the sutures.

# D. Avoiding, Recognizing, and Managing Complications

## 1.  Bleeding from abdominal wall

a.  **Cause and prevention**. This problem usually manifests itself as a continuous stream of blood dripping from one of the trocars, and/or as blood seen on the surface of the abdominal viscera or omentum. Less commonly, delayed presentation as a hematoma of the abdominal wall or rectus sheath may occur. This source of bleeding is usually the inferior epigastric artery or one of its branches. Abdominal wall hemorrhage may be controlled with a variety of techniques, including application of direct pressure with the operating port, open or laparoscopic suture ligation, or tamponade with a Foley catheter inserted into the peritoneal cavity (Fig. 5.12).

b.  **Recognition and management**. To determine the point at which the vessel is injured, cantilever the trocar into each of four quadrants until the flow of blood is noted to stop. Then, place a suture in such a manner that it traverses the entire border of the designated quadrant. Specialized devices have been made that facilitate placement of a suture, but are not always readily available. The needle should enter the abdomen on one side of the trocar and exit on the other side, thereby encircling the full thickness of the abdominal wall. This suture can either be passed percutaneously using a large curved #1 absorbable suture as monitored endoscopically, or using a straight Keith needle passed into the abdomen and then back out using laparoscopic grasping forceps. The suture, which encircles the abdominal wall, is tied over a gauze bolster to tamponade the bleeding site.

## 2.  Visceral injury

a.  **Cause and prevention**. Careful observation of the steps just enumerated will minimize the chance of visceral injury. However, placement of the Veress needle is a blind maneuver,

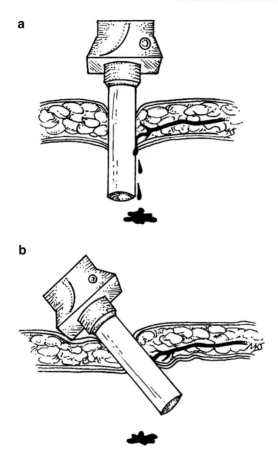

Fig. 5.12 (**a**) Bleeding from a trocar site. (**b**) Cantilevering the sheath into each quadrant to find a position that causes the bleeding to stop. When the proper quadrant is found, pressure from the portion of the sheath within the abdomen tamponades the bleeding vessel, thus stopping the bleeding. A suture can then be passed under laparoscopic guidance.

and even with extreme care puncture of a hollow viscus is still possible.

b. **Recognition and management**. If aspiration of the Veress needle returns yellowish or cloudy fluid, the needle is likely in the lumen of the bowel. Due to the small caliber of the needle itself, this is usually a harmless situation. Simply remove the needle and repuncture the abdominal wall.

After successful insertion of the laparoscope, examine the abdominal viscera closely for significant injury.

If, however, the laparoscopic trocar itself lacerates the bowel, there are four possible courses of action, depending on the surgeon's experience: formal open laparotomy and bowel repair or resection; laparoscopic suture repair of the bowel injury; laparoscopic resection of the injured bowel and reanastomosis; minilaparotomy, using an incision just large enough to exteriorize the injured bowel segment for repair or resection and reanastomosis (similar to the technique of laparoscopic-assisted bowel resection). If possible, leave the trocar in place to assist in identifying the precise site of injury.

## 3.    *Major vascular injury*

a.    **Cause and prevention**. Major vascular injury can occur when the sharp tip of the Veress needle or the trocar nicks or lacerates a mesenteric or retroperitoneal vessel. It is rare when the open (Hasson cannula) technique is used.

b.    **Recognition and management**. If aspiration of the Veress needle reveals bloody fluid, remove the needle and repuncture the abdomen. Once access to the abdominal cavity has been achieved successfully, perform a full examination of the retroperitoneum to look for an expanding retroperitoneal hematoma.

If there is a central or expanding retroperitoneal hematoma, laparotomy with retroperitoneal exploration is mandatory to assess for and repair major vascular injury. Hematomas of the mesentery and those located laterally in the retroperitoneum are generally innocuous and may be observed. If during closed insertion of the initial trocar there is a rush of blood through the trocar with associated hypotension, leave the trocar in place (to provide some tamponade of hemorrhage and assist in identifying the tract) and immediately perform laparotomy to repair what is likely to be an injury to the aorta, vena cava, or iliac vessels.

# Selected References

Baadsgaard SE, Bille S, Egeblad K. Major vascular injury during gynecologic laparoscopy: report of a case and review of published cases. Acta Obstet Gynecol Scand. 1989;68:283–5.

Chapron CM, Pierre F, Lacroix S, Querleu D, Lansac J, Dubuisson J-B. Major vascular injuries during gynecologic laparoscopy. J Am Coll Surg. 1997;185:461–5.

Deziel DJ, Millikan KW, Economou SG, Doolas A, Ko ST, Arian MC. Complications of laparoscopic cholecystectomy: a national survey of 4,292 hospitals and an analysis of 77,604 cases. Am J Surg. 1993;165:9–14.

Oshinsky GS, Smith AD. Laparoscopic needles and trocars: an overview of designs and complications. J Laparoendosc Surg. 1992;2:117–25.

Riza ED, Deshmukh AS. An improved method of securing abdominal wall bleeders during laparoscopy. J Laparoendosc Surg. 1995;5:37–40.

Soper NJ. Laparoscopic cholecystectomy. Curr Probl Surg. 1991;28:585–655.

Soper NJ, Odem RR, Clayman RV, McDougall EM, editors. Essentials of laparoscopy. St. Louis: Quality Medical Publishing; 1994.

Wolfe WM, Pasic R. Instruments and methods. Obstet Gynecol. 1990;75:456–7.

References

# 6. Generation of Working Space: Extraperitoneal Approaches

*David M. Brams, M.D.*
*Amila Husic, M.D.*

## A. Indications

**Extraperitoneal endoscopic surgery (EES)** was first described by Bartel in 1969. Wickham and Miller described the use of carbon dioxide ($CO_2$) and videoscopic control in 1993 while performing a ureterolithotomy. The initial difficulties using this approach mainly related to inability to create a sufficient pneumoretroperitoneum. Gaur introduced balloons for retroperitoneal dissection in 1993, and Hirsch and coworkers described the use of a trocar mounted balloon for extraperitoneal dissection in 1994.

Over the past 10 years, there has been increasing development in the use of extraperitoneal approach for urologic and gynecologic surgery such as in endoscopic extraperitoneal radical prostatectomy (EERPE), hysterectomy, adrenal, renal, and bladder surgery and in pelvic and retroperitoneal lymph node dissection. Recently, there has been an increasing interest in laparoscopic approach to spine surgery as well as aortoiliac procedures including aortobifemoral bypass. The major challenges involve steep learning curve and evolving technology. Today, the EES is most commonly utilized for totally extraperitoneal (TEP) inguinal herniorrhaphy.

There are both advantages and disadvantages to this approach (Table 6.1).

N.J. Soper and C.E.H. Scott-Conner (eds.), *The SAGES Manual: Volume 1*    79
*Basic Laparoscopy and Endoscopy*, DOI 10.1007/978-1-4614-2344-7_6,
© Springer Science+Business Media, LLC 2012

Table 6.1. Advantages and disadvantages of extraperitoneal endoscopic surgery.

| Advantages | Disadvantages |
|---|---|
| • Decreased risk of bowel injury | • Small working space |
| • Decreased problems with bowel retraction | • Orientation can be confusing |
| • Less postoperative ileus | |
| • Less chance of adhesion formation leading to small bowel obstruction | • Inadvertent entry into peritoneum causes loss of working space |
| • Closure of peritoneum not required when mesh implanted retroperitoneally | • Retractors often needed to displace peritoneal sac |
| • Less adverse hemodynamic effects from retroperitoneal insufflation | • Prior extraperitoneal dissection is a contraindication to this approach |

## B.  Anatomic Considerations

Knowledge of anatomic landmarks is essential to orientation in the extraperitoneal space, which can be divided into the following:

1.  Preperitoneal space—between the transversalis fascia and parietal peritoneum of anterior abdominal wall. The inferolateral border includes the space of Bogros which is lateral to the epigastric vessels and dissected in the TEP inguinal herniorrhaphy
2.  Retroperitoneal space—containing the aorta, vena cava, and the retroperitoneal organs
3.  Subperitoneal space—surrounds the pelvic organs anteriorly beginning at the space of Retzius between the pubic bone and the bladder and posteriorly with the pararectal spaces
4.  The lumbar retroperitoneal space is the posterior continuation of the space of Bogros bounded by the vena cava and aorta medially, the psoas dorsally, the colon ventrally, and transversalis fascia laterally. This space contains the kidney, adrenal, ureter, and Gerota's fascia.

## C.  Access to the Extraperitoneal Space

Depending on the type of procedure, the patient is either placed in supine or lateral decubitus position. There are three basic ways to gain access to the extraperitoneal space. For TEP approach, the incision is typically periumbilical, on the opposite side of the hernia. For access to retroperitoneal organs, the incision is usually 2 cm above iliac crest in posterior axillary line.

1. The **open approach**
   a. Make a 2-cm incision overlying the space to be developed.
   b. Bluntly dissect down to the preperitoneal space and develop this space.
   c. Place a Hasson cannula or a structural balloon trocar
   d. Continue dissection with laparoscope or balloon dissector (see Sect. D).

2. Use of a **lens-tipped trocar**
   a. Make a 12-mm skin incision over the desired location.
   b. Place a 0° laparoscope into a lens-tipped trocar.
   c. Use this to penetrate the layers of the abdominal wall under direct vision.
   d. Once the correct plane is achieved, place a Hasson cannula or structural balloon trocar and continue dissection (see Sect. D).

3. The closed approach using the **Veress needle**
   a. Insert a Veress needle suprapubically through the fascial layers into the preperitoneal position. The needle will traverse two palpable points of resistance (the anterior rectus sheath and transversalis fascia).
   b. Insufflate 1 L of $CO_2$.
   c. Make a skin incision lateral to the midline.
   d. Insert a 10-mm trocar, directed caudad, until the gas-filled space is entered.
   e. Place the laparoscope into the trocar and use it to dissect the space while insufflating $CO_2$.
   f. The major **disadvantage** is that this procedure is relatively "blind" and risks visceral and vascular injury as well as penetration of the peritoneum. If this technique is used to develop the lumbar retroperitoneal space, fluoroscopic control with ureteral and nephric imaging is essential.

# D.  Dissection of Extraperitoneal Space

Just as there are several techniques for obtaining access, there are several methods of dissecting the extraperitoneal space to create working room.

1.  **Operating laparoscopes** have a 5-mm instrument channel (in a 10-mm laparoscope). These allow dissection under direct vision during insufflation of $CO_2$.
2.  Alternatively, a **30° laparoscope** can be used alone to open the space by sweeping tissue away while insufflating $CO_2$.
3.  **Balloon dissection** is the most popular, if most expensive, method of developing the extraperitoneal space. It *may* be beneficial, particularly early in the surgeon's experience with this procedure. Spherical balloon dissectors are most useful. Kidney-shaped balloon dissectors are available for lateral dissection in bilateral hernia repair. There are a variety of commercially available balloons, with inflatable volumes up to 1,000 cc, although cheaper glove balloons have been used with equal success (Fig. 6.1).

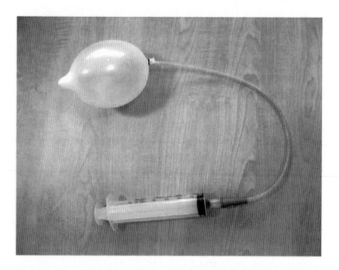

Fig. 6.1.  Balloons are made from the middle finger of a size eight surgical glove and a 14-F Nelaton catheter tied with silk suture, attached to a 50-mL inflator (Reproduced with permission from Ozgok Y, et al. Two-glove-finger-balloon dissection of retroperitoneal space for laparoscopic urology. J Chin Med Assoc. 2009;72(12):625–8. Fig. 1).

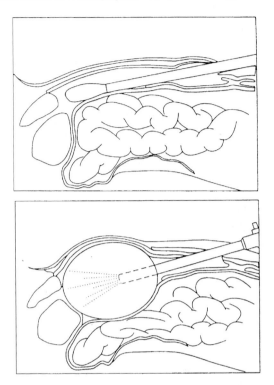

Fig. 6.2. Balloon used to dissect extraperitoneal space (Reproduced with permission from Tsoi EKM, Organ CH, Jr, eds. Abdominal access in open and laparoscopic surgery. New York: Wiley, 1996).

    a.   Insert an air-inflated, trocar-mounted clear plastic dissection balloon into the space to be developed.

    b.   Place a 0° laparoscope into the balloon and inflate the balloon while identifying landmarks (Fig. 6.2). Identify blood vessels, such as the inferior epigastrics, and avoid injury by controlled insufflation. The balloon is typically left inflated for several seconds during which direct pressure improves the hemostasis.

4.   Insert additional trocars under direct vision after creating the initial space. Develop and enlarge the extraperitoneal space with blunt dissection and atraumatic graspers, "peanut" dissection, and cautery scissors. A 30° laparoscope can facilitate exposure.

# E.  Maintenance of Extraperitoneal Space

There are several ways to maintain an extraperitoneal working space.

1.  Insufflation to 8–10 mmHg $CO_2$ will maintain a working space while avoiding excessive subcutaneous emphysema.
2.  Planar abdominal wall-lifting devices, allow gasless extraperitoneal endoscopy using conventional instruments.
3.  In TEP hernia repairs, the structural balloon trocar replaces a Hasson cannula and displaces peritoneum posteriorly while providing a seal between skin and fascia and providing access for the laparoscope (Fig. 6.3).
4.  Peritoneal retraction devices are necessary to displace the peritoneal sac for lumbar and iliac extraperitoneal laparoscopy. These instruments can be used in a gasless or gas extraperitoneal laparoscopic procedure.
5.  In retroperitoneal approaches to the kidney and adrenal, **laparoscopic ultrasound** can be used to help identify structures.

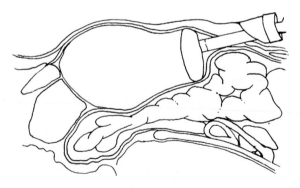

Fig. 6.3. Structural balloon trocar provides access for gas insufflation and laparoscope while the peritoneum is retracted posteriorly.

# F. Potential Problems

1. **Penetration into the peritoneal cavity** during access or dissection may necessitate conversion to a transabdominal laparoscopic or open procedure. Occasionally, relocation of the dissecting balloon trocar into the opposite rectus sheath will allow access into the extraperitoneal space.

2. **Peritoneal holes** allow $CO_2$ to leak, creating a pneumoperitoneum that decreases the extraperitoneal space. Close peritoneal holes with pretied suture.

3. **Venous bleeding** can be controlled with cautery and will usually stop spontaneously in the limited extraperitoneal space.

4. Cautery, clips, harmonic scalpel or suture ligation can also be used to control **arterial hemorrhage**. Suction and irrigation should be available.

5. **Prior retroperitoneal dissection** obliterates the potential space and is a contraindication to the extraperitoneal approach.

6. **Prior intra-abdominal surgery** will fuse the peritoneum to the abdominal wall. Begin the dissection away from old scars and leave dissection of these areas for last. This will diminish the risk of peritoneal violation.

7. This procedure is more difficult in **obese patients**, as excess adipose tissue in the extraperitoneal space will obscure planes and landmarks.

# Selected References

Carver BS, Sheinfeld J. The current status of laparoscopic retroperitoneal lymph node dissection for non-seminomatous germ-cell tumors. Nat Clin Pract Urol. 2005 Jul;2(7):330–5.

Coptcoat MJ. Overview of extraperitoneal laparoscopy. Endosc Surg Allied Technol. 1995;3:1–2.

Di Centa I, Coggia M, Cerceau P, Javerliat I, Alfonsi P, Beauchet A, Goëau-Brissonnière O. Total laparoscopic aortobifemoral bypass: short- and middle-term results. Ann Vasc Surg. 2008 Mar;22(2):227–32.

Eden CG. Alternative endoscopic access techniques to the retroperitoneum. Endosc Surg Allied Technol. 1995;3:27–8.

Farinas LP, et al. Cost containment and totally extraperitoneal laparoscopic herniorrhaphy. Surg Endosc. 2000;19:37–40.

Gaur DD. Laparoscopic operative retroperitoneoscopy. Use of a new device. J Urol. 1993;148:1137–9.

Gazzeri R, Tamorri M, Galarza M, Faiola A, Gazzeri G. Balloon-assisted endoscopic retroperitoneal gasless approach (BERG) for lumbar interbody fusion: is it a valid alternative to the laparoscopic approach? Minim Invasive Neurosurg. 2007 Jun;50(3):150–4.

Himpens J. Techniques, equipment and exposure for endoscopic retroperitoneal surgery. Semin Laparosc Surg. 1996;3(2):109–16.

Hirsch IH, Moreno JG, Lotfi MA, et al. Controlled balloon dilatation of the extra- peritoneal space for laparoscopic urologic surgery. J Laparoendosc Surg. 1994;4:247–51.

Kavallaris A, Hornemann A, Chalvatzas N, Luedders D, Diedrich K, Bohlmann MK. Laparoscopic nerve-sparing radical hysterectomy: description of the technique and patients' outcome. Gynecol Oncol. 2010;119(2):198–201.

McKernan JG, Laws HL. Laparoscopic repair of inguinal hernias using a totally extraperitoneal prosthetic approach. Surg Endosc. 1993;7:26–8.

Mirilas P, Skandalakis JE. Surgical anatomy of the retroperitoneal spaces part II: the architecture of the retroperitoneal space. Am Surg. 2010 Jan;76(1):33–42.

Ozgok Y, Kilciler M, Istanbulluoglu MO, Piskin M, Bedir S, Basal S. Two-glove-finger-balloon dissection of retroperitoneal space for laparoscopic urology. J Chin Med Assoc. 2009 Dec;72(12):625–8.

Stolzenburg JU, Truss MC, Do M, Rabenalt R, Pfeiffer H, Dunzinger M, Aedtner B, Stief CG, Jonas U, Dorschner W. Evolution of endoscopic extraperitoneal radical prostatectomy (EERPE)—technical improvements and development of a nerve-sparing, potency-preserving approach. World J Urol. 2003;21(3):147–52.

Tsoi EKM, Organ Jr CH, editors. Abdominal access in open and laparoscopic surgery. New York: Wiley; 1996.

Ullah MZ, Bhargava A, Jamal-Hanjani M, Jacob S. Totally extra-peritoneal repair of inguinal hernia by a glove-balloon: technical innovation. Surgeon. 2007 Aug;5(4):245–7.

Wickham JEA, Miller RA. Percutaneous renal access. In: Payne SR, Webb DR, editors. Percutaneous renal surgery. New York: Churchill Livingstone; 1983. p. 33–9.

Yanbo W, Xiaobo D, Yuchuan H, Yan W, Fengming J, Haifeng Z, Chunxi W. Retroperitoneal laparoscopy rather than an open procedure for resection of pheochromocytomas could minimize intraoperative blood pressure fluctuations and transfusion events. Int Urol Nephrol. 2010;43:353–7.

# 7. Single-Site Access Surgery

*James A. Dickerson II, M.D.*
*Chan W. Park, M.D.*
*Aurora D. Pryor, M.D.*

## A. Background

Laparoscopic surgery has been widely accepted as an alternative to open surgery across a myriad of surgical disciplines. Its benefits of diminished pain, faster recovery, improved cosmesis, and shorter hospitalization have been well documented across a spectrum of surgical procedures.

As a means to further minimize the invasiveness of laparoscopy, the concept of Natural Orifice Transluminal Endoscopic Surgery (NOTES) was created with the elusive goal of "incision-free" abdominal surgery. However, concerns over contamination, closure of the visceral access site, need for specialized equipment, and a steep learning curve have limited its widespread clinical application. As an alternative to NOTES, single-site access surgery has become one of the new frontiers in minimally invasive surgery. It serves as an alternative more closely resembling standard laparoscopy with similar cosmetic benefits and no obvious added risks.

The concept is not new. Over 40 years ago, Wheeless and Thompson reported the successful completion of 2,600 transumbilical tubal ligations. Despite its feasibility, the technique was not widely adopted. Not until 1992 was the first case series of 25 patients undergoing single-incision appendectomies reported by Pelosi and Pelosi. Navarro et al. published the first single-incision cholecystectomy in 1997, but the procedure failed to gain acceptance due to the lack of proper instrumentation.

The adoption of laparoscopy for the performance of more advanced surgical procedures coupled with advancements in technology has resulted in the resurgence of single-site surgery. Widespread enthusiasm by surgeons, patients, and the media has led to rapid incorporation of the

N.J. Soper and C.E.H. Scott-Conner (eds.), *The SAGES Manual: Volume 1 Basic Laparoscopy and Endoscopy*, DOI 10.1007/978-1-4614-2344-7_7, © Springer Science+Business Media, LLC 2012

technique into clinical practice. Consequently, there have been a variety of differing monikers employed throughout the literature leading to confusing terminology. Some of the more common acronyms include the following:

- Single-incision laparoscopic surgery (SILS™).
- Single-site laparoscopy (SSL).
- Single-port access (SPA™).
- Laparoendoscopic single site (LESS).
- One-port umbilical surgery (OPUS).
- Transumbilical endoscopic surgery (TUES).
- Embryonic NOTES (eNOTES).
- Single laparoscopic incision transabdominal surgery (SLIT).
- Single-instrument port laparoscopic surgery (SIMPL).

Numerous other terms have also been coined to describe single-site laparoscopy. As a means to both advance the field and standardize terminology, the Laparoendoscopic Single-Site Surgery Consortium for Assessment and Research (LESSCAR) assembled in 2008 by leaders in the field. LESSCAR unanimously concluded that the term laparoendoscopic single-site (LESS) surgery most "accurately conveys the broad philosophical and practical aspects of the field," and it is subsequently utilized in this chapter.

## B. Indications

At this time, there are no clear indications for single-site surgery. However, the technique has gained tremendous momentum, and its applicability and feasibility have been demonstrated throughout many of the surgical disciplines. The implementation of this technique has been witnessed in the fields of urologic, gynecologic, gastrointestinal, pediatric, thoracic, and bariatric surgery.

## C. Patient Selection

Patient selection is paramount to the successful implementation of LESS surgery. Consider the following:

1. **Key operative steps**. How will each step be impacted by the limitations of LESS?

2. **Unique patient characteristics and issues inherent in the pathophysiology**. Previous abdominal surgery, an acute inflammatory process, and obesity can potentially impact the successful completion of single-site laparoscopy.

3. **Patient habitus**. Obesity, as mentioned above, may render the procedure difficult. In addition, consider distance from the umbilicus (the preferred entry site given its overall cosmetic benefit) to the operative site. Thus, umbilical entry site may not be suited for upper abdominal surgery in patients with a long torso (and/or a low-lying umbilicus).

4. **Physiologic reserve**. Also consider whether the patient can tolerate a potentially longer operation with prolonged exposure to pneumoperitoneum and its adverse physiologic consequences.

# D. LESS Access Technique

1. **Multiple Port Technique**: Access is typically obtained via a single incision at the umbilicus, as it affords the greatest ability to hide the incision. A limited subcutaneous flap allows the introduction of multiple standard trocars to be placed 1–2 cm apart, resulting in greater freedom of movement. Separate fascial punctures limit the loss of pneumoperitoneum. Typically, a 2–3 cm incision can accommodate 3–4 working ports, one of which serves for optics. A benefit of this technique is that no specialized equipment is required, and costs similar to standard laparoscopy are incurred. One potential concern is the fascial weakening associated with closely placed trocars, and the creation of a "Swiss-Cheese" hernia defect. Although individually placed dilating-tip trocars are associated with a low incidence of incisional hernias, placement of multiple trocars in close proximity may result in a higher incidence of incisional hernias. A recommended solution is the communication of all defects with fastidious fascial closure.

2. **Multiport Access System**: Commercial systems are now available that are designed specifically for single-site surgery (Table 7.1). Access is typically obtained through an umbilical incision. In contrast to the multiport technique, a single, albeit larger, fascial incision is required. The length of the incision

Table 7.1. Examples of multiport devices.

- Triport® (Advanced Surgical Concepts, Wicklow, Ireland)
- SILS™ Port (Covidien, Norwalk, CT)
- GelPOINT® (Applied Medical, Rancho Santa Margarita, CA)
- Single-Site Laparoscopy (SSL) Access System (Ethicon Endo-Surgery, Cincinnati, OH)
- AirSeal™ (Surgiquest, Orange, CT)
- Uni-X™ Single-port Laparoscopic System (Pnavel Systems, Morganville, NJ)
- Octo™ Port (Dalim Surgnet, Seoul, Korea)

varies with the specific device employed, but typically ranges from 2 to 3 cm in length. Once the platform is deployed, it allows for the introduction of 2 or 3 working instruments and a laparoscope. Multiport systems often include interchangeable low-profile trocars that minimize valve clashing. Alternative systems have eliminated the need for trocars and provide varying sized ports. If additional instruments are required, a standard trocar may often be placed adjacent to the system. This technique, however, is often limited by either the incision length or size of the platform. The larger fascial opening facilitates the removal of specimens, but may also result in a higher hernia rate. The resulting fascial defect is closed in standard fashion (Table 7.1).

3. **Single-incision Platforms**: The loss of triangulation resulting from LESS has led biomedical companies to develop platforms to offset this limitation. TransEnterix™ (Durham, NC) has brought to market the Single Port Instrument Delivery—Extended Reach System (SPIDER™), a unique platform employing the combination of flexible and rigid instruments to achieve triangulation through a single incision (Fig. 7.1). Another option is provided by da Vinci® Surgical System (Intuitive Surgical, Sunnyvale, CA) which employs robotics and articulating arms to increase freedom of movement through a single incision.

# E. Limitations and Solutions

1. **Triangulation**: The single greatest impediment of LESS surgery is the loss of triangulation. Wide spacing of ports is a basic tenet of standard laparoscopy. In contrast, the introduction of

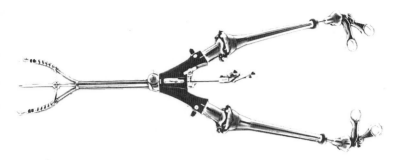

Fig. 7.1. Single Port Instrument Delivery—Extended Reach (SPIDER™, TransEnterix, Durham, NC). A single-incision platform that combines rigid and flexible instruments to achieve triangulation.

parallel devices through a single access site makes triangulation exponentially more difficult. "Sword-fighting" and disruption of the surgical view occur when the telescope and/or camera head collide with the surgeon's instruments (Fig. 7.2). A common way to minimize this sparring is to cross hands. Articulating or bent graspers can sometimes compensate for in-line surgery, but may require counterintuitive external hand movements. Instruments of differing shaft lengths can lessen clashing and offer some degree of triangulation. As the field of LESS surgery continues to mature, several techniques and instruments have been developed with the goal of minimizing these inherent limitations.

2. **Trocars**: Colliding instruments or trocar heads present another common problem, whether a single-incision with multiple trocars or multiport system is in use. Modern trocars have been enhanced to facilitate the replacement of instruments and introduction of the insufflant while minimizing the loss of pneumoperitoneum. Unfortunately, this enhancement has led to an increase in the external profile of these ports. While rarely an issue with standard laparoscopy, it imposes severe limitations on degrees of freedom during LESS surgery. Low-profile trocars, often without insufflation valves, allow greater instrument mobility. Placing trocars at different levels or "stair-stepping" can be helpful. In patients with a thicker abdominal wall, trocars of varying length can assist in staggering of the heads. When using multiple trocars through a single incision, it is always best to maximize trocar spacing.

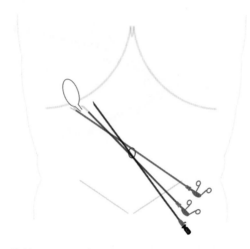

Fig. 7.2.   Parallel instrumentation and optics results in limited freedom of movement and instrument crowding.

3.  **Camera**: Another common restriction is imposed by interaction of the laparoscope and operative instruments. An oblique lens of 30° or greater can significantly improve the operative view. The light source and camera cables on standard laparoscopes frequently interfere with working instruments. A cost-effective solution is the use of a 45-cm telescope with a 90° light-cord adaptor. The added length and adaptor removes the camera head and light cord from the surgeon's field. Recently developed deflectable-tip laparoscopes further reduce collisions during LESS surgery. Articulation at the camera tip allows the camera to be moved from the surgeon's way while still providing the customary downward view (Fig. 7.3).

4.  **Retraction**: The common fulcrum between instruments constrains the hand separation that is typically needed to provide proper retraction. Also, a restricted number of working channels may alter traditional methods of retraction. Fixation or sling sutures can provide retraction that is normally offered by an assistant. Transabdominal percutaneous sutures introduced via a straight needle can be manipulated extracorporeally and result in adjustable degrees of tension. Alternatively, intra-abdominal stay sutures between peritoneal surfaces can often retract or displace organs to improve visualization. A novel

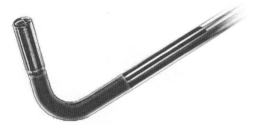

Fig. 7.3. Deflectable-tip laparoscope.

approach involves creation of a pulley system. An uncut suture is placed between the tissue to be retracted and the lateral peritoneum; the suture can then be exteriorized adjacent to or through an existing port. Increasing the amount of tension on the suture translates into greater retraction. The EndoGrab™ (Virtual-ports, Israel) (Fig. 7.4) is a retrievable retraction system with two opposed hooks that allows tissue retraction to an intra-abdominal surface. Use of this device frees an otherwise dedicated port or reduces the total number of required trocars.

5.  **Instruments**: New graspers and dissectors that articulate at the handle and/or tip are presently available (Fig. 7.5). These instruments can provide increased mobility at the tips, but can accentuate the need for external hand-crossing (Fig. 7.6). This technique is commonly practiced in LESS surgery, but requires an added degree of experience and dexterity. Prebent instruments can counter this drawback but may require the use of specialized trocars that could lead to increased costs. As previously mentioned, the introduction of flexible instrumentation through a rigid shaft is an alternative to conventional rigid instrumentation.

An alternative to pure single-incision surgery is the liberal use of mini- or micro-instrumentation. Similar in diameter to a Veress needle, these instruments can be used for dissection, cautery, and retraction while resulting in a virtually undetectable scar. Similar percutaneous options can serve as a bridge between standard laparoscopy and single-site surgery, while critical LESS skills are developed. Although in their infancy, magnetic anchors, motorized instruments and wireless cameras may ultimately serve to further propel LESS surgery.

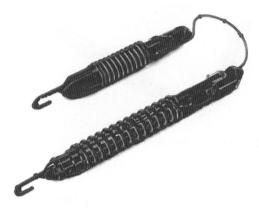

Fig. 7.4. EndoGrab™ (Virtual Ports®, Israel). A double end, retrievable grasper can provided intra-abdominal retraction without need for an additional port.

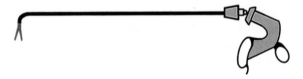

Fig. 7.5. Articulating grasper.

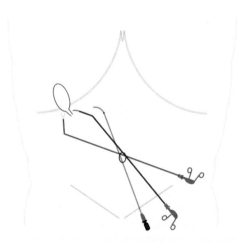

Fig. 7.6. The use of articulating instruments reduces "sword-fighting," but often leads to external hand-crossing and counterintuitive movements.

# F. Potential Advantages and Disadvantages

A variety of potential advantages to LESS surgery have been purported. The most evident benefit conferred is that of cosmesis. A single, well-placed incision within the umbilical ring can completely conceal a surgical scar. This affords patients an added degree of privacy, can have a positive psychological impact, and may result in greater patient satisfaction. Future diagnostic dilemmas may result from the lack of a visible scar.

A limited number of published studies have demonstrated that incisional pain after laparoscopic surgery is improved by diminishing the size of the incisions. This premise serves as one of the principal objectives of single-site surgery.

Because each separate entry portal gives potential for increased operative morbidity, limiting access to a single site theoretically should result in fewer iatrogenic injuries. Conversely, the need for multiple or larger fascial incisions coupled with greater torque at that site may lead to a higher incidence of incisional hernias.

In contrast to the specialized equipment and advanced endoscopic skills required for NOTES, the relative ease for an experienced laparoscopic surgeon to transition to LESS surgery has made it an attractive option. The simple conversion to standard laparoscopy for difficult cases or during the initial learning phase is an added benefit. Conventional access techniques are employed, and difficulties with closure of a hollow viscous are negated. Although technically feasible with existing laparoscopic instrumentation, dedicated single-incision platforms and instrumentation are becoming more prevalent. While minimizing some of the inherent difficulties of LESS surgery, they may result in greater equipment costs. The increased degree of complexity may also result in greater operative times. With mounting clinical experience, practiced LESS surgeons are demonstrating times comparable to standard laparoscopy.

Despite the debated advantages and disadvantages of LESS surgery, it is important to highlight the lack of high-level evidence to either support of refute these claims. To date, the only proven benefit of single-site surgery is cosmesis. In an era of evidence-based medicine, the fate of single-site surgery will ultimately be decided by well-designed comparative studies clearly defining its safety and the advantage over standard laparoscopy (Table 7.2).

Table 7.2. Potential advantages and disadvantages of LESS surgery.

| Advantages | Disadvantages |
|---|---|
| • Improved Cosmesis<br>• Familiar anatomic views<br>• Skills readily acquired by laparoscopic surgeons<br>• Easy conversion to standard laparoscopy<br>• Feasibility with existing instrumentation<br>• ? Decreased pain<br>• ? Decrease in access injuries | • Loss of triangulation<br>• In-line viewing and instrumentation<br>• "Sword-fighting" and hand-crossing<br>• Retraction may be problematic<br>• Decreased freedom of movement<br>• Increased complexity<br>• ? Increased costs<br>• ? Longer operative times<br>• ? Increased incidence of hernias |

# G. Future Direction

The future direction of single-site surgery is unclear. Technological advances will play a significant role in the progression of LESS surgery. The rapid deployment of platforms and instruments designed solely for use in single-site surgery is matched only by an increasing number of procedures applicable to this technique. Further refinements in wireless optical systems and magnetic anchors will diminish the limitations imposed by in-line surgery. Robotic-assisted technologies are emerging as another potential solution to these inherent limitations. The eventual acceptance of single-site surgery will likely result from a combination of improvements in technology, technique, and outcome.

The ability to safely perform increasingly complex operations through an "invisible" scar remains the ultimate goal of minimally invasive surgeons. Despite a myriad of feasibility studies, the implementation of single-site surgery is in its infancy with no widely accepted standards. To further propagate the concept, carefully designed studies to prove any possible advantages regarding post-operative morbidity are mandatory. These protocols should be done under institutional review board regulation with clearly defined goals. As prescribed by the LESSCAR committee, procedural details should be clearly described, leading to standardized techniques. Patient safety and improved clinical outcomes should remain the goal of LESS surgery. Regardless of whether single-site surgery is the next evolution in minimally invasive surgery, the technical skills developed will enhance standard laparoscopic surgery.

# H.  Technical Tips for LESS Surgery

There are a few things to keep in mind when embarking upon LESS.

- Proper patient selection—in the beginning, avoid: obesity, acute inflammatory process, and previous abdominal surgery.
- Attend wet and simulation labs or minifellowships early in experience.
- 45 cm scope with 90° light cord adaptor or deflectable tip laparoscope.
- Low-profile and "stair-stepping" of trocars.
- Instruments of differing shaft lengths decrease sword-fighting.
- Articulating instruments may enhance triangulation.
- "Minilaparoscopy" instruments as adjuncts.
- Percutaneous or internal sutures to provide retraction.
- Small movements result in less instrument clashing.
- Use additional trocars liberally.
- Low threshold to convert to standard laparoscopy or open procedure.
- Fastidious fascial closure.
- IRB regulatory procedures should be followed.
- Patient safety far outweighs cosmesis.

# Selected References

De la Fuente SG, DeMaria EJ, Reynolds JD, et al. New Developments in surgery Natural Orifice Transluminal Endoscopic Surgery (NOTES). Arch Surg. 2007;142(3): 295–7.

Gill IS, Advincula AP, Aron M, et al. Consensus statement of the consortium of laparoendoscopic single-site surgery. Surg Endosc. 2010;24:762–8.

Navarra G, Pozza E, Occhionorelli S, et al. One-wound laparoscopic cholecystectomy. Br J Surg. 1997;84(5):695.

Pfluke JM, Parker M, Stauffer JA, et al. Laparoscopic surgery performed through a single incision: a systematic review of the current literature. J Am Coll Surg. 2011;212(1): 113–8.

Podolsky ER, Rottman SJ, Poblete H, et al. Single Port Access (SPA™) cholecystectomy: a completely transumbilical approach. J Laparoendosc Adv Surg Tech. 2009;19(2): 219–22.

Ponsky TA. Single port laparoscopic cholecystectomy in adults and children: tools and techniques. J Am Coll Surg. 2009;209:e1–6.

Raman JD, Cadeddu JA, Rao P, et al. Single-incision laparoscopic surgery: initial urological experience and comparison with natural-orifice transluminal endoscopic surgery. BJU Int. 2008;101(12):1493–6.

Rao PP, Rao PP, Bhagwat S. Single-incision Laparoscopic Surgery – current status and controversies. J Minim Access Surg. 2011;7(1):6–16.

# 8. Hand-Assisted Laparoscopic Surgery[*]

*Carol E.H. Scott-Conner, M.D., Ph.D.*

## A. Background

Hand-assisted laparoscopic surgery (HALS) or handoscopic surgery was described in the 1990s as a means of overcoming the obstacles presented by laparoscopic procedures at that time. Surgeons first introduced the gloved hand into the abdomen via a mini laparotomy incision to improve depth perception, regain tactile sensation, aid in tissue extraction, and reduce operative time. HALS also provided a means to avoid conversion to an open procedure in some difficult situations.

The method initially described relied upon tight apposition of the abdominal wall tissues against the surgeon's forearm to maintain pneumoperitoneum. Difficulty with air leak and the inability to advance or withdraw the hand without sudden loss of pneumoperitoneum led necessarily to the development of hand-assist devices.

A variety of hand-assist devices are available. All require a small (7–10 cm) incision to insert the device. The device then provides a seal against the abdominal wall and a portal through which the surgeon's gloved hand can be inserted. Figures 8.1 and 8.2 show one such device and its placement. The device has two components; one fits in the wound, holding it open and mating with a second part mounted on the surgeon's forearm. The actual size of the device and hence the incision depend upon the size of the surgeon's gloved hand.

---

[*] This chapter was contributed in the previous edition by Benjamin E. Schneider M.D.

N.J. Soper and C.E.H. Scott-Conner (eds.), *The SAGES Manual: Volume 1 Basic Laparoscopy and Endoscopy*, DOI 10.1007/978-1-4614-2344-7_8,
© Springer Science+Business Media, LLC 2012

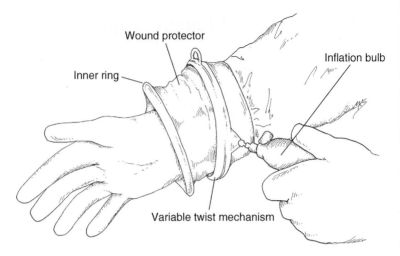

Fig. 8.1. The Omniport: its two flexible rubber rings that straddle the abdominal wall after insertion are connected to a double-layer spiral cuff that closes on the surgeon's wrist and expands over the wound edges when inflated.

The limitations of this technique include the obvious need for an additional incision in the abdominal wall. With current trends toward smaller incisions and single-incision techniques, this approach has become less desirable. A less-obvious disadvantage is the space occupied within the abdomen by the surgeon's hand, and the attendant potential for difficult visibility.

# B. Indications

HALS may be useful when a large fascial defect is required for tissue extraction, tactile feedback is required, or the laparoscopic approach is not progressing and otherwise would require conversion to an open procedure. The advantages and disadvantages of HALS are listed in Table 8.1. For some procedures, the nondominant hand is the gentlest retracting device available. HALS has been applied to procedures in all the following areas:

1.  Nephrectomy (particularly living donor nephrectomy).
2.  Colorectal surgery.
3.  Splenectomy for massive splenomegaly.

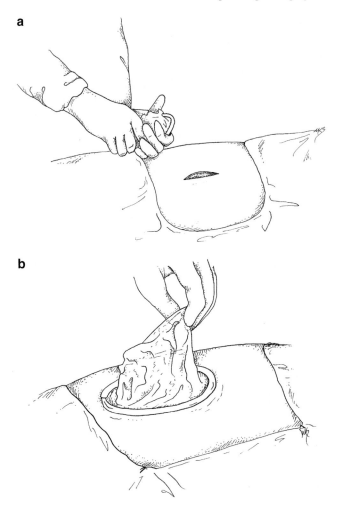

Fig. 8.2. (**a**) Insertion of Omniport; (**b**) Omniport in place.

4.  Gastroesophageal surgery.
5.  Gynecology.
6.  Aortoiliac surgery.
7.  Pancreatic surgery.
8.  Hepatic resection.

Table 8.1.  Advantages and disadvantages of hand-assisted laparoscopic surgery (HALS).

| Advantages | Disadvantages |
| --- | --- |
| • Allows for tactile sensation | • Hand encroaches upon intra-abdominal working space |
| • Specimen retrieval and anastomosis may be performed through hand port site | • May reduce benefit of laparoscopic procedure secondary to larger hand port |
| • Rapid control of bleeding by direct pressure | • Large incision at risk for incisional hernia |
| • Improved depth perception and shortened learning curve | • Device-dependent air leak |
| • Avoidance of conversion to open approach | • Ergonomically unfavorable, leading to shoulder and forearm fatigue and strain |

For most of these procedures, alternative techniques have superseded HALS techniques. Applications to specific procedures are discussed and illustrated in the chapters that follow.

## C.  Devices

A number of hand port devices are commercially available. Among the commonly used devices reported in the literature are the following:

GelPort (Applied Medical, Rancho Santa Margarita, CA).
Lap Disc (Ethicon Endosurgery, Cincinnati, OH).
HandPort System (Smith & Nephew, Inc., London, England).
Dexterity Pneumo Sleeve device (Dexterity Inc., Roswell, GA).
Omniport (Advanced Surgical Concepts, Dublin, Ireland).
Intromit Device (Medtech Ltd, Dublin, Ireland).

## D.  Technical Tips for HALS

Strategic placement of the hand port is critical to avoid obstruction of the laparoscopic view and to improve ergonomics. Concepts crucial to HALS success include the following:

1.  Remember the concept of triangulation and place the incision in a location that allows the nondominant hand to assist much like a standard laparoscopic instrument.

2. For procedures involving dissection in several abdominal quadrants, placement of the port centrally or in the midline will improve the range over which the hand may function.

3. For procedures centered upon a single quadrant, place the hand port at the periphery.

4. For certain cases, consider placing the hand port so that the incision is oriented to facilitate conversion to an open approach or for specimen extraction.

5. Follow the manufacturer's recommendations and make an incision just long enough to accommodate the port appropriate for the size of your gloved hand.

6. Use a darker colored glove to reduce reflective glare in the operative field.

# Selected References

Darzi A. Hand-assisted laparoscopic colorectal surgery. Surg Endosc. 2000;14:999–1004.

Gandhi DP, Ragupathi M, Patel CB, Ramos-Valadez DI, Pickron TB, Haas EM. Single-incision versus hand-assisted laparoscopic colectomy: a case-matched series. J Gastrointest Surg. 2010;14:1875–80.

HALS Study Group. Hand-assisted laparoscopic surgery vs standard laparoscopic surgery for colorectal disease: a prospective randomized trial. Surg Endosc. 2000;14:896–901.

Hanna GB, Elamass M, Cuschieri A. Ergonomics of hand-assisted laparoscopic surgery. Semin Laparosc Surg. 2001;8:92–5.

Leahy PF, Bannenberg JJ, Meijer DW. Laparoscopic colon surgery: a difficult operation made easy. Surg Endosc. 1994;8:992.

Meijer DW, Bannernberg JJ, Jakimowicz JJ. Hand-assisted laparoscopic surgery. Surg Endosc. 2000;14:891–5.

Patel CB, Ragupathi M, Ramos-Valadez DI, Haas BM. A three-arm (laparoscopic, hand-assisted, and robotic) matched-case analysis of intraoperative and postoperative outcomes in minimally invasive colorectal surgery. Dis Colon Rectum. 2011;54:144–50.

Southern Surgeon's Club. Handoscopic surgery: a prospective multicenter trial of a minimally invasive technique for complex abdominal surgery. Arch Surg. 1999;134:477–85.

Swanson TW, Meneghetti AT, Sampath S, Connors JM, Panton ON. Hand-assisted laparoscopis splenectomy versus open splenectomy for massive splenomegaly: 20 year experience at a Canadian centre. Can J Surg. 2011;54:189–93.

Targarona EM, et al. Hand-assisted laparoscopic surgery. Arch Surg. 2003;138:133–41.

Vogel JD, Liag L, Kalady MF, de Campos-Labeta LF, Alves-Ferreira PC, Rernzi FH. Hand-assisted laparoscopic right colectomy: how does it compare to conventional laparoscopy? J Am Coll Surg. 2011;212:367–72.

Wadstrom J, Biglarnia A, Gjertsen H, Sugitani A, Fronek J. Introducing hand-assisted retroperitoneoscopic live donor nephrectomy: Learning curves and development based on 413 consecutive cases in four centers. Transplantation. 2011;91:462–9.

Wolf Jr JS, Moon TD, Nakada SY. Hand assisted laparoscopic nephrectomy: comparison to standard laparoscopic nephrectomy. J Urol. 1998;160:22–7.

# 9. Laparoscopic Hemostasis: Energy Sources[*]

*James G. Bittner IV, M.D.*
*Michael M. Awad, M.D., Ph.D., F.A.C.S.*
*J. Esteban Varela, M.D., M.P.H, F.A.C.S.*

While the benefits of laparoscopy include more precise visualization of tissues, less postoperative pain, and shorter hospital length of stay among others, laparoscopic operations are not without their challenges. Namely, the need for rapid and secure control of vessels and hemorrhage is critical to maintain adequate visualization and avoid conversion to an open operation. The surgeon must understand the general principles of energy-induced hemostasis and appreciate currently available equipment and devices designed for laparoscopy. Laparoscopic energy-dependent technologies for hemostasis have their own unique complications. Consequently, the surgeon should be aware of the various strategies to prevent and address these issues.

## A. General Principles of Energy-Induced Hemostasis

1. **Thermal tissue destruction**. Even before the laparoscopic revolution, surgeons relied on energy sources, rather than mechanical means such as sutures and clips, to aid in hemostasis in the operating room. Electricity, ultrasonic waves, and laser energy are the energy sources most often employed.

[*]This chapter was contributed by Richard M. Newman, M.D., and L. William Traverso, M.D. in the previous edition and cited herein

These modalities all function by the same mechanism, i.e., an energy source is delivered to tissue, resulting in hemostasis via a predictable pattern of coagulation and thermal tissue destruction. The temperature attained in the tissues may predict the changes observed:

a. **At 45°C**, collagen uncoils and may reanneal, allowing apposed edges to form covalent bonds and fuse.

b. **At 60°C**, irreversible protein denaturation occurs and coagulation necrosis begins. This is characterized by a blanching in color.

c. **At 80°C**, carbonization begins and leads to drying and shrinkage of tissue.

d. **From 90 to 100°C**, cellular vaporization occurs and vacuoles form and coalesce, leading to complete cellular destruction. The surgeon observes a plume of gas and smoke that represents water vapor.

e. **Above 125°C**, complete oxidation of protein and lipids leads to carbon residue or eschar formation.

2. Variations in the rate of tissue heating and the degree of thermal spread accounts for the differences seen between the various energy sources. A basic understanding of how each energy source functions, as well as its limitations and potential complications, allows the surgeon to make careful choices of operative settings and avoid potential problems.

# B. Electrical Energy Sources Used in Laparoscopy

1. **Definitions**. Electrosurgery has evolved into the gold standard of energy sources for achieving laparoscopic hemostasis because of familiarity, cost, and versatility. Therefore, it is important to understand the meaning of the terms commonly used to describe properties of electrosurgical systems.

   a. **Circuit** is the pathway for the uninterrupted flow of electrons.

   b. **Current** is the flow of electrons during a period of time (amperes).

   c. **Voltage** is the force pushing current through the resistance (volts).

d. **Resistance** is the obstacle to the flow of direct current (ohms).

e. **Impedance** is the resistance to flow of alternating current (ohms).

f. **Capacitance** is the stored electrical charge that occurs when two conductors are separated by an insulator (farad).

g. **Power** is the rate at which heat energy is produced (watts).

h. **Active electrodes** are connected to an electrosurgical generator and concentrate the flow of electrons to allow for directed application of current to a specific point thereby producing a tissue effect in a concentrated area.

i. **Grounding (patient return) electrodes** are low-resistance conductors that accept electrons from active electrodes and facilitate their return to the electrosurgical generator.

j. **Electrocautery** is a surgical tool or device (active electrode) that connects to an electrosurgical generator and allows the performance of electrosurgery.

k. **Electrosurgery** describes the surgical use of a tool or device that employs heat generated by a high-voltage, high-frequency alternating current passed through an active electrode to dissect and/or coagulate tissue. Because nerve and muscle stimulation cease at 100,000 cycles/s, electrosurgery uses "radio" frequencies over 200,000 cycles/s. This allows energy to pass through the patient with minimal neuromuscular stimulation and no risk of electrocution.

l. **Current density** is the ratio of current intensity to area, perpendicular to current direction, through which current is flowing (current density = amperes/cm$^2$). Reducing the surface area of the active electrode increases the current density.

m. **Temperature** is a measure of heat produced as a result of electrosurgery. The heat produced is directly proportional to the resistance of the tissue and inversely proportional to the cross-sectional area of tissue through which the current is flowing (temperature = current density$^2$).

2. **Electrosurgery systems**

a. **Grounded electrosurgical generators** are a source of high-voltage, high-frequency alternating current and voltage. They require an active electrode and a grounding electrode to function properly. Burns can occur at the site of the grounding electrode (which is usually hidden under surgical drapes). To lessen this risk, most grounded electrosurgical systems monitor the level of impedance at the patient/pad interface and deactivate the generator before an injury can occur. Additionally, many of these systems continuously monitor changes in tissue resistance and adjust maximum voltage to reduce capacitive coupling and video interference.

b.  **Isolated electrosurgical generators** also produce high-voltage, high-frequency alternating current and voltage. However, in isolated electrosurgical systems, the circuit is completed by the generator rather than by the ground. Current from an isolated electrosurgical generator recognizes the patient return electrode as the preferred pathway back to the generator, thereby eliminating certain hazards inherent in grounded systems, most importantly current division and alternate site burns.

c.  **Closed-loop, isolated electrosurgery generators** are a source of high-voltage, high-frequency alternating current and voltage capable of including tissue feedback data in every mode available. The tissue sensing energy platform is a computer controlled system that senses impedance in patient tissues and adjusts output voltage, electrical current, and generator power. This provides consistent electrosurgical effect across a wide range of varying patient tissue resistance/impedance.

1.  **Examples**: Force FX™ and Force EZ™ with Instant Response™ technology (Covidien), Aaron 3250™ with BovieFDFS™ technology (Bovie Medical Corporation), and System 7550™ and System 5000™ with Dynamic Response technology (ConMed Corporation).

3.  **Monopolar electrosurgery** is frequently used during laparoscopy for cutting and coagulating tissues to facilitate dissection and ensure hemostasis of raw surfaces, small vessels, and ill-defined sources of bleeding (Table 9.1).

a.  **Alternating current** from a grounded electrosurgical generator is transmitted to an active electrode, which concentrates the flow of electrons in a desired area. The grounded electrosurgical generator can produce two types of current

Table 9.1. Selected electrical and ultrasonic energy devices used in laparoscopy.

| Energy type | Laparoscopic device | Company[a] | Available tips | Shaft length (cm) | Shaft diameter (mm) | Max Blade temp (°C) | Thermal spread (mm)[c] | Average[b] Arterial burst (mmHg) | Burst failure (%)[d] | Max Vessel sealing (mm)[e] |
|---|---|---|---|---|---|---|---|---|---|---|
| Monopolar | ENDOPATH® | Ethicon | Spatula, J/L hooks | 29, 34 | 5 | – | – | – | – | – |
| | Opti2™ | Covidien | Spatula, J/L/flat hooks | 36, 45 | 5 | – | – | – | – | – |
| | Opti4™ | Covidien | Spatula, J/L/flat hooks | 28, 36 | 5 | – | – | – | – | – |
| | PKS™ | Olympus | Spatula, J/L/flat hooks, needle | 28, 35 | 5 | – | – | – | – | – |
| Monopolar+ Argon | ArgonPlus™ | Covidien | Spatula, flat, needle | 28 | 5 | – | – | – | – | – |
| | APC™ | ERBE | Spatula, hook, needle | 32, 50 | 5 | – | – | – | – | – |

(continued)

Table 9.1. (continued)

| Energy type | Laparoscopic device | Company[a] | Available tips | Shaft length (cm) | Shaft diameter (mm) | Max Blade temp (°C) | Thermal spread (mm)[c] | Average[b] Arterial burst (mmHg) | Burst failure (%)[d] | Max Vessel sealing (mm)[e] |
|---|---|---|---|---|---|---|---|---|---|---|
| Bipolar | ENSEAL® TRIO | Ethicon | Straight, curved, rounded | 14, 25, 35, 45 | 5 | 87 | 1 | 255–891 | 0–2 | 7 |
| | LigaSure™ | Covidien | Straight, curved | 32, 34, 37, 44 | 5, 10 | 35, 97 | 0–4.5 | 380–885 | 0–5 | 7 |
| | HALO PKS™ | Olympus | Straight | 15, 24, 33, 45 | 5 | – | – | 614 | 10 | 7 |
| | OMNI PKS™ | Olympus | Curved | 15, 24, 33, 45 | 5 | – | – | – | – | 7 |
| | Trissector PKS™ | Gyrus | Curved | 15, 24, 33, 45 | 5 | 36 | 3.6 | 291–418 | 43–92 | 7 |
| | BioClamp® | ERBE | Straight, curved | 34 | 5 | – | – | – | – | – |

| | | | | | | | | | |
|---|---|---|---|---|---|---|---|---|---|
| Ultrasonic | HARMONIC® ACE | Ethicon | Curved | 14, 23, 36, 45 | 5 | 105 | 1–2.4 | 204–908 | 8–22 | 5 |
| | HARMONIC® LCS | Ethicon | Curved | 45 | 5 | 96 | 3.1 | 363 | 39 | 5 |
| | SonoSurg® | Olympus | Straight, curved | 34, 45 | 5, 10 | – | – | 647–1,071 | 11 | 5 |

[a] Ethicon Endo-Surgery, Inc., Cincinnati, OH; Covidien, Mansfield, MA; Olympus Surgical and Industrial America, Inc., Center Valley, PA; ERBE USA, Inc., Marietta, GA; and Gyrus ACMI, Inc., an Olympus Company, Southborough, MA were invited to provide relevant data and/or references

[b] Data are compiled from multiple, independent, in vivo and ex vivo animal studies in which vessel sealing devices were tested on arteries of various diameters (≤7 mm for bipolar and ≤5 mm for ultrasonic devices) according to manufacturer specifications. Reported averages vary by device and vessel diameters tested, electrosurgery generators used, and study methodology employed (see "Selected References")

[c] Average lateral thermal spread distances are derived by thermography and/or histopathology

[d] Average arterial burst failure incidence is based on incomplete sealing or burst pressures of <50 mmHg in some studies and <360 mmHg in others

[e] United States Food and Drug Administration-approved maximum vessel sealing diameters

(cutting and coagulating), which vary depending on the waveform. After passing through tissue in the surgical field, the electrons travel an unpredictable course along the path of least resistance toward ground, which may not always be the grounding (patient return) electrode. However, the path of electrons from active to grounding electrodes will be more direct as the grounding electrode gets closer to the operative site. To minimize the risk of burn at the return electrode, utilize an isolated electrosurgical system, avoid excessively high current concentrations, and ensure the skin surface impedance is not compromised by excessive hair, adipose tissue, bony prominences, fluid invasion, adhesive failure, scar tissue, or other variables.

1. **Cutting current** (continuous waveform, high frequency, low voltage) produces a focal and rapid tissue heating and cutting effect. Cutting current divides tissue with electric sparks that focus intense heat at the surgical site. To create this spark the surgeon should hold the electrode slightly away from the tissue to produce maximum current concentration. This will produce the greatest amount of heat over a very short period of time, thereby vaporizing tissue. Heating occurs so rapidly that there is minimal associated coagulation necrosis and therefore no hemostasis. In laparoscopic procedures, owing to a limited visual field, the immediate control of all bleeding is desirable; therefore, pure cutting current is rarely employed.

   a. **Vaporization** (sparking with the cutting current) heats cells very rapidly converting water to steam, which in turn disrupts the cell causing it to explode (Fig. 9.1).

   b. **Desiccation** occurs when the active electrode is in direct contact with the tissue and cutting current is employed. The cells heat more slowly and form a coagulum rather than vaporize and explode (Fig. 9.1).

2. **Coagulating current** (pulse waveform, low frequency, high voltage) produces a slower heating that causes protein denaturation. Hemostasis occurs via coagulative necrosis in and around the target tissue.

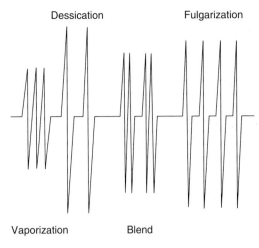

Fig. 9.1. Duty cycles of monopolar cutting (vaporization, dessication), blending, and coagulating (fulgarization) current.

a. **Fulguration** (sparking with the coagulating current) coagulates the tissue over a wide area and produces less heat. The result is a hemostatic coagulum and eschar. Due to the high impedance of air, sparking with the coagulating current requires higher voltage. In minimally invasive surgery, fulguration has implications related to carbon dioxide pneumoperitoneum (Fig. 9.1).

3. **Blended current** (continuous waveform, intermediate frequency, intermediate voltage) is not a pure combination of cutting and coagulating currents. Only the cutting current is altered so that the duty cycle is reduced by approximately 50% to provide more hemostasis compared to pure cutting current. Setting the electrosurgical generator to blended current does nothing to alter the coagulating current (Fig. 9.1).

a. **Benefits** of monopolar electrosurgery are several.

1. **Low voltage** is available as cutting current.

2. **Hemostasis** can be achieved for bleeding tissues not amenable to bipolar electrosurgery or ultrasonic devices.

3. **Rapid** cutting and coagulating of tissue is possible.

4. **Bipolar electrosurgery** is increasingly employed during laparoscopy, especially for sealing vascularized tissue pedicles and blood vessels (Table 9.1).

   a. **Alternating current** from a grounded electrosurgical generator is transmitted to an active electrode, which concentrates the flow of electrons in a desired area. Bipolar electrosurgery employs forceps with two tines. One tine of the forceps serves as the active electrode while the other functions as the return electrode; therefore, no patient return electrode is required. Flow of current beyond the surgical field is minimal.

      1. **Vessel sealing devices** are low voltage, high amperage bipolar electrosurgery instruments that, in combination with optimal pressure delivery by the instrument, fuse vessel walls and create a permanent seal. The output is feedback-controlled in a continuous manner so that a seal is achieved in minimal time, independent of the type or amount of tissue in the jaws. The result is sealing of vessels ≤7 mm in diameter with minimal thermal spread.

   b. **Benefits** of bipolar electrosurgery are multiple.

      1. **Hemostasis** and division of unsupported vascular tissues ≤7 mm in diameter using coagulating mode.

      2. **Versatility** as a laparoscopic tool that grasps, dissects, cuts, and coagulates tissue. This versatility may result in fewer instrument exchanges during procedures.

      3. **Less thermal injury** occurs compared to monopolar electrosurgery devices.

      4. **No capacitive coupling** occurs and inadvertent direct coupling is unlikely.

      5. **Fewer accessories** are required such as grounding electrodes, eliminating the possibility of alternate site burns.

      6. **Safety** of the technology for use in laparoscopy has been established.

5. **Radiofrequency electrosurgery** is employed primarily for ablative therapy.

   a. **Alternating current** through the tissue increases intracellular temperature and generates localized interstitial heating. Above 60°C, proteins irreversibly denature and tissue begins to coagulate.

b.   **Radiofrequency ablation systems** are made up of a unique active electrode and a generator designed to monitor tissue impedance through a feedback algorithm and adjust the output accordingly. The generator delivers pulsed current at increasing frequencies over time (10–12 min), limiting tissue impedance that might minimize effect on tissues.

6.   **Argon-enhanced electrosurgery** is utilized in open and laparoscopic operations, most frequently for procedures involving solid organs (Table 9.1).

a.   **Argon gas** can enhance the effectiveness of monopolar electrosurgery. The benefit is that ionized, pressurized argon gas completes the circuit between the active electrode and the target tissue, resulting in denaturation of surface tissue proteins and formation of a shallow eschar. At the same time, argon gas pressure displaces oxygen from the combustion area so that heat is confined to a lower temperature range. This pressurized gas stream also displaces blood and fluid away from the bleeding source and allows for more precise fulguration.

b.   The significantly limited cutting ability, lack of tactile feedback, and concerns about gas embolism limit routine use in laparoscopy.

# C.  Ultrasonic Energy Sources Used in Laparoscopy

1.   **Ultrasonic shears** employ both compression and friction to efficiently deliver mechanical energy to target tissues resulting in a predictable pattern of thermal destruction. Due to these forces acting on target tissue, amino acids unwind and reshape and hydrogen bonds break resulting in a sticky coagulum that seals vessels (Table 9.1).

a.   **Friction** is created in target tissues by ultrasonic shears, which contain piezoelectric diskes that convert generated electrical energy to mechanical energy. The mechanical energy is amplified by silicone elements then transferred to the instrument blade, which vibrates at high frequency. Ultrasonic shears have one active blade that can be rotated to expose the tissue to a sharp edge, a rounded edge, or a flat edge. Hemostatic tissue effect can be enhanced by blade configuration and tissue traction in a manner analogous to electrode design for electrosurgery (i.e., the broader the blade, the more coagulation effect). A nonactivated pad opposes the active blade and acts as an anvil to hold tissue, enabling the creation of frictional and shearing forces necessary for cutting and coagulating.

1. **Cutting mode** (max) generates rapid cycling of the active blade resulting in more precise cutting of tissue and less thermal spread but minimal hemostasis.

2. **Coagulating mode** (min) generates slow cycling of the active blade resulting in less precise cutting of tissue but more thermal spread and hemostasis. Select ultrasonic shears are approved to seal vessels measuring $\leq 5$ mm in diameter.

b. **Benefits** of ultrasonic shears for use in laparoscopy are multiple.

1. **Hemostasis** and division of unsupported vascular tissues $\leq 5$ mm in diameter using coagulating mode.

2. **Versatility** as a laparoscopic tool that grasps, dissects, cuts, and coagulates tissue. This versatility may result in fewer instrument exchanges during procedures.

3. **Monopolar utility** of the device is possible using the active blade alone.

4. **No tissue sticking** occurs because of the vibrations of the active blade on the tissue and the lower heat generated at the blade-tissue interface.

5. **Minimal thermal injury** occurs as a function of the energy type and mechanics of the ultrasonic shears.

6. **Fewer accessories** are required such as grounding electrodes, eliminating the possibility of alternate site burns.

7. **No capacitive coupling** occurs and inadvertent direct coupling is unlikely.

8. **Safety** of the technology for use in laparoscopy has been established. In fact, a recent review article suggests use of ultrasonic shears for laparoscopic cholecystectomy may improve outcomes compared to monopolar electrosurgery.

# D. Complications of Electrical and Ultrasonic Energy Sources Used in Laparoscopy

1. **Monopolar electrosurgery complications** include those listed below.

   a. **Current concentration** can occur when cutting connective tissue between structures with varying current density.

      1. **For example**, when cutting an adhesive band between the gallbladder and duodenum with monopolar electrosurgery, if the band is wider near the gallbladder than duodenum, the current density will be greater on the duodenum. Such current concentration can inadvertently injury the duodenum and may go unrecognized during the procedure.

      2. **Safety methods** include paying close attention to structures on either side of tissue before the use of electrosurgery and avoiding electrosurgery to adhesions already transected, as this will concentrate current further.

   b. **Insulation failure** occurs when the insulation surrounding the laparoscopic instrument breaks. This allows the transmission of electrical current to an undesired and often unrecognized target such as an instrument, trocar, or tissue. Even imperceptible insulation failures may result in significant injury. In fact, the smaller the break the greater the likelihood of injury if contact with tissue occurs.

      1. **Safety methods** to limit this source of patient injury include routine inspection of the insulation covering all electrosurgical instruments. Further protection against insulation failure is provided by an active electrode monitoring system, a conductive sheath that covers laparoscopic instruments, that collects stray energy resulting from insulation failure and returns this current to the electrosurgical generator.

   c. **Direct coupling** occurs when an active electrode is in contact with a conductive instrument or material.

      1. **For example**, it is possible to use direct coupling to coagulate tissue grasped in one instrument by touching it with a different active electrode.

       2.   **Safety methods** to reduce direct coupling include using only insulated instruments and paying careful attention to electrosurgery devices within and outside the visual field. Furthermore, avoid direct coupling near metal objects such as clips, staples, and laparoscopes, as this generates heat and damages surrounding tissue.

    d.  **Capacitive coupling** occurs when an active electrode with intact insulation passes through a conductor without insulation. The capacitively coupled current is stored until the electrosurgical generator is turned off or until the stored electrons complete the circuit through a noninsulated conductor or tissue.

       1.   **Examples** of possible capacitive coupling include electrosurgery cables wrapped around metallic towel clamps, metallic prostheses, sweating skin within a surgical glove, a retractable active electrode within an insulated suction-irrigator device, and a metallic trocar around an insulated electrosurgery instrument. In these examples, the patient's skin serves as a conductor.

       2.   **Safety methods** to limit or eliminate capacitive coupling include utilizing cutting current whenever feasible (capacitance is greatest with coagulating current), keeping electrodes free of eschar (lowers resistance), employing larger diameter trocars and smaller diameter electrodes (lowers capacitance), inserting all metal trocars for use with insulated electrosurgery instruments, using a specially designed suction-irrigator device (eliminates capacitance), and/or connecting an electrode monitoring system.

    e.  **Tissue sticking** occurs when eschar accumulates on the active electrode and increases resistance to current flow.

       1.   **Safety methods** to reduce tissue sticking include using a Teflon-coated electrode and keeping the electrode clean.

  2.  **Bipolar electrosurgery complications** are fewer than monopolar electrosurgery.

    a.  **Incomplete coagulation** arises when desiccation of the outer tissue layers increases resistance to current flow and ceases coagulation before it is complete. This results in a lack of correlation between the visual, external end point of tissue coagulation and what has occurred internally.

Table 9.2. Differences between electrosurgery devices and ultrasonic shears.

| Category | Electrosurgery | Ultrasonic shears |
|---|---|---|
| Grounding electrode | Yes | No |
| Smoke generation | Yes | No |
| EKG, pacemaker interference | Yes | No |
| Current travels through patient | Yes | No |
| Heat generation | Constant | Time dependent |
| Thermal spread | Moderate | Minimal |
| Cost | Low/intermediate | Intermediate/high |
| Complications | Current concentration | Minimal |
|  | Direct coupling |  |
|  | Capacitive coupling |  |
|  | Tissue sticking |  |

*EKG* electrocardiogram

1.  **For example**, incomplete coagulation of fallopian tubes using bipolar electrosurgery can result in ineffective tubal ligation and subsequent pregnancy.
2.  **Safety methods** to eliminate incomplete coagulation include the use of an ammeter, which registers the presence of current and signals complete coagulation of tissue.
b.  **Tissue sticking** occurs when eschar accumulates on one or both electrodes and increases resistance to current flow.
    1.  **Safety methods** to reduce tissue sticking include using sufficient irrigation and keeping the electrodes clean.
3.  **Ultrasonic device complications** are fewer still than complications associated with monopolar and bipolar electrosurgery devices. General differences between electrosurgery devices and ultrasonic shears are listed in Table 9.2.

# Selected References

Airan MC, Ko ST. Electrosurgery techniques of cutting and coagulation. In: Arregui ME, Fitzgibbons RJ, Katkhouda N, McKernan JB, Reich H, editors. Principles of Laparoscopic Surgery. New York, NY: Springer; 1995. p. 30–5.

Amaral JF. Electrosurgery and ultrasound for cutting and coagulating tissue in minimally invasive surgery. In: Zucker KA, editor. Surgical laparoscopy. 2nd ed. Philadelphia, PA: Lippincott Williams & Wilkins; 2001. p. 47–76.

Campbell PA, Cresswell AB, Frank TG, Cuschieri FA. Real-time thermography during energized vessel sealing and dissection. Surg Endosc. 2003;17:1640–5.

Clements RH, Paiepu R. In vivo comparison of the coagulation capability of SonoSurg and Harmonic Ace on 4 mm and 5 mm arteries. Surg Endosc. 2007;21:2203–6.

Gandsas A, Adrales GL. Energy sources. In: Talamini MA, editor. Advanced Therapy in Minimally Invasive Surgery. Lewiston, NY: BC Decker; 2006. p. 3–9.

Harrell AG, Kercher KW, Heniford BT. Energy sources in laparoscopy. Semin Laparosc Surg. 2004;11:201–9.

Hruby GW, Marruffo FC, Durak E, et al. Evaluation of surgical energy devices for vessel sealing and peripheral energy spread in a porcine model. J Urol. 2007;178:2689–93.

Lamberton GR, His RS, Jin DH, Lindler TU, Jellison FC, Baldwin DD. Prospective comparison of four laparoscopic vessel ligation devices. J Endourol. 2008;22:2307–12.

Macaluso A, Larach SW. Laparoscopic instrumentation. In: MacFadyen BV, Arregui ME, Eubanks WS, Olsen DO, Peters JH, Soper NJ, Swanstrom LL, Wexner SD, editors. Laparoscopic surgery of the abdomen. New York, NY: Springer; 2004. p. 335–51.

Newcomb WL, Hope WW, Schmelzer TM, et al. Comparison of blood vessel sealing among new electrosurgical and ultrasonic devices. Surg Endosc. 2009;23:90–6.

Newman RM, Traverso LW. Principles of laparoscopic hemostasis. In: Scott-Conner CEH, editor. The SAGES Manual: Fundamentals of Laparoscopy, Thoracoscopy, and GI Endoscopy. 2nd ed. New York, NY: Springer; 2006. p. 49–59.

Person B, Vivas DA, Ruiz D, Talcott M, Coad JE, Wexner SD. Comparison of four energy-based vascular sealing and cutting instruments: a porcine model. Surg Endosc. 2008;22:534–8.

Phillips CK, Hruby GW, Durak E, et al. Tissue response to surgical energy devices. Urology. 2008;71:744–8.

Pietrow PK, Weizer AZ, L'Esperance JO, et al. PlasmaKinetic bipolar vessel sealing: burst pressures and thermal spread in an animal model. J Endourol. 2005;19:107–10.

Sasi W. Dissection by ultrasonic energy versus monopolar electrosurgical energy in laparoscopic cholecystectomy. JSLS. 2010;14:23–34.

Scott DJ, Goova MT. New and evolving laparoscopic instrumentation. In: Soper NJ, Swanstrom LL, Eubanks WS, editors. Mastery of endoscopic and laparoscopic surgery. 3rd ed. Philadelphia, PA: Lippincott Williams & Wilkins; 2009. p. 24–33.

Wu MP, Ou CS, Chen SI, et al. Complications and recommended practices for electrosurgery in laparoscopy. Am J Surg. 2000;179:67–73.

# 10. Laparoscopic Hemostasis: Hemostatic Products and Adjuncts

*Thadeus L. Trus, M.D.*

## A. Introduction

The field of laparoscopic surgery continues to develop at a rapid pace, with surgeons performing increasingly complex procedures. Laparoscopy demands a bloodless field, as the surgeon does not have direct manual access to the operative field. Furthermore, visualization is easily lost as blood absorbs the light of the laparoscope. The use of suction can drastically diminish the volume of pneumoperitoneum, also limiting visualization. Obviously, proper patient selection and thorough preoperative preparation are essential to a good surgical outcome. Meticulous surgical technique, including precise tissue dissection and proper identification of vascular anatomy, will help avoid bleeding complications. A wide variety of hemostatic tools exist to assist the surgeon should bleeding occur. This chapter focuses on two major hemostatic modalities: mechanical devices and tissue sealants. Thermal hemostatic modalities are discussed elsewhere.

## B. Mechanical Methods of Hemostasis

### 1. Laparoscopic Clips

a. *Titanium clip appliers* have been developed for use in laparoscopic surgery and allow for the ligation of small vascular structures. Both disposable and reusable clip appliers are available in 5 and 10 mm sized instruments. Titanium clips are most often

N.J. Soper and C.E.H. Scott-Conner (eds.), *The SAGES Manual: Volume 1 Basic Laparoscopy and Endoscopy*, DOI 10.1007/978-1-4614-2344-7_10, © Springer Science+Business Media, LLC 2012

used, but locking polymer clips have gained popularity with many surgeons. Reusable clip appliers require each clip be loaded individually, limiting their use in emergency situations. On the other hand, disposable clip appliers contain up to 20 clips and can be fired repeatedly.

Although titanium clips are useful in sealing blood vessels, and easier to apply than laparoscopic suture ligatures, there are limitations to their use. In order to prevent inadvertent injury to surrounding structures, the target vessel should be fully dissected and both ends of the clip visualized before firing. Titanium clips can dislodge with further dissection of the surrounding tissue. Therefore, a minimum of two to three clips are required for vascular control. Additionally, titanium clips can interfere with the application of endoscopic staplers and should not be used on or near major vascular structures or on hollow viscera that may require stapling.

b. *Polymer clips* contain a self-locking mechanism when applied correctly, making them less likely to slip. They are available in a variety of sizes, including 15 mm, and can be used on major vessels like the renal artery or vein. The clip is configured with a "hook-like" lock; if the structure to be ligated is not fully and circumferentially dissected, this "hook" can catch and perforate tissue. In the case of vascular structures, this can cause major bleeding by itself. Always visualize both ends of the clip around the vessel before locking to help prevent this complication as well. Additionally, when using polymer clips on larger vessels, leaving two to three clips on a significant vascular stump may help prevent slippage. Reports of slippage when one such clip device was used to secure the renal artery during living donor nephrectomy have led the FDA to issue an advisory (see "Selected References").

## 2. Laparoscopic Vascular Staplers

These staplers allow for the simultaneous ligation and division of major vessels, vascular pedicles, or highly vascular tissue under nonemergent conditions. Vascular endostaplers deploy parallel rows of 2.5 mm staples while approximating the target tissue between the stapler and its anvil; the tissue is then divided, leaving two to three rows of staples on each side of the linear incision. Reticulating staplers are available and advantageous when the working space is limited. Adequate instruction on proper use of the device is advisable, given the potential for devastating hemorrhagic complications. Both distal ends of the stapler should be visualized around the entire target before closing the stapler and time should be allowed for hemostatic compression of the tissue before firing. Again, any metallic clips must be removed from the tissue to be stapled because they will interfere with the cutting device.

## 3. Pretied Suture Loops

Ready-to-use suture loops are available for controlling already transected tissue or vascular structures. Although less time consuming and less complicated than laparoscopic suturing, deploying a pretied suture loop (EndoLoop™ Ethicon Endo-Surgery Corp) requires some laparoscopic skill. The structure to be ligated must first be completely transected. The transected tissue is then gently elevated with a laparoscopic grasper for temporary control. The grasper must be briefly released while encircled by the suture loop. Once the pretied suture loop is positioned appropriately, the tissue is again grasped and gently elevated, and the loop cinched around the target using the prefashioned slip knot. Care must be taken not to avulse the target tissue with excessive traction.

## 4. Suturing

As in open surgery, sutures are very effective hemostatic tools in laparoscopy. Suture ligation is achieved by either extra- or intracorporeal tying. There is a learning curve for both methods. Care must be taken with extracorporeal knot-tying to avoid excessive traction and "sawing" through the tissue. Intracoporeal knot-tying and suturing are more complex task and require practice and training to achieve technical proficiency.

## C. Tissue Sealants

A wide variety of tissue sealants are available for use in laparoscopic surgery (Table 10.1), although it must be emphasized that these products are adjuncts and do not replace traditional means of hemostasis. Tissue

Table 10.1. Available products, characteristics, and recommendations for use.

| Product | Constituent elements | Mechanism of action | Comments |
|---|---|---|---|
| *Fibrin sealants* | | | |
| Tisseal™, Evicel™ | Thrombin and fibrinogen from pooled plasma | Thrombin cleaves fibrinogen to form fibrin clot | Requires thawing. Mixed at time of application. Apply to relatively dry surfaces. |
| Costasis™/Vivostat™ | Autologous plasma/fibrinogen and bovine thrombin | Thrombin cleaves fibrinogen to form fibrin clot | Utilizes 120 mL of patient's blood processed overnight. Mixed at time of application. |
| Tacholsil™ | Thrombin/fibrinogen from pooled plasma | Thrombin cleaves fibrinogen to form fibrin clot | Ready to use, coated, collagen fleece. Good for sealing parenchymal defects. |
| *Gelatin based products* | | | |
| FloSeal™ | Thrombin from pooled plasma and bovine gelatin matrix | Gelatin matrix swells, thrombin cleaves fibrinogen to form fibrin clot | Requires contact with blood for autologous fibrinogen. |
| *Oxidized cellulose* | | | |
| Surgicel™ | Regenerated oxidized cellulose | Scaffold for clot formation | Best applied as dry fabric. Low pH prohibits use with other hemostatic agents. May cause inflammatory adhesions. |
| *Microfibrillar collagen* | | | |
| Endoavitene™ | Bovine corium | Platelet aggregation/activation | Good for large areas of parenchymal bleeding. Requires functional platelets to work. |

sealants are designed to augment or promote the physiologic clotting cascades, the end point of which is formation of the fibrin plug from fibrinogen cleavage by thrombin.

## 1. Fibrin Glues

The use of fibrin for hemostasis dates back to the early 1900s, when bovine thrombin was combined with human plasma for topical application. The modern product is largely unchanged, containing human fibrinogen, bovine or human thrombin, ionized calcium, and an anti-thrombolytic agent. The human components are mainly derived from pooled blood and can be associated with viral transmission, although products now exist that utilize autologous blood. The bovine elements can result in coagulopathies, anaphylaxis, or prion transmission. A completely human based product is available to avoid potential complications from the bovine components.

Fibrin glues are the most common tissue sealant used in laparoscopic surgery and are applied via a long applicator connected to a two cylinder syringe system containing fibrinogen and thrombin. The two components are thus combined in situ and form a fibrin plug. Of note, fibrin sealants work best on a relatively dry field.

## 2. Gelatin Based Adjuncts

Gelatin based hemostatic agents originated in the 1940s. Dry sponges were made from purified animal skin gelatin for use in open surgery. Its hemostatic properties seem to be physical and largely due to its capacity to absorb blood and/or fluids; it can swell to double its volume. A liquid variant has been developed, consisting of bovine or human based thrombin and bovine derived gelatin matrix, with obvious applicability in laparoscopic surgery. The two components are mixed in a syringe before use and the product has a two hour shelf life. Because the fibrinogen required to form the fibrin clot must come from the patient's own blood, this product requires a moist field for effective hemostasis. The gelatin matrix absorbs surrounding blood/fluid, swells, and acts as a tamponade, while the fibrin clot hardens. Although there are risks of viral transmission and allergic reaction with this bovine based product, it is usually well tolerated.

## 3. Fibrinogen and Thrombin Fleece

This ready to use product consists of a dry collagen fleece coated with fibrinogen and thrombin. The flexible dry fleece is deployed on tissue with a fan-like, laparoscopic applicator and can be layered on parenchymal bleeding areas of spleen, liver, and kidney. Constant compression of the fleece while moistening it with saline is required for it to seal tissue; this process takes 3–5 min. Advantages of this product include its anti-adhesive nature and its ability as a sealant to withstand the application of additional hemostatic measures, i.e., bipolar coagulation or sutures.

## 4. Oxidized Cellulose

This plant-based topical hemostatic was first developed in the 1960s. The hemostatic fabric is made from regenerated cellulose which is then oxidized. It can be easily used laparoscopically as the material is soft, flexible, and can be cut to fit any size. It can be used to hold direct pressure on bleeding tissue but it also serves as a scaffold for platelet aggregation and clot formation. Final hemostasis however, is dependent on the patient's own clotting ability. Oxidized cellulose creates an acidic environment; red blood cell lysis occurs on contact with the material which accounts for the brown discoloration of the fabric. Because of this acidity, however, oxidized cellulose cannot be used with other hemostatic agents like thrombin. Of note, oxidized cellulose does cause a foreign body reaction with granuloma formation, which may cause adhesion formation in the area of use.

## 5. Microfibrillar Collagen

This product was developed in the 1970s, originally as a powder derived from bovine corium. Its fibrils act as a platform for platelet adherence, activation, and aggregation, with subsequent thrombus formation. This process takes 2–5 min. It is also available as a sheet, sponge, or pad and is best used to control oozing from raw surfaces, such as the retroperitoneum. A prerolled sheet is available for laparoscopic procedures and can be deployed through an applicator designed to fit through a standard trocar.

# D.  Laparoscopic Management of Active Hemorrhage

Active bleeding will occur despite the surgeon's best efforts to carefully dissect and identify structures prior to division. Mechanical means of hemostasis will fail. When bleeding does occur, the laparoscopic surgeon must remain calm and proceed systematically to gain control of the hemorrhage. Blind application of clips is dangerous and can lead to unintended injury to vital structures. Although conversion to an open procedure is always an option, it is not necessarily the best first step when active bleeding is encountered. The first step should be to maintain or establish exposure of the presumed bleeding source. Suction should be judiciously used in order to clear the operative field while maintaining adequate pneumoperitoneum. The tip of the suction device can be used to hold pressure on the identified bleeding source while additional trocars or instruments are being introduced into the field. Care should be taken not to obscure the scope with blood or irrigation fluid. Once the bleeding target is identified, control it with a nontraumatic grasper or a fine-tip dissector. If the bleeding stems from a vascular structure, clips can be used to control the bleeding. Again, the surgeon must be able to place clips entirely around the vessel under direct visualization. If a parenchymal injury has occurred, compression with a hemostatic product may be all that is needed or provide the time to prepare for intracorporeal suture ligatures. If the bleeding structure cannot be adequately controlled as described above, or if there is question of inadvertent injury to surrounding structures, the surgeon should convert to an open procedure.

## Selected References

De la Torre RA, Bachman SL, Wheeler AA, Barlow KN, Scott JS. Hemostasis and hemostatic agents in minimally invasive surgery. Surgery. 2007;142(4 Suppl):S39–45.

FDA and HRSA Joint Safety Communication: Weck Hem-o-Lok ligating clips contraindicated for ligation of renal artery during laparoscopic living-donor nephrectomy. http://www.fda.gov/MedicalDevices/Safety/AlertsandNotices/ucm253237.htm. Accessed 20 July 2011.

Sileski B, Achneck H, Ma L, Lawson JH. Application of energy-based technology and topical hemostatic agents in the management of surgical hemostasis. Vascular. 2010; 18:197–204.

Spotnitz WD. Fibrin sealant: past, present, and future, a brief review. World J Surg. 2010; 34:632–4.

Spotnitz WD. Active and mechanical hemostatic agents. Surgery. 2007;142(4 Suppl):S34–8.

# 11. Principles of Tissue Approximation[*]

*William C. Beck, M.D.*
*Michael D. Holzman, M.D., M.P.H.*

## A. Laparoscopic Suturing and Intracorporeal Knot Tying: General Principles

As techniques for minimally invasive surgery have advanced so much that technically more challenging procedures are performed, the ability to suture proficiently has become even more important for the successful laparoscopic surgeon. The ability to suture delicate tissues such as the vascular system and biliary tree allows a surgeon to perform more advanced surgical procedures without compromising patient outcomes. The technical challenges of intracorporeal maneuvers include the nontraditional visual image, limited movement, and awkward instrumentation. These challenges can be overcome by practicing a mental choreography of step-by-step maneuvers, and by working slowly, precisely, and patiently to master this new skill in dry labs and simulators.

In laparoscopic tissue approximation, intracorporeal suturing and knot tying are generally the preferred methods because they are highly adaptable, flexible, economical and use available equipment. Sometimes extracorporeal knotting may be preferred (even when intracorporeal knotting is possible). In either instance, learning to suture requires special attention to the setup, visual perception, eye–hand coordination, and motor skill. These factors are described and illustrated individually.

1. **Position of the surgeon and primary monitor** are determined by relationship of the instruments and the orientation of the intended suture line. Position of the laparoscope and instrument ports is based on the principle of triangulation. Position the camera midway or parallel to the two suturing instrument

---

[*]This chapter was contributed by Zoltan Szabo, Ph.D. in the previous edition.

N.J. Soper and C.E.H. Scott-Conner (eds.), *The SAGES Manual: Volume 1 Basic Laparoscopy and Endoscopy*, DOI 10.1007/978-1-4614-2344-7_11, © Springer Science+Business Media, LLC 2012

port(s); mimicking the normal relationship between the eyes and two hands. Shift these three ports/instruments in unison when attempting to suture in a different location. Proper port positioning relative to the suture line provides the optimum angle of access and a fulcrum for the instruments. The laparoscopic surgical suite must accommodate proper patient, monitor, and instrument positioning. An ergonomically poor ergonomics setup may cause repetitive motion injury.

2. **Visual perception** is a significant factor because the operative field is viewed indirectly through a closed-circuit video system. Ideally the monitors are viewed from a distance of no more than 5–6 ft and are placed at eye level or slightly lower. One of the challenges of this procedure is that the visual field is inversely proportional to the magnification power; hence, greater magnification decreases the size of the visual field. Additional magnification also demands a proportionate reduction of the speed and range of instrument movement to maintain control. Visualization is affected by the following:

   a.  Use of optical instrument (laparoscope).
   b.  Flat two-dimensional (2D) image on the video monitor.
   c.  Ability of the surgeon to adjust to the new viewing perspective.
   d.  Triangulation (see below).
   e.  The assistant's ability to manipulate the camera in order to follow the surgeon's motions in a fluid manner.

   At best, this setup presents significant challenges. As details are magnified, the visual field becomes proportionately smaller and depth of field shallower. The surgeon must adjust eye–hand coordination and adapt to the speed of instrument movement. Excellent visual memory and a trained eye are essential.

3. **Eye–hand coordination**: Triangulation is critical to the success of laparoscopic suturing (Fig. 11.1). Correct triangulation, incorporating position of surgeon, ports, and the monitor, allows the surgeon to use the monitor as a reference point to locate and fix points in space. Movements in laparoscopic surgery should be slower than in open surgery. A general principle is that the speed of movements should be inversely related to the degree of magnification. Magnified images on a screen shows how quickly instruments are perceived to move, even at a normal pace. Slow

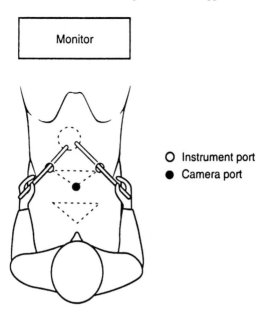

Fig. 11.1. Position of the surgeon for visual path coaxial alignment. Note the triangulation of camera and operating ports, which corresponds to triangulation of the surgeon's eyes and two hands. The surgeon, target tissue, suture line, and monitor are aligned.

the pace of movement to restore control and allow sufficient time to process the visual information. Eliminate unnecessary movements and tightly choreograph your technique. This allows the most efficient use of time, by increasing precision and eliminating unnecessary movements. Proper training courses and practice improve the overall success and efficiency of laparoscopic suturing.

4. **Motor skill** determines the performance of a successful surgical procedure. Balance and coordination of perception, decision making, and motor skill orchestrate the ideal procedure. Motor skills developed over a lifetime of everyday practice during open surgery require modification to be used in the magnified 2D field of laparoscopic surgery. The imbalance created by magnification and the use of foot-long instrumentation can be overcome by using the same principles employed during microsurgery.

# B. Equipment and Instrumentation

1. **Video equipment**. While laparoscopic surgeons typically express a preference for high definition (HD) video systems used in laparoscopy, actual quantitative analysis indicates that HD monitors do not offer a statistically different advantage over their standard definition counter parts.

2. **Suturing instruments** come in various designs. The handle can have either a pistol grip or an in-line, coaxial handle, with or without a ring to hold it securely. Ringless handles afford greater maneuverability. The **assisting grasper**, used by the nondominant hand, handles the tissue and thus should be atraumatic. This grasper needs to have a narrower tip than traditional graspers to assist with needle handling and knot tying. The **needle holder**, used by the dominant hand, handles the needle and suture material. The length of the laparoscopic needle driver results in the transmission of reduced force from the surgeon's hands to the instrument jaws. This decreases needle control. Though numerous instruments are commercially available, most surgeons prefer ratcheted instruments, with a curved and blunt tip (see point 8 below).

3. **Trocars** should be slightly longer than the thickness of the abdominal wall, with a preferred diameter of 5–10 mm. Trocars that are too long interfere with instrument mobility and function by preventing the opening of the instrument jaws and minimizing movement in the abdomen. Particularly in the obese patient, the angle in which the port is placed can greatly affect the torque on the suturing instruments.

4. **Geometry of the needle tip** controls the characteristics of the tissue penetration and size and shape of the tunnel cut. To minimize tissue trauma, ease of penetration is important in laparoscopic surgery. Stronger, sturdier needles are required to penetrate thicker tissue layers; smaller, thinner needles are required to penetrate delicate tissues. A needle tip with a high tapering ratio, or "taper cut" tip, penetrates tissue layers more readily.

5. **Suture material** is selected based upon favorable tissue response, handling characteristics, and visibility, and for its particular attributes such as absorbability, strength, and tissue reaction as in open procedures. Light colored or colorless sutures can be more difficult to visualize in laparoscopic surgery and

their use may be limited. The handling characteristics of the braided materials, such as silk, polygalactan 910, braided polyester, or braided nylon, are more optimal due to more flexibility and less memory. Alternatives such as monofilament polypropylene, polydioxanone, and nylon can be stiff and be more difficult to tie intracorporeally.

6. **Needle handling and passage**. Bicurve geometry affects the handling and scooping characteristics of the needle and can be adapted easily to particular tissues and their access requirements. In difficult situations, take the time necessary to reexamine simple movements to execute them efficiently. Entrance and exit bites and knot tying are the main movements repeated during tissue approximation. The needle follows the tip in passing through tissue layers with the least amount of trauma and effort if the tissue resistance, needle tip, grasping point, and direction of force are assembled on the same axis. The directions of (1) the needle tip and (2) the needle-driving force must be identical; the optimal direction for both is 90°, head-on against tissue resistance (Fig. 11.2). If these directions are dissimilar, the needle will be deflected within the instrument jaws or create unnecessary tissue trauma when passing through the desired location, potentially damaging or tearing fragile tissues when performing delicate laparoscopic procedures.

7. **A high level of concentration** is integral to performing even simple needle-driving maneuvers when one is working in a magnified field. Indirect tissue manipulation further complicates this.

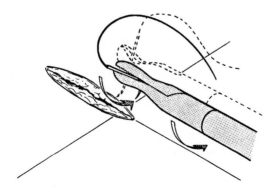

Fig. 11.2. Pushing the needle head-on against tissue resistance.

8. **Needle holder design**. To compensate, surgeons seek instruments with more powerful jaws and features such as the self-righting jaws (which facilitate proper orientation of the needle within the jaws of the needle holder). As mentioned previously, needle control is accomplished by correctly directing the needle tip as well as the needle-driving force. Without awareness of these factors, application of increased force can easily result in tissue damage or a poorly constructed suture line. Instruments designed to hold the needle more forcefully tend to have a more cumbersome lock mechanism, and deployment of this locking mechanism may increase tissue trauma. A self-righting design automatically locks the needle into one position, perpendicular to the instrument shaft. This is helpful when the suture line is aligned perpendicular to the resulting needle plane; when it is not, this feature can be counterproductive. Therefore, it is important to develop and learn needle-driving techniques that depend more on skill than on gadgetry.

## C. Needle Positioning

Needle positioning can present difficulties as surgeons learn to work in the 2D image. Initially straight needles were frequently used just to overcome the issue, but with increased experience most advanced surgeons prefer standard needles and suture. Several techniques have evolved to pass the needle and suture into the abdominal cavity and position it in the jaws of the needle holder.

1. **Suture first, needle trailing**. The needle may be passed into the abdominal cavity through the trocar of the dominant hand by grasping the *suture* a couple of millimeters beyond the swage. Once the needle and suture have been introduced into the peritoneal cavity, use the grasper in the nondominant hand to secure the needle and position it in the needle holder, midway along the needle curvature.

2. **Needle first, suture trailing**. Alternatively, grasp the needle rather than the suture itself (Fig. 11.3). The authors routinely use a technique in which the needle swage is grasped with the jaws of the needle holder, and the needle is positioned in parallel with the instrument, with the needle tip lying against the shaft of the needle holder. The needle holder is introduced

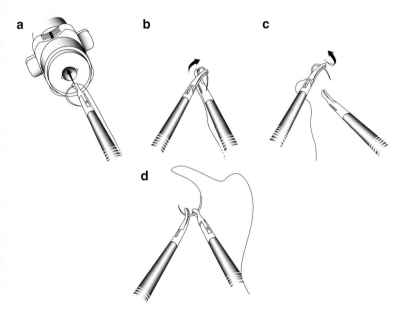

Fig. 11.3. (**a**) Right handed technique. The needle is backloaded and introduced through the trocar. (**b**) The needle holder rotates in a clockwise direction, so the needle concavity points toward 6 o'clock. (**c**) The left handed instrument grasps the needle at its midpoint and rotates counterclockwise. The needle concavity now points toward 12 o'clock. (**d**) the needle is grasped and ready for suturing (Reprinted from Brody F, Rehm J, Ponsky J, Holzman M. A reliable and efficient technique for laparoscopic needle positioning. Surg Endosc. 1999;13:1053–54, with kind permission of Springer Science+Business Media).

into the trocar of the dominant hand. Use a grasper in the nondominant hand to push the needle, positioning it within the jaws of the needle holder into the desired position.

## D. Suturing Techniques

Suturing and intracorporeal knotting are among the final challenges of a laparoscopic procedure, and the surgeon's skill and endurance. A surgeon's skill level can be measured to some degree, e.g., by the ability to tie a square knot correctly in 30 s or less. Facility with these techniques can be achieved with confidence and skill only after 20–40 h of formal training (as observed by the author). Intracorporeal knotting can be the beginning and finishing points of continuous and interrupted suture lines.

Prepare and position the tissues in anticipation of either interrupted sutures, continuous sutures, or a combination of both types so that minimal tension exists.

1. **Interrupted suturing**. When constructing a linear suture line, the factors involved in creating entrance and exit bites include length of incision or laceration, type of tissue layers to be approximated and their function, needle and thread combination selection, and length of suture.

   a. Place the instrument port positions so the laparoscope port is aligned with the suture line, with the instrument ports triangulated for the surgeon's dominant and nondominant hands (see Triangulation, above).

   b. Place the needle perpendicular to the suture line. The entrance and exit scooping motion should follow a 3 o'clock-to-9 o'clock direction relative to the surgeon's frontal plane.

   c. Use interrupted sutures with a suspension slip-knot technique if tension is present or visibility or access is poor. Place these sutures evenly, approximating the tissue precisely without tension.

2. **Continuous suturing**. This type of suture is more rapid, yet more difficult to accomplish correctly. The technique begins and ends with an anchoring knot, the last of which can be tied to the loop of the last stitch. Tissue edges must be identified by shifting the tension on the suture loops carefully as the approximation continues.

3. **Suture choice** is a necessary component, because monofilament and braided materials behave differently. Monofilament is stiff, springy, but slides smoothly through tissue. This property may contribute to loss of adequate tension on the suture line. Braided material is less prone to slip but may drag through the tissue and lock unexpectedly. It can be more cumbersome to work with because each stitch must be taut before proceeding to the next.

4. **Anastomosis**. Laparoscopic anastomosis of hollow viscera is a challenge that can be accomplished by using methods from microvascular anastomoses and duplication of open surgical techniques. It can be performed end to end, end to side, or side to side.

a. **End-to-end anastomosis** is the preferred method for approximating tubes or ducts of equal caliber and wall thickness. The number of stitches, their configuration, and size of the bites are calculated depending on the function of the structure. Either interrupted or continuous sutures can be used. Interrupted sutures provide better precision and control; continuous sutures are performed more rapidly, but are less forgiving.

b. Conduits with different lumina and wall thickness can be joined with an **end-to-side anastomosis**.

c. **Side-to-side anastomosis** is a practical method for conduits that lie side by side. This method of approximation is similar to the end-to-side anastomosis.

# E. Knot Tying

Both intracorporeal and extracorporeal knot tying techniques have an important role in laparoscopic surgery. For most purposes, intracorporeal knot tying is preferred. **Intracorporeal knots** are placed by a process that duplicates the methods used during open surgical procedures. Intracorporeal tying is faster and requires less suturing. **Extracorporeal tying** involves knots designed to slip in only one direction; both categories of knotting methods are illustrated in Figs. 11.4 and 11.5.

An **extracorporeal knot** is tied externally and slid down to the tissue with the aid of a knot pusher. Although it may appear to be a simpler procedure, it requires long threads and a systematic and careful application to avoid traumatizing the tissues and contaminating or damaging the suture. Extracorporeal knot tying has been shown to be faster and easier for the novice, but is equivalent to intracorporeal knot tying for the experienced laparoscopic surgeon.

While other types of extracorporeal knots have now been introduced for laparoscopic surgery, the **Roeder knot** was the first and is the most widely used. It was developed around the turn of the century and incorporated into laparoscopic practice before intracorporeal knotting was developed. This knot is also used in commercially available, pretied suture ligatures. The method is described and illustrated in Fig. 11.4. Another common method of extracorporeal knot tying uses a modified square knot, with each throw tied extracorporeally and pushed down using a knot pushing device.

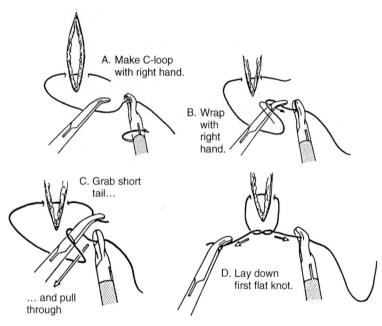

A. Make C-loop with right hand.

B. Wrap with right hand.

C. Grab short tail…

… and pull through

D. Lay down first flat knot.

**Fig. 11.4. A. Square and surgeon's knot. overhand flat knot**. (1) *Starting position*: Create a C-loop as the right instrument reaches over to the left side of the field, grasps the long tail, and brings it back to the right below the short tail. This loop must be in a horizontal plane; otherwise it will be difficult to wrap the thread. If a monofilament material is used, the right instrument can rotate the thread counterclockwise until it lies flat against the tissue. The right instrument holds the long tail, and the left instrument is placed over the loop. The short tail should be so long that it cannot be pulled out of the tissue accidentally, but not so long that its end requires additional effort to locate it. A large loop should be used to allow ample space to maneuver both instruments, and movements should be slowed to retrieve the short tail without disturbing the setup. Use the right instrument to wrap the long tail around the stationary tip of the left instrument. Rotate the right instrument forward (clockwise) to create an arch in the suture and assist the wrapping motion. Keep the jaws of the instruments retrieving the short tail closed until ready to grasp the tail. In the inset, the right instrument is shown wrapping the suture around the left instrument twice, which creates a surgeon's knot. (2) *Grasping the short tail*: Both instruments should move together toward the short tail. This process prevents a tight noose from forming around the instrument, making it difficult to reach the short tail. Grasping the short tail near the end avoids formation of an extra loop (or "bow tie") when one is pulling the suture through. (3) *Completing the first flat knot*. Pull the short tail through the loop and hold it still, while the long tail continues to be pulled, parallel to the stitch, until the knot is cinched down. The end will be hard to find if the tail is too long. The left instrument then drops the short tail, and the right instrument keeps its grasp on the long tail. This illustrates the surgeon's knot that has been created.

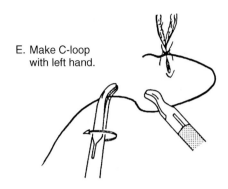

E. Make C-loop
with left hand.

Fig. 11.4.  (continued)

**B. Second opposing flat knot**. (1) *Creating the reversed C-loop, wrapping the thread, and grasping the short tail.* The reversed **C-loop** is created as the right instrument is brought to the left side of the field under the short tail and rotated clockwise 180°. The right instrument transfers the long tail to the left instrument. The right instrument is placed over the reversed C-loop and the left instrument wraps the thread around the right instrument. The tips of both instruments are moved in unison toward the short tail, which is grasped with the right instrument. (2) *Completing the second knot.* Pull the short tail through the loop; then pull both tails in opposite directions, parallel to the stitch, with equal tension. Verify that the knot is configured correctly as the knot cinches up.

**C. Slip knot for the square knot**. (1) *Starting position and pulling.* To convert the square knot (locking configuration) to a slip knot (sliding configuration), both instruments must grasp the suture on the same (ipsilateral) side. One instrument grasps the thread outside the knot and the other in the suture loop (between the knot and issue). Both instruments pull in opposite directions (perpendicular to the stitch). A snapping or popping sensation often can be felt, and the short tail may flip up. The knot now resembles a pretzel. If the conversion does not occur after several attempts, try the maneuver on the other side of the knot. Conversion is easier on monofilament suture. (2) *Pushing the slip knot.* The right instrument maintains its grasp on the tail and pulls tightly. The left instrument now assumes the role of a knot pusher and advances the knot to the tissue by sliding on the tail. A common error is caused by the surgeon inadvertently grasping the knot or tail, rather than solely pushing the knot forward. (3) *Cinching down.* Cinch down the slip knot until the tissue edges have been approximated to the desired tension. Recenter the knot and recheck the tension. Before making additional overhand throws, reconvert the slip knot to a square knot as follows: both instruments regrasp the tails in opposite directions, parallel to the stitch in the same way as when the square knot was tried originally. An additional overhand knot is necessary on top, and is tied in the same manner as the first throw [Fig. 11.3.A(1)–(3)].

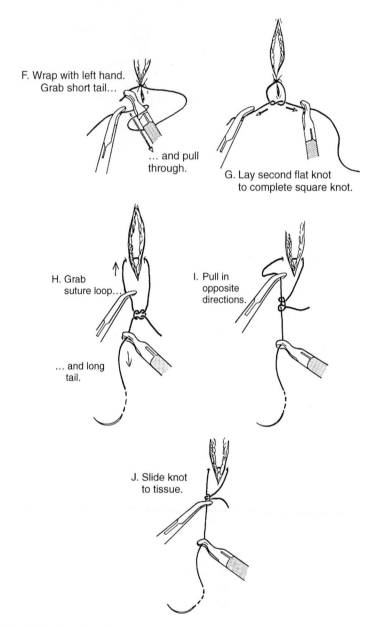

F. Wrap with left hand.
Grab short tail…

… and pull
through.

G. Lay second flat knot
to complete square knot.

H. Grab
suture loop…

… and long
tail.

I. Pull in
opposite
directions.

J. Slide knot
to tissue.

Fig. 11.4. (continued)

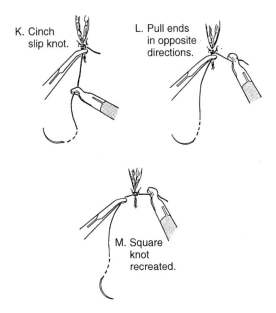

K. Cinch slip knot.

L. Pull ends in opposite directions.

M. Square knot recreated.

Fig. 11.4.  (continued)

# F.  Laparoscopic Simulation

The increasing prevalence and complexity of laparoscopic procedures has prompted the development of numerous laparoscopic simulation models to develop complex motor skills, such as laparoscopic knot
tying, prior to implementing these skills in the operating room. Simulation
models used for the development of laparoscopic skills include simple
and inexpensive box trainers, computerized models designed to demonstrate common procedures such as cholecystectomy and fundoplication,
to the reproduction of operative suites. Numerous studies have validated
the utility and transference of simulation based training to the performance of basic and complex laparoscopic procedures to the operating
room prompting the integration of formalized laparoscopic training into
surgical residency programs nationwide. In 2009, the American Board of
Surgery mandated the completion of the Fundamentals of Laparoscopic
Surgery (FLS) course prior to taking the general surgery board examination. Successful completion of the FLS course requires manual tasks in
peg transfer, pattern cutting, pretied loop ligature placement, extracorporeal suturing, and intracorporeal suturing.

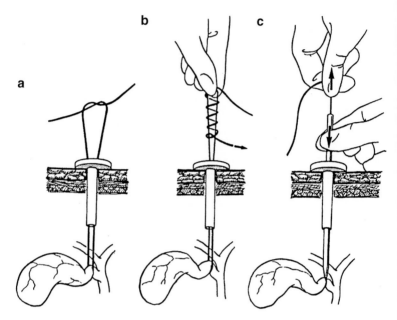

Fig. 11.5. **Extracorporeal knot**. Bring a long suture into the laparoscopic field, leaving its tail outside the port. Place the stitch; then bring the needle end out through the same port. Create a Roeder knot by tying an overhand knot and then wrapping the suture tail back around both arms of the loop three times. Lock the suture by bringing the tail back through the large loop, between the last two twists of the wrap. Slide the knot down with a plastic applicator rod or knot pusher.

## Selected References

Bowyer DW, Moran ME, Szabo Z. Laparoscopic suturing in urology: a model for vesicourethral anastomosis following radical prostatectomy. Min Invas Ther. 1993; 4(2):165–70.

Buncke HJ, Szabo Z. Introduction to microsurgery. In: Grabb WC, Smith JW, editors. A concise guide to plastic surgery. Boston: Little, Brown; 1980. p. 653–9.

Cuchieri A, Szabo Z. Tissue approximation in endoscopic surgery. Oxford: Isis Medical Media; 1995.

Guthrie CC. Blood vessel surgery and its application: a reprint. Pittsburgh: University of Pittsburgh; 1959. p. 1–69.

Szabo Z. Laparoscopic suturing and tissue approximation. In: Hunter JG, Sackier JM, editors. Minimally invasive surgery. New York: McGraw-Hill; 1993. p. 141–55.

Wolfe BM, Szabo Z, Moran ME, Chan P, Hunter JG. Training for minimally invasive surgery: need for surgical skills. Surg Endosc. 1993;7:93–5.

# 12. Other Devices for Tissue Approximation

*Byron F. Santos, M.D.*
*Eric S. Hungness, M.D.*

## A. Introduction

Techniques and instruments for tissue approximation have evolved dramatically since the dawn of surgical history. For millennia, surgical needles and thread were some of the only tools available to surgeons for approximating tissues and closing wounds. While these basic tools still occupy a crucial role in current surgical practice, modern surgeons have a variety of additional sophisticated tissue approximation devices at their disposal. This chapter presents an overview of currently available laparoscopic tissue approximation devices and discusses considerations for the proper selection and use of these devices.

## B. Staplers

### 1. Intended Function and Indications

   i.   Surgical staplers are used as an alternative to suturing for hollow-organ resections, creation of anastomoses, ligation of ductal or vascular structures, as well as for pulmonary or solid organ resections.

   ii.  While staplers are frequently used in modern surgical practice and can make certain procedures more efficient or convenient for the surgeon, they are not intended to replace surgical judgment, basic surgical principles (e.g., hemostasis, proper tissue

N.J. Soper and C.E.H. Scott-Conner (eds.), *The SAGES Manual: Volume 1 Basic Laparoscopy and Endoscopy*, DOI 10.1007/978-1-4614-2344-7_12, © Springer Science+Business Media, LLC 2012

apposition, elimination of tension in an anastomosis) or the knowledge and technical skill required to perform a conventional, hand-sewn procedure. It is imperative that surgical trainees gain familiarity and experience performing hand-sewn procedures, as well as facility in use of staplers.

iii.   Conventional staplers are widely available and frequently used. These staplers use the mechanical force applied to the instrument by the surgeon's hand to deploy the staples into the tissue.

## 2. Selection Considerations

i.   **Staple height** is an important consideration to ensure proper functioning of the stapler. Staples come in a variety of heights in order to accommodate both thin tissues such as blood vessels and thicker tissues such as the stomach or rectum. Staplers for different tissue thicknesses are usually color-coded and marked by a specified staple height. The choice of the correct staple height is important, as the use of a staple height that is too small for a given tissue can lead to incomplete tissue penetration or result in a malformed staple shape leading to staple line leakage or failure. Conversely, the use of staples with an excessive height can result in an inadequately compressed staple line that may bleed or leak. Unfortunately, there is no universal standard for labeling stapler cartridges by color. Thus, users of surgical staplers are advised to refer to the specific manufacturer's instructions in choosing a cartridge with an appropriate staple height.

ii.   **Linear** staplers are easily recognized by their straight, elongated jaws which are clamped across the tissue to be stapled. These staplers typically deploy multiple rows of staples along the length of the jaws, compressing and joining the tissues in contact with both jaws (Fig. 12.1).

1.   **Stapler handle length** is an important consideration when selecting a laparoscopic stapler, as both standard and bariatric lengths are typically available. Standard length staplers may be inadequate to traverse the thick abdominal wall in bariatric patients, resulting in inability to reach the operative site. When in doubt, it is always better to overestimate length requirements when choosing a surgical stapler.

2.   **Articulating versus straight** jaws on a stapler determine the angle with which a stapler can be deployed. Depending

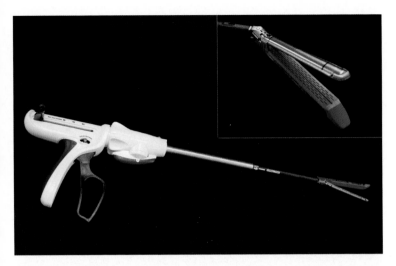

Fig. 12.1. Linear stapler with articulating capability. A close-up view of the jaws reveals how the stapler seals and transects tissue by deploying three rows of staples on either side and cutting in between (*inset*).

on the manufacturer, the jaws of a linear stapler may be articulated up to approximately 45° in order to help achieve a transversely oriented staple line in a difficult to reach area such as the pelvis or near the esophageal hiatus.

3. **Cutting and noncutting** linear staplers are both available, with cutting linear staplers being the most common. Cutting linear staplers typically deploy multiple rows of staples on either side of a central blade which transects tissue in a linear fashion along the length of the stapler. These staplers effectively transect tissue and seal both sides of the incision with multiple rows of staples. Noncutting linear staplers deploy multiple rows of staples but do not transect the tissue.

4. **Cartridge length** Cartridge length is also an important consideration, generally varying from 30 to 60 mm. The deployment of a cartridge that is too short can require additional cartridge deployments to ensure completion of a staple line. However, these shorter cartridge lengths may be easier to deploy in narrow areas such as the pelvis. Conversely, the use of an excessively long cartridge may leave a large number of free staples in the operative field, or may be difficult to articulate in a narrow area such as the pelvis.

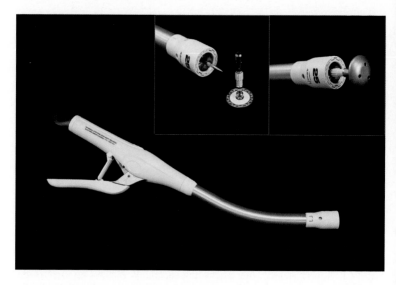

Fig. 12.2. Circular stapler. *Inset views* show the stapler head along with the detachable anvil. This type of stapler deploys a double, circular row of staples and cuts the tissue within the circle to create an anastomosis.

iii. **Circular staplers**, in contrast, consist of a detachable circular anvil, which is attached to a corresponding circular stapler head at the end of a typically curved, elongated stapler handle (Fig. 12.2).

1. **Mechanism**: The tissues that are clamped between the stapler anvil and head are joined by two circular rows of staples, with the excess tissue inside the circle excised to create a circular anastomosis.

2. **Anvil diameter** is also an important consideration. Larger anvils create larger anastomoses, less prone to stricturing however, an anvil that is too large for the lumen of the bowel may excessively dilate and damage it. Anvil diameters typically vary from 21 to 34 mm. The choice of anvil size will vary by procedure (e.g., gastric bypass v. proctectomy) and also should be a function of the patient's anatomy.

iv. **Suture line buttressing** involves the addition of a thin strip of reinforcement material to each side of a stapled piece of tissue. This reinforcement material helps to more tightly compress the tissue in between and has been proposed to help reduce the

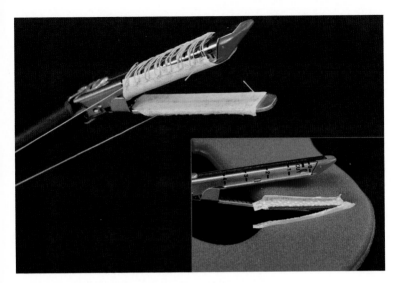

Fig. 12.3.  Suture-line reinforcement material loaded onto the jaws of a linear stapler. The stapler is fired across tissue and the suture strands are pulled to release the reinforcement material, which remains to help further compress the tissue that has been stapled (*inset*).

incidence of suture line leaks and bleeding, although there is considerable controversy as to its actual benefits in the literature. Suture line reinforcement material can be absorbable or nonabsorbable, biologic or synthetic in origin, and is available for both linear and circular staplers. The material is added to the jaws of a linear stapler or to the head of a circular stapler prior to deployment (Fig. 12.3).

v.  **Powered or conventional staplers** may be used. Powered staplers are driven using either a mechanical drive-shaft or with gas-operated mechanisms with or without computer-aided control. Some of these staplers may have sensing mechanisms to optimize stapler deployment given differences in tissue thickness, with the ultimate goal of making staple deployment more reliable and consistent in achieving tissue apposition. However, to date there is no evidence of superior outcomes as a result of using these more advanced, automated stapling systems. The use of these staplers requires familiarity with their deployment mechanisms, may require an on-site technician, and may introduce higher costs.

## 3. Considerations During Use

i. **Become familiar with the controls** and rehearse the firing mechanism and reloading mechanism of the specific stapler to be used prior to use in a real setting. Ideally, this should be done in a skills lab environment, or with nonsterile demonstration units, given that stapler designs are in constant evolution. Stapler cartridges are expensive, thus it is desirable to minimize demonstration or trial-and-error in the operating room. In addition, most disposable staplers are designed to be safely fired only a limited number of times prior to replacement with a new unit. Exercise similar precautions when "improved" staplers are used, or if your hospital changes vendors.

ii. **Proper port selection and placement** is important to ensure that surgical staplers will be able to reach the operative site. All linear staplers currently require a port size of at least 12 mm, with some staplers requiring up to a 15-mm port for introduction of cartridges with the largest staple height.

iii. **Insert the staplers** into the body under laparoscopic visualization, with the stapler jaws closed and the stapler in a nonarticulated configuration. Likewise, remove the stapler with the jaws closed in a nonarticulated configuration to prevent dislodgement of the laparoscopic trocar. The entire active part of the stapler (jaw hinge, articulating mechanism) must be seen to exit the trocar in order for the stapler to function properly. It may be necessary to partially withdraw the trocar to accomplish this.

iv. **Use of a stapler as a tissue grasper, retractor, or temporary bowel clamp** may sometimes be useful. However, it should be noted that some stapler jaws are designed to compress the tissue between the jaws prior to deploying staples, and may exert excessive compression forces to fragile tissues.

v. **The importance of ensuring adequate perfusion** of the tissues to be stapled is worth noting. Staplers are designed to approximate healthy tissue and will result in suture line failure when used on ischemic or necrotic tissues. Unfortunately, suture line failure due to ischemic or necrotic tissue is usually a process which may not manifest until several days after a patient's operation. Similarly, care should be taken to avoid the creation of a bridge of tissue between two staple lines as this may increase the risk of ischemic necrosis at that site.

vi. **Tissue compression** is a factor affecting the safe firing of staplers. Depending on the design of the stapler, tissue compression may occur when the jaws of the stapler are closed (prior to staple deployment), or during the process of staple deployment. In the latter, staple deployment should be done in a slow, controlled manner to allow tissue compression to occur. Allowing adequate time for tissue compression results in a normal egress of fluid from the tissues and ensures proper staple formation and tissue penetration after deployment. Inadequate tissue compression may result in inadequate staple penetration or malformed staples, leading to bleeding or staple line failure. Given the importance of tissue compression on staple line integrity, it is important to verify the correct firing instructions for each stapler type prior to use.

vii. **Prior to staple deployment, it is important to properly position the stapler on the tissues**. The tissue to be stapled should lie within the cutting and stapling range of the stapler jaws (usually marked on the side of the stapler cartridge). Blood vessels to be sealed should lie entirely within the stapling and cutting range to prevent partial sealing and transection. Tissues that are not intended to be cut and stapled should lie free of the tips of the stapler.

viii. **Ensuring hemostasis of staple lines** is important, as postoperative bleeding from the site of an anastomosis is not an uncommon complication. Inspection of a staple line may be done laparoscopically (everted staple line) or with endoscopic visualization (inverted staple line). The bleeding may be addressed by placing a suture ligature at a focal bleeding site, judicious use of electrocautery, or by refashioning the staple line using a cartridge with a smaller staple height or buttress material.

ix. **Inspect and test the staple line**, whenever feasible, to rule out a technical error or stapler misfire. The laparoscope should be used to inspect the external aspect of a staple line and ensure proper staple configuration along the entire length of the staple line. Likewise, intraluminal inspection using an endoscope can be used to inspect staple lines for defects or iatrogenic stricturing, as well as to rule out intraluminal bleeding. Saline leak-testing is recommended for select high-risk anastomoses such as gastrojejunal anastomoses during gastric bypass or colorectal anastomoses. This testing is generally performed by submerging the anastomosis under saline while insufflating the lumen with air to look for bubbling, indicating an anastomotic defect.

x.  **Reinforcement or inversion of staple lines** using additional suture placement is an option to address intraoperative technical errors with a suture line. However, the routine reinforcement or inversion of all staple lines is a practice that is largely surgeon or operation dependent, not advocated by stapler manufacturers, and which is not based on currently available literature.

## 4. Pitfalls and Dealing with Misfires

i.   **The possibility of stapler failures or misfires** should always be considered, especially in high-risk situations such as vascular ligation. The surgeon should be prepared to use backup measures to achieve vascular control should a problem occur during stapler use.

ii.  **Refashion any staple line** that is observed to have improperly formed staples or immediate staple line failure, indicating the use of a cartridge with a staple height that is too short for the thickness of the tissue. Likewise, a staple line created using a cartridge with an excessively tall staple height may result in bleeding or leaking, and should be refashioned.

iii. **Avoid using staplers in the setting of ischemic, necrotic, or severely inflamed or edematous tissues**, as this may lead to immediate or delayed staple line failure.

iv.  **A hand-sewn anastomosis** may be performed as a backup in the case of a failed stapled anastomosis.

# C. Specific Devices and Techniques: Tissue Fastener Devices

## 1. Intended Function and Indications

i.   Tissue fastener devices deploy individual tissue fasteners with each actuation and are intended to facilitate approximation of mesh to the abdominal wall during hernia repairs.

ii.  These devices are intended to complement, but not replace the use of multiple, well-placed, transfascial sutures.

## 2. Selection Considerations

i. **Helical fasteners** (Fig. 12.4) **or staples** (Fig. 12.5) are deployed by tissue fastener devices, depending on the specific model. No studies have studied the comparative safety or efficacy of these different types of fasteners.

ii. **Nonabsorbable (titanium) as well as newer absorbable helical fasteners are available**. The theoretical benefits of absorbable fasteners may include less acute or chronic postoperative pain, as well as a reduction in fistula or adhesion formation. However, these potential benefits have not been proven in the literature and thus the choice of absorbable versus nonabsorbable helical fasteners for mesh fixation is currently surgeon-dependent.

iii. **Applier length and diameter varies** according to the type of tissue fastener used. Staple appliers are only available in 12 mm sizes, versus helical fastener appliers which are 5 mm in diameter.

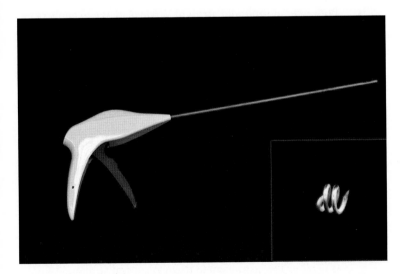

Fig. 12.4. Tissue fastener device (helical fastener type). This device may also be used to approximate hernia mesh to the abdominal wall. Close-up view shows the helical fastener deployed into the tissue with each actuation of the handle.

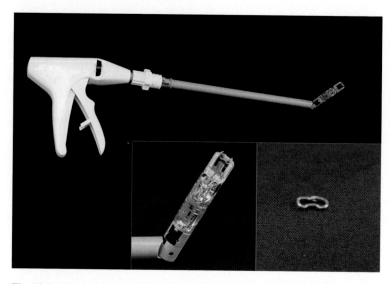

Fig. 12.5. Tissue fastener device (staple type). This device is used to approximate hernia mesh to the abdominal wall. Close-up views show the stapler head and final configuration of staple. The device deploys a single staple with each actuation of the handle and has an articulating capability.

iv.  **Both articulating and straight** versions of staple appliers are manufactured. Articulating instruments may facilitate placing fasteners perpendicular to the plane of the mesh surface to ensure maximum tissue penetration. Currently, only straight appliers are available for deploying helical tissue fasteners. However, proper use of abdominal wall pressure using the contralateral hand can be used to facilitate perpendicular deployment of helical tissue fasteners.

v.  **Staple heights and helical fastener lengths vary**, and determine the depth of tissue fastener penetration.

## 3. Considerations During Use

i.  **Select and place ports** to allow the introduction of 5 or 12 mm tissue fastener devices (depending on the device used), as well as to allow the instrument to reach the operative site.

ii.  **The tip of the device should compress the mesh against the underling abdominal wall** during deployment. This can be done by using the opposite hand to create counterpressure on the abdominal wall.

iii. **Take care to ensure that tissue fasteners are not deployed over major vessels or nerves** to prevent injuries to these structures.

iv. **The deployed tissue fastener should lie near, but not on the edge of the mesh**, to prevent the mesh from fraying and becoming detached.

v. **Remove individual metallic helical tacks or staples**, if necessary, using a blunt grasper under careful visualization. Treat these removed fasteners as potentially hazardous to prevent sharps-related injuries or damage to tissues.

# D. Specific Devices and Techniques: Clip Appliers

## 1. Intended Function and Indications

i. Laparoscopic clip appliers are indicated to ligate appropriately sized vascular or ductal structures (e.g. cystic duct or artery) by compressing tissues between U-shaped clips, which remain in place after deployment.

ii. They are not intended to securely ligate large vessels, fallopian tubes, or close hollow viscera.

## 2. Selection Considerations

i. **Disposable or re-usable clip appliers** (Fig. 12.6) are both available, with the major differences being the diameter of the applier (re-usable clip appliers are generally available only with a 10 mm shaft diameter), cost (may be higher for disposable instruments), and the ability to deploy multiple clips without the need to remove the instrument (a feature more common for disposable clip appliers).

ii. **Clip length and jaw span** vary and are important considerations depending on the size of the structure that is to be ligated. Clip lengths may vary from 6 to 11 mm. Clip appliers with larger diameters may have also have larger jaw spans, allowing clip placement on larger diameter structures.

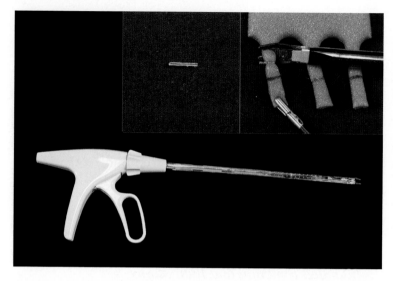

Fig. 12.6. Laparoscopic clip applier. This device is used for ligating tubular structures such as the cystic duct or artery. *Inset* shows final shape of clip as well as proper visualization of both clip applier tips prior to clip deployment.

   iii.   **Clip applier material** may be either metallic or nonabsorbable plastic depending on the manufacturer. Plastic clip appliers are only available as single-fire devices, whereas metallic clip appliers can be either single-fire or multifire devices.

   iv.   **Clip applier diameter** determines the diameter of ports that are needed for clip applier use, ranging from 5 to 11 mm.

## *3. Considerations During Use*

   i.   **Select and place ports** sufficient for the diameter of the clip applier shaft, and that allow the clip applier to reach the operative site.

   ii.   **Dissect vessels or ducts circumferentially** to reduce the risk of clip dislodgement once placed.

   iii.   **Insert multifire clip appliers** in an unloaded configuration (no clip present in the jaws) to prevent dislodgement of the clip during insertion. In contrast, single-fire clip appliers need to be inserted in a loaded configuration (clip present in the jaws), after partially closing the jaws to allow passage of the clip applier through the port.

iv.   **Load the jaws of the clip applier** before positioning the jaws across the structure to be ligated. This prevents jamming or improper loading of the clip prior to deployment.

v.   **Ensure that the distal jaws of the clip applier are free of tissue or previously placed clips, and that the tips can be seen to extend beyond the structure to be ligated** prior to clip deployment. This can be visualized with the laparoscope, and may be facilitated with a slight rotation of the clip applier jaws.

vi.   **Deploy clips perpendicular to the long axis of the structure to be ligated** in a smooth, controlled fashion, without excessive rotational torque on the clip applier jaws, and ensuring full compression of the tissue.

vii.   **Inspect clips** to verify that the diameter of the ligated structure is completely traversed and sealed by the length of the clip. If necessary, place additional clips to reinforce closure of the structure.

viii.   **Withdraw clip appliers** either after having deployed the clip, or with the jaws in a closed position to prevent clip dislodgement into the abdomen during removal of the instrument.

# 4.  Pitfalls

i.   **Failure to verify that the distal jaws of the clip applier are free of tissue** prior to clip deployment may lead to inadvertent injury to adjacent structures, insecure clip placement, or ineffective sealing of structures.

ii.   **Blind clip deployment** is frequently ineffective and may lead to inadvertent injuries. Clips should only be deployed under adequate visualization, after vascular control has been achieved (e.g., by grasping a vessel with an atraumatic grasper).

iii.   **Deploying clips on top of or overlapping previously placed clips may result in ineffective, malformed clips**.

# E. Ligating Loops

## 1. Intended Function and Indications

i.   Ligating loops (Fig. 12.7) are devices which deploy a pre-tied suture ligature onto a previously divided vascular, ductal or lumenal structure (i.e., appendix). Typically, they can be used as an alternative to clips for ligating the cystic duct or as an alternative to a linear stapler to secure the appendiceal stump.

ii.  Ligating loops should be used similarly to the way a suture tie might be used in open surgery. With this in mind, they may not be adequate to secure larger vessels, in which case linear staplers or conventional suturing may be preferable.

## 2. Selection Considerations

i.   **Suture material may be absorbable or nonabsorbable**, and should be chosen depending on the structure to be ligated (e.g., cystic duct versus blood vessels).

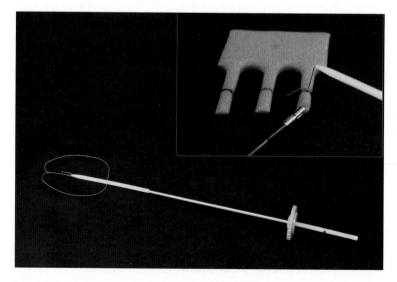

Fig. 12.7.  Ligating loop. This device may be used to place a suture ligature on a tubular structure such as the cystic duct or appendiceal stump. It is important to use a grasper as shown to stabilize the structure being ligated.

## 3. Considerations During Use

i. **Any port 5 mm or larger may be used** to introduce ligating loops. However these devices are generally slightly shorter than a standard length instrument. Thus, the port through which the ligating loop will be used should be close to the operative site.

ii. **Technique for deploying ligating loops**:

1. **The structure to be ligated** should either already be transected (e.g., cystic duct) or short enough to allow placement of a ligating loop over the tip and hence around its circumference (e.g., appendix).

2. **Pass a separate grasper through the loop to hold the structure to be ligated**. The surgeon may use one hand for the ligating loop and the other hand to operate the grasper. Alternatively, an assistant may hold the grasper, allowing the surgeon to use both hands to operate the ligating loop.

3. **Place the rigid tip of the ligating loop device (knot pusher) at the site of intended ligation**. Bend and separate the external end of the ligating loop from the knot pusher. Hold the knot pusher against the structure to be ligated while slowly pulling the external end of the suture to gradually constrict the suture loop knot around the intended structure. Next, withdraw the knot pusher slightly to expose the excess suture outside of the loop. Trim this to desired length with laparoscopic scissors. Finally, remove the knot pusher and excess suture.

4. **Verify the location and tightness of the suture loop** to ensure a secure ligature and the absence of a leak.

## 4. Pitfalls

i. **It is essential to use a grasper while deploying a ligating loop** to ensure the loop remains on the intended target.

ii. **It is important to ensure an adequate tissue stump remains** so that the ligating loop does not easily become avulsed and result in bleeding or a leak.

## F. Tissue Glues

### 1. Intended Function and Indications

    i.   Topical agents have been developed as adjuncts to existing surgical techniques to improve tissue sealing. Some of these agents have additional hemostatic activity which may help to stop or prevent bleeding from surfaces such as the spleen, liver, or vascular anastomoses.

    ii.   Some of these agents may also be used on gastrointestinal anastomoses with the goal of helping to prevent leaks. Some agents have an approved indication for use in colostomy reversal as tissue sealing adjuncts.

    iii.   Some tissue adhesives have approved indications for closure of skin incisions.

    iv.   Hernia mesh fixation has also been a reported use for some of these topical agents, however, this type of use is off-label and investigational.

### 2. Types of Tissue Adhesives

    i.   **Fibrin sealants** have combined hemostatic and tissue adhesive activity and are composed of fibrinogen plus thrombin, which interact to form a fibrin clot at the site of use.

    ii.   **Cyanoacrylates** are tissue adhesives made from *n*-butyl-2-cyanoacrylates, the precursor of which is commonly known as "super glue."

    iii.   **Albumin and glutaraldehyde combinations** have also been developed for use as tissue sealants for vascular anastomoses.

### 3. Selection Considerations

    i.   **Internal or external use depends on the type of tissue adhesive**. Fibrin sealants and albumin/glutaraldehyde adhesives are meant for internal use, whereas cyanoacrylates should only be used externally to close skin incisions. Internal use of cyanoacrylates may result in foreign body reactions, tissue damage as a result of exothermic polymerization reactions, or tattooing in the case of histoacryl blue.

ii.   **Tissue adhesives may be of synthetic or donor-derived origin**. Fibrin-based sealants are donor-derived formulations of either pooled human plasma or autologous plasma. Products made from pooled human plasma undergo processing to inactivate or remove many viruses. However, there may still be a theoretical risk of infection from agents such as the Creutzfeldt Jakob disease agent or small, nonlipid enveloped viruses such as Parvoviruses. Synthetic or autologous tissue adhesives do not have these disease-transmission risks.

iii.  **Bovine-derived** compounds or polypeptide additives such as aprotinin (found in some fibrin sealants) may increase the risk of allergic or anaphylactic reactions when these products are used.

iv.   **Hemostatic effects** may be desirable for some adhesives such as fibrin sealants. However, these agents should not be allowed to enter devices used for autologous blood salvage or cardiac bypass circuits as they may cause clotting.

v.    **Preparation and storage** instructions vary by product but should be reviewed ahead of time, as many require thawing prior to use.

## 4. Considerations During Use

i.    **Laparoscopic spray applicators** may be used to apply internal tissue adhesives such as fibrin sealants. Some of these applicators are gas-driven to facilitate a continuous and even distribution of sealant.

ii.   **Use tissue adhesives or fibrin sealants as adjuncts, not substitutes** for proper surgical control of bleeding or anastomotic techniques.

iii.  **Apply tissue sealants as the final step** when used as an adjunct for gastrointestinal anastomoses (after the anastomoses has been tested and inspected).

iv.   **Maintain a high level of vigilance** to recognize the uncommon but serious adverse effects associated with these agents.
   1.  **Anaphylactic or hypersensitivity reactions** manifest as unexplained hypotension, tachycardia, or urticaria.
   2.  **Air embolisms** may occur with gas-driven applicators that are used at higher than recommended pressures or too close to the tissues.

# G. Less Commonly Used and Experimental Tissue Approximation Devices

## 1. Anastomotic Ring Devices

i.  Devices for performing suture-less gastrointestinal anastomoses have a long history, having been first described in the 1800s. Although there are commercially available biofragmentable anastomotic rings on the market, their use is not as widespread, likely due to the success and ease of use of surgical staplers.

## 2. Laser Tissue Welding

i.  Bonding of tissue margins to create anastomoses has also been described experimentally using computer-controlled laser energy, with adjuncts such as albumin as soldering agents. Although this technology has not yet reached the clinical arena, it may be a promising modality used for tissue approximation in the future.

## Selected References

Brown SL, Woo EK. Surgical stapler-associated fatalities and adverse events reported to the Food and Drug Administration. J Am Coll Surg. 2004;199(3):374–81.

Chu T, Chandhoke RA, Smith PC, Schwaitzberg SD. The impact of surgeon choice on the cost of performing laparoscopic appendectomy. Surg Endosc. 2011;25(4):1187–91.

Finks JF, Carlin A, Share D, et al. Effect of surgical techniques on clinical outcomes after laparoscopic gastric bypass-results from the Michigan Bariatric Surgery Collaborative. Surg Obes Relat Dis. 2011;7(3):284–9.

Giannopoulos GA, Tzanakis NE, Rallis GE, Efstathiou SP, Tsigris C, Nikiteas NI. Staple line reinforcement in laparoscopic bariatric surgery: does it actually make a difference? A systematic review and meta-analysis. Surg Endosc. 2010;24(11):2782–8.

Kaidar-Person O, Rosenthal RJ, Wexner SD, Szomstein S, Person B. Compression anastomosis: history and clinical considerations. Am J Surg. 2008;195(6):818–26.

Lovisetto F, Zonta S, Rota E, et al. Use of human fibrin glue (Tissucol) versus staples for mesh fixation in laparoscopic transabdominal preperitoneal hernioplasty: a prospective, randomized study. Ann Surg. 2007;245(2):222–31.

Silecchia G, Boru CE, Mouiel J, et al. The use of fibrin sealant to prevent major complications following laparoscopic gastric bypass: results of a multicenter, randomized trial. Surg Endosc. 2008;22(11):2492–7.

Spector D, Rabi Y, Vasserman I, et al. In vitro large diameter bowel anastomosis using a temperature controlled laser tissue soldering system and albumin stent. Lasers Surg Med. 2009;41(7):504–8.

Spotnitz WD, Burks S. Hemostats, sealants, and adhesives: components of the surgical toolbox. Transfusion. 2008;48(7):1502–16.

# 13. Documentation

*Minh B. Luu, M.D.*
*Daniel J. Deziel, M.D.*

## A. General Considerations

Modern video technology converts the optical image from a laparoscopic lens to an electronic signal that can be displayed, transmitted, and recorded. Electronic images can be archived in a variety of formats as videos or as still images. These recorded images are invaluable ways to convey information for clinical, scientific, educational, and medicolegal purposes. Improved image resolution, increased sense of depth in three-dimensional (3D) effects, and equipment integration are ongoing goals of manufacturers. New formats for video imaging and laparoscopic documentation will continue to become available as technology develops. Cost, equipment, storage requirements, and general availability of a particular format are important practical considerations. Digital images, signal processing, and recording technology have replaced standard analog systems.

## B. Components of Video Imaging

The basic components for laparoscopic imaging are the telescope, light cable, light source, camera head, video signal processor, video cable, and monitor. In modern practice, additional recording components, such as digital capture devices and photo printers, are usually appended. In general, the best pictures come from the fewest devices that the video signal has to pass through. Therefore, for best image quality these components should be arranged in a distributed configuration as opposed to a chain configuration (Figs. 13.1 and 13.2). The components are usually housed in mobile towers or in dedicated endosuites (Figs. 13.3 and 13.4).

N.J. Soper and C.E.H. Scott-Conner (eds.), *The SAGES Manual: Volume 1*    163
*Basic Laparoscopy and Endoscopy*, DOI 10.1007/978-1-4614-2344-7_13,
© Springer Science+Business Media, LLC 2012

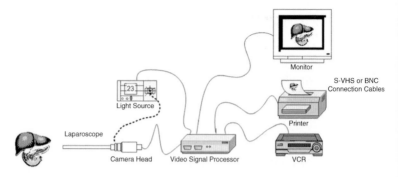

Fig. 13.1. Standard video setup utilizing a distributed approach to the video signal array.

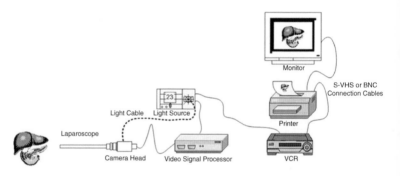

Fig. 13.2. Standard video setup with sequential "pass-through" of the video signal through each of the video components. This arrangement degrades the signal at each step of the chain.

The development of the Hopkins rod-lens system used in modern laparoscopes was a key to allowing photographic and video documentation (Fig. 13.5 top). Light is transmitted through a series of glass rods with lenses at the ends rather than through air, as in previous lens systems. This provides improved light transmission with higher resolution, a wider viewing angle, and a larger image than previously available. Currently, rigid laparoscopes range from 10 mm to 2 mm in size with lens angles of 0°, 30°, and 45°. Standard telescope lengths are 35 cm, but longer (50 cm) scopes have been developed for bariatric and single incision laparoscopic surgery. Flexible endoscopes with an image sensor at the tip (Fig. 13.5 bottom) permit variable viewing angles compared to the fixed angles of rigid rod-lens scopes.

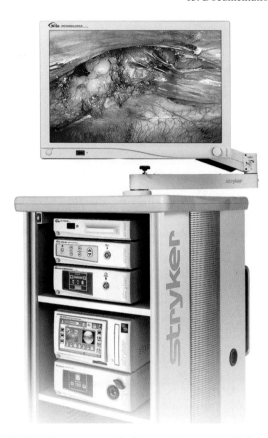

Fig. 13.3.  Mobile video towers typically contain a monitor, light source, video signal processor, digital recorder, insufflator with carbon dioxide tanks, and printer (Courtesy of Stryker, San Jose, CA).

Three-dimensional laparoscopes are designed with single or dual channels. Single channel laparoscopes are smaller in diameter and can be angled but often produce a weaker 3D effect than dual channel scopes. The wider the distance between each channel, the more pronounced the 3D effect. Dual channel 3D laparoscopes are used in the robotic da Vinci® Surgical System (Intuitive Surgical, Sunnyvale CA) but have yet to gain wide acceptance in laparoscopic surgery.

The problem of insufficient illumination for laparoscopic documentation was overcome by the development of the high-intensity halogen (150 W), metal halide (250 W), and xenon lamps (300 W). Xenon bulbs are currently used in most modern light sources due to the improved

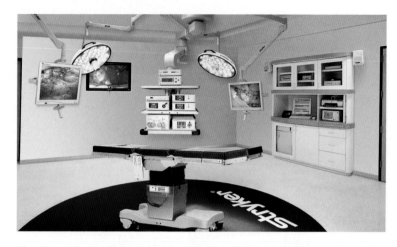

Fig. 13.4.  Modern dedicated endosuite with ceiling mounted flat panel monitors and towers (Courtesy of Stryker, San Jose, CA).

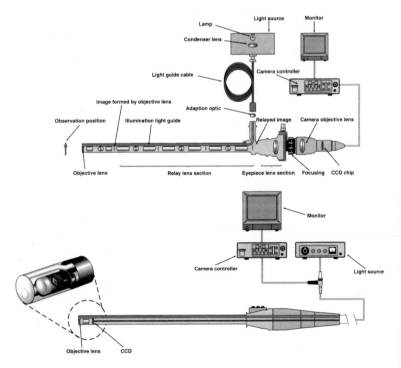

Fig. 13.5. Traditional rod-lens compared to digital laparoscopes (From Preminger, 2007, with permission).

durability and performance over metal halide bulbs. Light is transmitted from the lamp to the laparoscope through cables. There are two types of cable: fiber-optic and fluid. Fiber-optic cables are constructed from a bundle of optical glass with fiber sizes ranging from 20 to 150 μm in diameter. They transmit light by internal reflection without generating heat, are flexible but are fragile. Fluid cables transmit more light, generate more heat, but are rigid due to the metal sheath and are also fragile. In addition, fluid cables require soaking for sterilization and cannot be gas sterilized. Fiber-optic cables are more commonly used because of their flexibility and ease of sterilization. Insufficient light can be the result of a failing light bulb, broken light bundle within the cable or laparoscope, auto-shutter malfunction, or mechanical occlusion of the scope or camera lenses.

Modern laparoscopic cameras are palm size and lightweight consisting of a light sensor, focusing ring, coupling ring (for attaching the telescope), water resistant casing, and an integrated cable. The basis of the sensor is the solid-state silicon computer chip or charge-coupled device (CCD) that consists of an array of light-sensitive silicon elements. Silicon emits an electrical charge when exposed to light. These charges can be amplified, transmitted, displayed, or recorded. Each silicon element contributes one unit (referred to as a pixel) to the total image. The resolution or clarity of the image depends upon the density of pixels or light receptors on the chip. High-resolution cameras may contain 450,000 pixels. Early video cameras used only one CCD sensor that required four silicon elements to generate the signal for one pixel. Resolution was enhanced fourfold by development of a three-chip CCD system. The image light is split into the primary colors by a prism and is directed onto three separate CCD sensors.

When rigid, rod-lens laparoscopes are used, the image is digitalized by the multiple CCD sensors after the image has been transmitted through a series of lenses. Flexible scope technology digitalizes the image immediately by placing a single CCD chip at the tip of the scope. In theory, this might offer better image quality by eliminating all non-digital components of the system and linking the digital signal processor, laparoscope and light cable as a single unit. Limitations of this arrangement are single chip processing, small size of the image sensor and lack of compatibility of flexible technology with nonproprietary systems. However, advances in miniaturization and chip design have enabled integrated videoendoscopes to produce high-quality images comparable to those produced by rod-lens systems with 3-chip CCD cameras.

Regardless of the camera capability and wiring format, the clarity of the image depends on the resolution capability of the monitor. For many years, the optical quality of images produced by endoscopes and CCD cameras far exceeded the display resolution of the monitors. Standard consumer-grade video monitors have 350 lines of horizontal resolution; monitors with about 700 lines are preferred for laparoscopic surgery. High-definition television (HDTV) monitors have more than 1,100 lines of resolution in a wide-screen format. Flat panel monitors have replaced cathode ray tube (CRT) monitors due to their lighter weight, space efficiency, and superior resolution. Eyestrain is decreased when the viewer is at a distance of 4–5 times the diagonal length of the screen. To allow the surgical team to view monitors up to 8 ft away, the monitor should be at least 19 in. in size. Ergonomics are also improved by ceiling or wall mounted monitors in dedicated endosuites.

The importance of the operator and of maintenance personnel for obtaining a quality video image cannot be underestimated. Besides assuring proper electronics, the operator must attend to mechanical details such as lens cleaning, focusing, and framing. No improvements in electronic signal processing can overcome the limitation of a scope that is damaged or a lens that is fogged, smeared, or out of focus. The ocular (proximal) and objective (distal) lenses of the laparoscope as well as the camera lens must be checked. The objective lens can be cleaned internally with irrigation and externally by wiping with dry gauze before applying antifogging solution. It is imperative that the cannulas be clean and that no tissue be in the way during introduction of the scope.

# C. Types of Video Signal

The optical or light image is converted into an electronic signal that can be scanned by a video monitor to produce a screen image. The electronic signal can be recorded as a voltage (analog) or as a binary code (0 or 1, digital). Analog signals are prone to noise and degradation (Fig. 13.6a). This effect is more pronounced when the signal is duplicated or copied. Digital signals, on the other hand, are more resistant to degradation (Fig. 13.6b).

Analog video systems initially used in laparoscopic surgery and elsewhere grew out of television broadcast technology. The National Television Systems Committee (NTSC) video signals combined both color (chrominance = C) and brightness (luminance = Y) information into

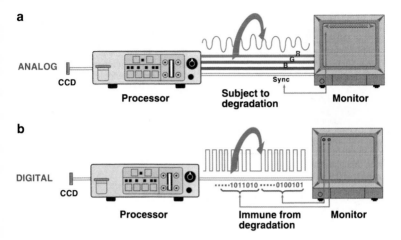

Fig. 13.6. Degradation of analog video signals (**a**) not seen in digital video signals (**b**) (From Preminger, 2007, with permission).

a single (composite) signal. The problem with this analog format was inferior resolution. In addition, these signals were recorded as voltages and therefore prone to error in subsequent recordings or duplication. Two additional analog video formats were developed that improved resolution. The first was the Y/C or Super VHS component signal that separated the luminance (Y) and color (C) thus reducing the cross noise that hampered the NTSC signals. The second format was the RGB (red, green, blue) that separated the signal into four separate components. In this format, color and luminance were separated into the three primary colors, each with their own luminance; the fourth signal was for synchronization. The RGB format required less electronic processing than the NTSC or Y/C formats and therefore resulted in superior image quality.

Digital converters translate video signals to binary codes (0 or 1) that are not prone to degradation as occurs with analog signals. Digital video signals can be processed to enhance images or can be merged with other formats (audio, text) for transmission and duplication without loss of information. A wide variety of analog and digital outputs (Fig. 13.7) are available from video signal processors. Digital Video Interface (DVI) and Serial Digital Interface (SDI) are standards that are used to carry high-quality, uncompressed, unencrypted digital video signals. The cables used in DVI transmission have length limitations that do not exist in SDI.

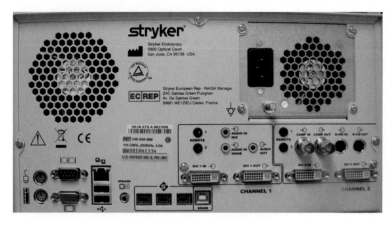

Fig. 13.7.  A variety of analog and digital outputs available from the video signal processor (camera controller unit).

## D.  Recording Media

Most video systems today are capable of recording still images or continuous recordings into their hard drives and exported to compact disk (CD), digital video disk (DVD), Media Cards, or universal serial bus (USB) flash drives (Fig. 13.8). DVD and USB are commonly used to store and transfer video files. DVDs are relatively inexpensive but only have a capacity of 4.7 gigabyte (GB), whereas USB flash drives can hold files up to 128 GB. Digitally captured material can be edited, stored, and exported with much greater ease than analog types. Captured still images are commonly stored as Bitmaps (BMP), Joint Photographic Experts Group (JPEG), Tagged Image File Format (TIFF), Portable Network Graphics (PNG), or Graphics Interchange Format (GIF) formats. Higher resolution pictures containing several megapixels are required for photo printing, while lower resolution images are adequate for Web pages or presentations. Videos are recorded as Moving Picture Experts Group (MPEG) or Audio Video Interleaved (AVI). Each minute of a video in an MPEG-2 format requires 42 MB of storage space, therefore, a DVD can store approximately 1 h and 50 min of video.

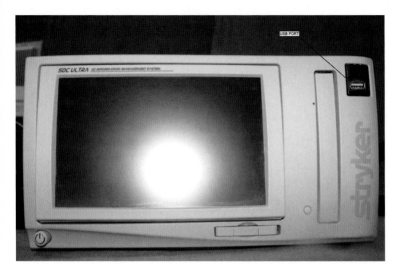

Fig. 13.8.  Video capture and storage system capable of exporting images to CD, DVD, and USB devices.

# Selected References

Berber E, Siperstein AE. Understanding and optimizing laparoscopic video systems. Surg Endosc. 2001;15:781–7.

Hagiike M, Phillips EH, Berci G. Performance differences in laparoscopic surgical skills between true high-definition and three-chip CCD video systems. Surg Endosc. 2007; 21:1849–54.

Kourambas J, Preminger GM. Advances in camera, video and imaging technologies in laparoscopy. Urol Clin North Am. 2001;28:5–14.

Preminger GM, Sur RL, Scales Jr CD. Video imaging and documentation. In: Smith A, Badlani G, Bagley D, Clayman R, Docimo S, editors. Smith's textbook of endourology. 2nd ed. Hamilton: BC Decker; 2007.

Schwaitzberg SD. Imaging systems in minimally invasive surgery. In: Soper N, Swanstrom L, Eubanks S, editors. Mastery of endoscopic and laparoscopic surgery. 3rd ed. Philadelphia: Lippincott Williams & Wilkins; 2009.

Szold A. Seeing is believing, visualization systems in endoscopic surgery (video, HDTV, stereoscopy, and beyond). Surg Endosc. 2005;19:730–3.

# 14. Laparoscopy During Pregnancy[*]

*Carmen L. Mueller, B.Sc., M.D.*
*Allan Okrainec, M.D., M.H.P.E., F.R.C.S.C., F.A.C.S.*

## A. Indications for Laparoscopy During Pregnancy

An estimated 1 in 635 pregnant patients will require nonobstetric abdominal surgery, with the most common diagnoses being acute appendicitis, biliary disease, ovarian torsion and intestinal obstruction. Approximately 1:1,500 pregnant women will develop acute appendicitis, and 3–8/10,000 pregnant patients require cholecystectomy. Intra-abdominal infection is associated with high fetal loss rates, with 1.5% reported for unperforated appendicitis, and as high as 20% in perforated appendicitis. Biliary disease harbors similar risks for mother and fetus, including 5% fetal loss rate for acute cholecystitis and 60% fetal loss and 15% maternal mortality with gallstone pancreatitis.

To prevent poor fetal and maternal outcomes, early diagnosis and treatment of surgical diseases in pregnancy are essential.

## B. Advantages and Feasibility of Laparoscopy During Pregnancy

Although the benefits of the laparoscopic approach for many surgical procedures have been well defined, it has been slow to gain acceptance during pregnancy because of concerns regarding fetal and maternal safety. Indeed, at the beginning of the laparoscopic era, pregnancy was viewed as a contraindication to utilizing the laparoscopic approach.

---

[*]This chapter was contributed by Miriam J. Curet M.D. in the previous edition.

N.J. Soper and C.E.H. Scott-Conner (eds.), *The SAGES Manual: Volume 1 Basic Laparoscopy and Endoscopy*, DOI 10.1007/978-1-4614-2344-7_14, © Springer Science+Business Media, LLC 2012

Over the past 15 years, a growing number of reports on the use of laparoscopy in the pregnant patient have demonstrated the same safety and advantages of laparoscopy in this patient population as in the nonpregnant patient.

1. Since 2000, there have been 16 retrospective case series published on laparoscopy in pregnancy for a variety of surgical diagnoses.

    a. One large population-based study by Kuy et al. reported the outcomes of 9,714 pregnant patients undergoing either laparoscopic or open cholecystectomy.

    b. No study has shown a significant difference in the rates of fetal loss, maternal and fetal complications and preterm labor in patients undergoing open versus laparoscopic surgery.

    c. In general, fetal losses are rare events, with a total of ten cases being reported in the last 10 years among all pregnant women undergoing nonobstetric abdominal surgery (five open and five laparoscopic).

    d. The rates of preterm labor average 5–18%, and no study has shown a difference in APGAR scores or fetal birth weight after open or laparoscopic surgery.

    e. Although the long-term effects of pneumoperitoneum and possible transient acidosis on the fetus are not known, a 2003 study by Rizzo followed 11 mothers and children for 1–8 years after delivery and reported no physical or developmental abnormalities in the children, and no adverse maternal outcomes.

2. Currently, laparoscopy is considered as safe as open surgery at any stage of pregnancy, and conveys the same benefits of laparoscopy as have been demonstrated in nonpregnant patients.

# C. Surgical Considerations

The following practice guidelines should be followed when performing laparoscopy in the pregnant patient. More information can be found in the SAGES GUIDELINES FOR LAPAROSCOPY DURING PREGNANCY (2011) (see Selected References).

## 1. Timing of Laparoscopy in Pregnancy

a. Laparoscopy is now considered safe and effective in any trimester of pregnancy.

b. The majority of reports on the use of laparoscopy in pregnancy involve patients in the first or second trimester, and historically the second trimester has been considered the safest time for any operation to avoid fetal complications (spontaneous abortion in the first trimester and premature labor in the third trimester).

c. No study has shown a clear difference in fetal loss rates or premature labor based on the timing of operative intervention, and delaying surgical treatment for intra-abdominal infections has its own risks with respect to fetal and maternal complications.

d. For patients with symptomatic cholelithiasis managed expectantly, recurrence of symptoms occurs in 92% of patients who present in the first trimester, 64% who present in the second, and 44% in the third, supporting the role of early surgical intervention.

e. Successful laparoscopic treatment of surgical diseases has been described at all stages of pregnancy and the decision to use the laparoscopic approach should be based on the surgeon's skill level and experience, and the availability of trained personnel and equipment, rather than the stage of pregnancy.

## 2. Perioperative Fetal Care

a. Always obtain obstetrical consultation and monitor perioperative fetal heart rate (if appropriate for gestational stage) in any patient undergoing surgery during pregnancy.

b. If signs of fetal distress develop, immediately decrease pneumoperitoneum and stabilize the mother's oxygenation and vital signs until fetal heart tracings return to normal.

c. In the majority of recent reports of laparoscopic surgery in pregnancy, routine prophylactic tocolytics have not been used, with no increase in the rates of preterm labor. As such, the prophylactic use of tocolytics is not currently recommended, although they should be administered under the guidance of an obstetrician should any signs of uterine irritability develop.

## 3. Patient Positioning

Position the pregnant patient in the left lateral recumbent position (supine with a wedge-shaped pillow underneath the right hip to displace the gravid uterus), to prevent caval compression and decreased venous return during surgery.

## 4. Perioperative Venous Thromboembolism Prophylaxis

a.  Pregnancy is a hypercoagulable state with increased levels of fibrinogen and factors VII and XII.

b.  This, in combination with pneumoperitoneum and reverse Trendelenburg position used in laparoscopy increases the risk of venous thromboembolism.

c.  Intraoperative and postoperative use of pneumatic compression devices is recommended until the patient is ambulating well, and early ambulation should be emphasized.

d.  Heparin has been shown to be safe in pregnancy and should be the agent of choice for medical prophylaxis.

e.  Although data in the pregnant population is lacking, preoperative subcutaneous administration of 5,000 U of UFH in other surgical patients has been shown to minimally increase bleeding risk and reduce VTE incidence for procedures lasting longer than 1 h.

## 5. Trocar Placement and Entry into the Abdomen

a.  Entry into the abdomen during pregnancy has been safely achieved by open Hasson, optical trocar and Veress needle techniques.

b.  However, the gravid uterus distorts intra-abdominal anatomy, and so the safest approach to minimize uterine, fetal, and maternal injury at any stage of pregnancy is the open Hasson technique; this approach is favored by the authors.

c.  Once initial entry to the abdomen has been achieved, place the remaining ports under direct vision as usual.

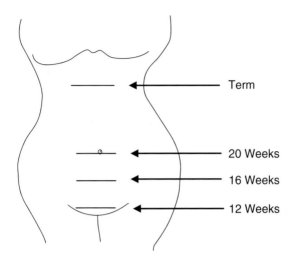

Fig. 14.1.  Fundal height at advancing stages of pregnancy.

d.  Take fundal height into account when placing trocars. This changes as the pregnancy develops. By generally accepted norms, the uterine fundus is palpable at the level of the pubic symphysis at 12 weeks, midway between the symphysis and umbilicus at 16 weeks, at the level of the umbilicus at 20 weeks, and 2–3 finger breadths beneath the xiphisternum at term (see Fig. 14.1).

e.  For any procedure, place the initial trocar to accommodate fundal height.

f.  For laparoscopic cholecystectomy, the remaining trocars can often be placed in their usual locations.

g.  For laparoscopic appendectomy, adjust trocar placement to accommodate the gravid uterus, (Figs. 14.2–14.4).

h.  In the third trimester, ports may need to be placed in the right upper and right lower quadrants to accommodate the dissection in the setting of an enlarged uterus (Fig. 14.4).

## 6. Insufflation Pressure

a.  Initial studies of $CO_2$ pneumoperitoneum in pregnant sheep demonstrated increased fetal acidosis with higher insufflations pressures, although this has not been shown in humans. Moreover, there have been no reports of long-term complications related

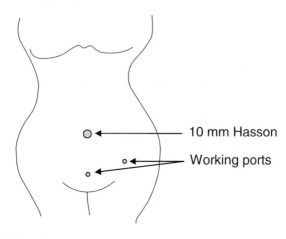

Fig. 14.2.  First trimester trocar placement for laparoscopic appendectomy.

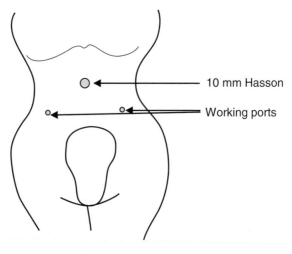

Fig. 14.3.  Second trimester trocar placement for laparoscopic appendectomy.

to temporary fetal acidosis in humans, and currently $CO_2$ pneumoperitoneum is considered safe in pregnancy.

b.  Considerations specific to the pregnant patient include reduced venous return due to caval compression, decreased uterine blood flow due to uterine compression, and difficulties with ventilation that can occur at higher insufflations pressures due to the physiologic changes of pregnancy.

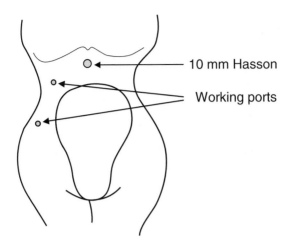

Fig. 14.4.   Third trimester trocar placement for laparoscopic appendectomy.

    c.    Despite these concerns, insufflation up to 15 mmHg has been safely used. Present guidelines recommend the use of the least insufflation pressure that still allows for adequate visualization, preferably at or below 12 mmHg.

    d.    Use capnography to monitor maternal $ETCO_2$ levels and acid–base status intraoperatively.

## 7. Intraoperative Cholangiogram

Choledocholithiasis in the pregnant patient is best treated with preoperative ERCP and sphincterotomy, followed by laparoscopic cholecystectomy. If intraoperative cholangiogram is required, perform this in the usual fashion but place lead to shield the fetus. Fluoroscopy delivers minimal radiation exposure, and no fetal complications have been described related to fluoroscopy exposure.

## D.  Summary

    1.    The growing body of evidence supports the use of laparoscopy in pregnancy, regardless of trimester.

    2.    The choice to use the laparoscopic approach should be based on the surgeon's experience and skill.

3.  Early intervention for acute appendicitis and acute cholecystitis has been shown to reduce fetal and maternal complications.
4.  Patients should be positioned in the left lateral recumbent position, and trocar placement should be planned to adjust for fundal height.
5.  Insufflation pressures that allow adequate visualization but do not impede maternal oxygenation and ventilation, and maintain $ETCO_2$ within the normal range should be used.
6.  Perioperative obstetrical consultation and fetal monitoring is recommended but should not delay treatment.
7.  Routine prophylactic tocolysis is not recommended. Venous thromboembolism prophylaxis should be employed, including use of pneumatic compression devices and preoperative unfractionated heparin administration for prolonged procedures, as well as early ambulation.

# Selected References

Bhavani-Shankar K, et al. Arterial to end-tidal carbon dioxide pressure difference during laparoscopic surgery in pregnancy. Anesthesiology. 2000;93(2):370–3.

Buser KB. Laparoscopic surgery in the pregnant patient–One surgeon's experience in a small rural hospital. JSLS. 2002;308:121–4.

Buser KB. Laparoscopic surgery in the pregnant patient: results and recommendations. JSLS. 2009;13(1):32–5.

Chohan L, Kilpatrick CC. Laparoscopy in pregnancy: a literature review. Clin Obstet Gynecol. 2009;52(4):557–69.

Comitalo JB, Lynch D. Laparoscopic cholecystectomy in the pregnant patient. Surg Laparosc Endosc. 1994;4(4):268–71.

Corneille MG, Gallup TM, Bening T, et al. The use of laparoscopic surgery in pregnancy: evaluation of safety and efficacy. Am J Surg. 2010;200(3):363–7.

Curet MJ, et al. Effects of $CO_2$ pneumoperitoneum in pregnant ewes. J Surg Res. 1996; 63(1):339–44.

Guidelines Committee of the Society of American Gastrointestinal and Endoscopic Surgeons, Yumi H. Guidelines for diagnosis, treatment, and use of laparoscopy for surgical problems during pregnancy. Surg Endosc. 2008;22(4):849–61. Updated on-line Jan, 2011. (http://www.sages.org/publications/publication.php?id=23).

Halkic N, Tempia-Caliera AA, Ksontini R, et al. Laparoscopic management of appendicitis and symptomatic cholelithiasis during pregnancy. Langenbecks Arch Surg. 2006; 391(5):467–71.

Hunter JG, Swanstrom L, Thornburg K. Carbon dioxide pneumoperitoneum induces fetal acidosis in a pregnant ewe model. Surg Endosc. 1995;9(3):272–7. discussion 277–9.

Kirshtein B, Perry ZH, Avinoach E, Mizrahi S, Lantsberg L. Safety of laparoscopic appendectomy during pregnancy. World J Surg. 2009;33(3):475–80.

Kuy S, Roman SA, Desai R, Sosa JA. Outcomes following cholecystectomy in pregnant and nonpregnant women. Surgery. 2009;146(2):358–66.

Lemieux P, Rheaume P, Levesque I, Bujold E, Brochu G. Laparoscopic appendectomy in pregnant patients: a review of 45 cases. Surg Endosc. 2009;23(8):1701–5.

Mathevet P, Nessah K, Dargent D, Mellier G. Laparoscopic management of adnexal masses in pregnancy: a case series. Eur J Obstet Gynecol Reprod Biol. 2003;108(2): 217–22.

Melnick DM, Wahl WL, Dalton VK. Management of general surgical problems in the pregnant patient. Am J Surg. 2004;187(2):170–80.

Moreno-Sanz C, Pascual-Pedreño A, Picazo-Yeste JS, Seoane-Gonzalez JB. Laparoscopic appendectomy during pregnancy: between personal experiences and scientific evidence. J Am Coll Surg. 2007;205(1):37–42.

Palanivelu C, Rangarajan M, Parthasarathi R. Laparoscopic appendectomy in pregnancy: a case series of seven patients. JSLS. 2006;10(3):321–5.

Park SH, Park MI, Choi JS, et al. Laparoscopic appendectomy performed during pregnancy by gynecological laparoscopists. Eur J Obstet Gynecol Reprod Biol. 2010;148(1): 44–8.

Richardson W, Apelgren K, Earle D, Fanelli R. Guidelines for deep venous thrombosis prophylaxis during laparoscopic surgery. Surg Endosc. 2007;21(12):2331–4.

Rizzo AG. Laparoscopic surgery in pregnancy: long-term follow-up. J Laparoendosc Adv Surg Tech A. 2003;13(1):11–5.

Rollins MD, Chan KJ, Price RR. Laparoscopy for appendicitis and cholelithiasis during pregnancy: a new standard of care. Surg Endosc. 2004;18(2):237–41.

Sadot E, Telem DA, Arora M, et al. Laparoscopy: a safe approach to appendicitis during pregnancy. Surg Endosc. 2010;24(2):383–9.

Schmidt SC, Henrich W, Schmidt M, et al. Laparoscopic appendectomy in pregnancy. Zentralbl Chir. 2007;132(2):112–7.

Scott LD. Gallstone disease and pancreatitis in pregnancy. Gastroenterol Clin North Am. 1992;21(4):803–15.

Soper NJ, Hunter JG, Petrie RH. Laparoscopic cholecystectomy during pregnancy. Surg Endosc. 1992;6(3):115–7.

Steinbrook RA, Brooks DC, Datta S. Laparoscopic cholecystectomy during pregnancy. Review of anesthetic management, surgical considerations. Surg Endosc. 1996;10(5): 511–5.

Upadhyay A, Stanten S, Kazantsev G, Horoupian R, Stanten A. Laparoscopic management of a nonobstetric emergency in the third trimester of pregnancy. Surg Endosc. 2007;21(8):1344–8.

Walsh CA, Tang T, Walsh SR. Laparoscopic versus open appendicectomy in pregnancy: a systematic review. Int J Surg. 2008;6(4):339–44.

Wang C-J, Yen C-F, Lee C-L, Soong Y-K. Minilaparoscopic cystectomy and appendectomy in late second trimester. JSLS. 2002;6(4):373–5.

the remainder of the cholecystectomy may be entirely uneventful. Unfortunately, however, adhesions are not always limited to the precise area of the incision, and may occupy a much greater expanse of the peritoneal membrane than the cutaneous scar would suggest. This is particularly true for Pfannenstiel incisions, where the peritoneal cavity is entered vertically, despite the low horizontal incision.

It is also important to know context of the previous operation as well as any potential complications. Emergent operations, those with excessive bleeding, or performed for peritonitis may lead to increased adhesion formation. Exercise particular caution when reoperating on these patients. Obtaining a copy of the previous operative report is sometimes helpful, especially if patients state there were complications after their prior operation.

Next, determine whether the old scar has healed properly or if an incisional hernia has developed. If a hernia is detected, the operative plan may include a laparoscopic hernia repair since laparoscopic techniques for incisional hernia repair are now widely accepted and applied. If a small hernia is in the general area of the anticipated laparoscopy (e.g., a periumbilical hernia in a patient being considered for laparoscopic cholecystectomy), it may be preferable to utilize that area for placement of a Hasson trocar with hernia repair at the time of closure. Large or extensive hernias, in the operative field, will require laparoscopic adhesiolysis and hernia reduction. If the intended operation is "clean," laparoscopic incisional hernia repair with permanent mesh may be considered. For "clean-contaminated" cases, placement a biologic mesh may be used (see Chap. 33—Laparoscopic Repair of Ventral Hernia).

Finally, consider patient positioning, operating table tilt and roll capabilities, and accessories (ankle straps, footboard) and assure that the benefits of gravity and shifting tissue–organ relationships may be exploited if necessary.

## C.  Access to the Peritoneal Cavity

Carefully plan the steps to achieve intra-abdominal access. Make the initial entry at a reasonable distance from any obvious scars. Possible access sites relative to common scars are illustrated in Fig.  15.1.

1. **Alternate-site Veress needle puncture technique** may be particularly useful for creation of pneumoperitoneum and subsequent access to the right or left subcostal, or the periumbilical

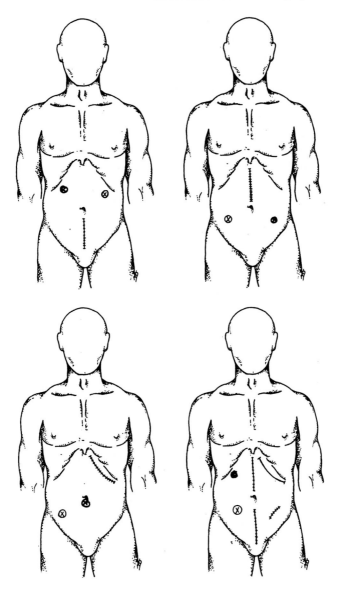

Fig. 15.1. Possible access sites for laparoscopic procedures in relationship to scars from previous abdominal incisions.

area. Aspiration to a saline filled syringe should be negative (except for possibly a few air bubbles), and the saline should freely flow into the abdomen with only gravity (saline drop test). The Veress needle is then attached to insufflator tubing and carbon dioxide is pumped into the peritoneal cavity. The initial pressure detected by the insufflator should be low. If not, the Veress needle should be repositioned or an alternate site should be chosen.

2. **Alternatively, use of Hasson trocar** is straightforward and possibly a safer means of gaining entrance to the peritoneal cavity. With practice, this will be found to be an expeditious means for entering any quadrant by making a miniature muscle-splitting incision in the subcostal, hypogastric, flank, or other region. Just as with open operations, however, bowel that happens to be adherent immediately under the chosen site of entry will be damaged by any blind cutting, spreading, or cauterization. If there is any question as to adherent underlying tissue, the initially chosen site may need to be abandoned and another one selected.

3. **Pass a small-diameter laparoscope** into the peritoneal cavity through this alternate site. Inspect all attempted access sites for potential injury after successful laparoscopic access is obtained. Inspect the abdomen for adhesions and choose secondary trocar sites to assist in any required adhesiolysis.

4. Achieving appropriate working distance is another reason for judicious selection of the entry site. Avoid ending up too close to any tissue of interest. The surgeon needs a comfortable working distance in order to properly manipulate instruments, either for lysing the interfering adhesions or for performing the primary procedure. Consider this issue when placing secondary trocars as well.

# D. Managing Adhesions

Once the peritoneal cavity has been accessed safely, the presence and extent of any adhesions will become apparent. Resist the common tendency to excessively eliminate adhesions. Only those adhesions that truly interfere with visualization of the area of interest or would prevent the placement of subsequent trocars, or subsequent instrument passage under vision should be dealt with. At times, the end of the laparoscope can be very easily manipulated around the edge of a sheet of omentum, suspended from the elevated body wall like a curtain, or fenestrated areas can be used as windows through which the scope can be advanced toward the operative area. If these maneuvers are not applicable, then adhesion lysis must be begun.

Safe adhesiolysis requires a combination of skillful technique and attention to visual cues. If the line of tissue adherence can be recognized, it will provide the most expeditious path to follow, with the least chance of causing significant bleeding or visceral injury. Principles of traction/countertraction are essential components of this phase of the operation, and the surgeon may occasionally need to experiment with varying directions of pull on the tissues to clearly display the boundary lines. For body wall adhesions, the combination of gravity pulling the tissues down while the distended abdominal wall moves in the opposite direction sometimes provides adequate stretch to allow the dissection to be done with only one working instrument. Frequently, however (and especially with viscera-to-viscera adherence), an assisting grasper is required, with its trocar being carefully positioned according to principles mentioned previously.

## E.  Instrument Considerations

The best tool to be used for adhesiolysis is determined by the circumstances and the characteristics of the adhesions and surrounding tissues. Naturally weak areas of areolar tissues appear "foamy" and can be swept away using techniques resembling finger dissection. Rounded graspers, the blunt edges of the scissors blades, and even the suction-irrigator all accomplish the same result with these types of adhesions. For more firmly adherent structures, however, scissors are usually the best choice. If the fusion of the tissues has not resulted in very much neovascularity, then as long as the proper plane of dissection is followed, adding cautery current to the scissors' action is not helpful.

Use of electrocautery during adhesiolysis requires diligence and respect for the potential tissue damage that may result from uncontrolled electrical energy. In addition, the surgeon's expectations for hemostasis must be realistic, using coaptive coagulation (pinching while applying current) for some vessels, but clips or ligatures for larger ones. Techniques for utilizing J- or L-shaped cautery devices commonly involve a hook-pull-burn sequence, but if the surgeon places sturdy traction on the tissues, and gently touches it with the elbow of the wire, a more precise and delicate separation of tissues will follow, as if the traction is actually performing the dissection, and the current is merely weakening the adherence. Although bipolar electrocautery instruments and ultrasonic dissectors are commercially available, their use is usually unnecessary and much more expensive in comparison to conventional monopolar instrumentation.

The loss of natural proprioceptive processes cannot be eliminated but can be minimized by careful attention to instrument design and function. The acceptability of the "feel" of a dissecting or grasping instrument is determined partly by personal preference. For example, some surgeons find rotatable instrument shafts to be very useful; however, others dislike the added bulk and the change in balance produced by the rotating mechanism. Other design features such as length, shaft flexibility, overall weight, and handle configurations must each be considered as a surgeon is determining whether adequate dexterity exists and whether careful tissue handling will be accomplished. It is particularly important for the closing and spreading movements of the jaws to be smooth and effortless; otherwise it will be impossible to sense how much force is being applied to the tissues.

The use of an **angled lens laparoscope** (e.g., a 30° laparoscope) is extremely helpful and recommended for these operations. Observing adhesions and abnormal tissue relationships from more than a single vantage point renders new, safer, or more productive dissection pathways apparent. Remember that although such lenses are conventionally thought of as "looking down," there may be great advantages to looking "up" or from a "sideways" perspective.

# F.  Complications

No operative procedure is risk free, particularly in a reoperative field. If an operation requires more than the usual efforts for tissue dissection or organ manipulation, there likely will be an increased opportunity for mishaps, so the surgeon must develop a keen sense of vigilance for any potentially dangerous situations. The two most serious complications that deserve discussion here are bleeding and visceral injury.

## 1.  Bleeding

a.  **Cause and prevention**. Although usually not life-threatening, bleeding during a laparoscopic procedure not only can be time-consuming to control but can add to the frustration and mental fatigue associated with an already difficult operation. In addition, if tissues become blood stained, the ability to recognize structures may be impaired, and illumination is less effective. Careful, painstaking dissection is the best preventive measure.

b.  **Recognition and management**. Minimize blood loss by rigorous attention to tissue planes, careful observation of tissue characteristics, and appropriate use of electrocautery or other hemostatic maneuvers. Such maneuvers, however, may cause injuries to adjacent structures if hurriedly applied, especially during efforts to control active bleeding. Remember that simple pressure—even with the scissors blades that created the problem—is an immediately available solution to consider when confronted with a spurting vessel (see Chaps. 9 and 10 for a more detailed discussion of hemostatic modalities).

## 2. *Visceral Injury*

a.  **Cause and prevention**. Injury to the viscera can result from excessive traction, as well as cutting, burning, or ligating misidentified structures. As previously described, careful controlled dissection in a bloodless field, with identification of all structures as the dissection progresses, is crucial to prevent these injuries.

b.  **Recognition and management**. With solid-organ injury (liver, spleen), bleeding is the immediate, as well as the obvious, consequence. Management of these injuries is primarily directed at obtaining hemostasis. Injuries to hollow viscera may be subtle and apparent only because of the appearance of luminal contents. The decision to perform a laparoscopic repair, in contrast to open conversion, should be influenced by the characteristics of the tissues and associated injury, as well as the surgeon's experience and capabilities. A "delayed" intestinal perforation, manifesting itself as postoperative peritonitis, may very well be an undetected intraoperative injury. For that reason, prior to removing the laparoscope, the mandatory final step of the operation should be a methodical inspection of all intra-abdominal areas that had been subjected to adhesiolysis, tissue manipulation, or actions to control bleeding.

# G. Conclusions

Today's laparoscopic surgeons must anticipate having to operate on patients with previous abdominal operations. Careful planning and precise technique are required to minimize a patient's morbidity and risk of complication.

## Selected References

Ahmad G, Duffy JM, Phillips K, Watson A. Laparoscopic entry techniques. Cochrane Database Syst Rev. 200816;(2):CD006583.

Caprini JA, Arcelus JA, Swanson J, et al. The ultrasonic localization of abdominal wall adhesions. Surg Endosc. 1995;9:283–5.

Chang FH, Chou HH, Lee CL, Cheng PJ, Wang CW, Soong YK. Extraumbilical insertion of the operative laparoscope in patients with extensive intraabdominal adhesions. J Am Assoc Gynecol Laparosc. 1995;2:335–7.

Chopra R, McVay C, Phillips E, Khalili TM. Laparoscopic lysis of adhesions. Am Surg. 2003;69:966–8.

Golan A, Sagiv R, Debby A, Glezerman M. The minilaparoscope as a tool for localization and preparation for cannula insertion in patients with multiple previous abdominal incisions or umbilical hernia. J Am Assoc Gynecol Laparosc. 2003;10:14–6.

Halpern NB. Access problems in laparoscopic cholecystectomy: postoperative adhesions, obesity, and liver disorders. Semin Laparosc Surg. 1998;5:92–106.

Patel M, Smart D. Laparoscopic cholecystectomy and previous abdominal surgery: a safe technique. Aust NZ J Surg. 1996;66:309–11.

Schirmer BD, Dix J, Schmieg RE, et al. The impact of previous abdominal surgery on outcome following laparoscopic cholecystectomy. Surg Endosc. 1995;9:1085–9.

Sigmar HH, Fried GM, Gazzon J, et al. Risks of blind versus open approach to celiotomy for laparoscopic surgery. Surg Laparosc Endosc. 1993;3:296–9.

Vilos GA, Ternamian A, Dempster J, et al. Laparoscopic entry: a review of techniques, technology, and complications. J Obstet Gynaecol Can. 2007;29(5):433–65.

Weibel MA, Majno G. Peritoneal adhesions and their relation to abdominal surgery: a post mortem study. Am J Surg. 1973;126:345–53.

Wongworowat MD, Aitken DR, Robles AE, Garberoglio C. The impact of prior intraabdominal surgery on laparoscopic cholecystectomy. Am Surg. 1994;60:763–6.

# 16. Robotics in Laparoscopic and Thoracoscopic Surgery

*W. Scott Melvin, M.D., F.A.C.S.*
*Andreas Kirakopolous, M.D.*

## A. Introduction

Every aspect of modern surgery is currently under technology-influenced transformation, including the following:

- **Training**: configuration and implementation of virtual reality simulators.
- **Diagnosis**: development of noninvasive diagnostic imaging modalities, micro-sized sensors, biologic imaging and new types of image overlay and patient specific data analysis.
- **Exchange of medical information and consultation**: Internet based data collections systems, social networking, and electronic medical records.
- **Surgeon–patient interface**: computer-enhanced and telerobotic surgery, distance learning and telerobotics and telementoring.

Behind these changes is revolutionary progress in computer science in conjunction with robotic systems development. After a long period in which research focused mainly on industrial robots, research groups turned their attention to building machines able to interface with humans in unstructured domains and to intelligently perform their assigned tasks. The introduction of robotics in the field of minimally invasive surgery came as no surprise, as the increased precision and improved quality associated with industrial robots stimulated the application of robots and computer systems in modern health-care systems. The practice that interposes this technology between the surgeon and the patient with an goal of enhancing the interaction is the focus of "Robotic Surgery." This term

N.J. Soper and C.E.H. Scott-Conner (eds.), *The SAGES Manual: Volume 1*    191
*Basic Laparoscopy and Endoscopy*, DOI 10.1007/978-1-4614-2344-7_16,
© Springer Science+Business Media, LLC 2012

remains imprecise and refers to a variety of interactions and technological application that encompass the broad scope of "Robotic Technology."

This chapter gives an overview and introduction to these emerging technologies and their applications.

# B. Robotics Overview

## 1. Historical Evolution

Czech writer Karel Čapek introduced the term *robot* in a play he wrote in 1920 called RUR (Rossum's Universal Robots), first performed in 1923. It is derived from the Czech word *roboto* meaning "compulsory labor."

Modern robots have been developed through a process that in the very first stages involved the configuration of numerous automated tools used mainly as industrial machinery addressing the demand for increased productivity and improved quality and product performance. From the initial attention devoted more toward flexible automation, the research shifted toward the development of systems that could operate in accordance to, or even without, human intervention, and interact in real time with dynamic environments. Today's robotic systems are mechanical systems controlled by computer processors and equipped with sensors and motors. Appropriate computer algorithms based on sophisticated software utilize environmental information and the operator input provided by sensors to determine appropriate motor movements to the associated mechanical system.

The application of robotics in the field of minimally invasive surgery represents the state of the art in surgery. The revolution began with the introduction of laparoscopic surgery, which changed the perception and the practice of surgery for both the patient and the surgeon. However, the ever-increasing complexity of the laparoscopic procedures and, especially, the performance of advanced laparoscopic operations, posed some serious demands on both the equipment and the personnel in the operating room. The goal of these systems is to relieve the limitations found in standard laparoscopic surgery, including two-dimensional perception of the operative field, an unstable camera platform, nonarticulated instruments inserted through fixed points resulting in limited movement, natural hand tremor, and difficult fine motor activity.

These inherent shortcomings gave impetus for the introduction and development of robotic systems in minimally invasive surgery.

Additionally, one of the initial concepts for the introduction of robotics in surgery was to develop the capability for operating remotely. The capability to perform a surgical procedure over a distance, transferring surgical expertise to a remote site (space station, developing country) seemed to be quite intriguing.

Advances in robotic engineering and computer technology soon allowed the development of several prototypes that eventually became commercially available. Current applications of robotics include surgical assistance, dexterity enhancement, systems networking, and image-guided therapy. Dexterity is enhanced by an interposed microprocessor between the surgeon's hands and the tip of the surgical instrument that allows downscaling of the gross hand movements and the physical hand tremor.

## 2. Current Status

The most advanced of today's robotic systems (daVinci™, Intuitive Surgical, Sunnyvale, CA, USA) makes use of a master–slave telemanipulator where all robotic movements are dictated from the surgeon through the use of an "on line" input device. The surgeon remains in control of the procedure while the movements of the instrument handles (master unit) are transformed into electronic signals filtered and transmitted in real time to the motorized robotic arm (slave unit) that controls the instrument tips. The term *computer-enhanced telesurgery* is the most descriptive term of the active functions of these devices. The different systems available today allow various operative tasks to be accomplished, with different levels of interface between the surgeon and the system established.

So far, the advantages that have been correlated with the initial use of the computer-enhanced robotics systems in surgical practice include the following:

- Allowance for increased degrees of freedom of movement, leading to significant improvement of intracavitary instrument articulations.
- Better visual control of the operative field due to three-dimensional (3D) view and the "immersing effect" to the surgeon.
- Filtering, modulation, and downscaling of the amplitude of the surgical motions resulting in more precise, hand-tremor-free operative manipulations, thus truly enhancing the ability of the operating surgeon.
- Ability to operate at a distance from the patient.

## 3. Definitions

- A robot is defined as (1) a mechanical device that sometimes resembles a human and is capable of performing a variety of often complex human tasks on command or by being programmed in advance and (2) a machine or device that operates automatically or by remote control.
- Davies (2000) describes a surgical robot as "a powered, computer controlled manipulator with artificial sensing that can be reprogrammed to move and position tools to carry out a wide range of surgical tasks."
  Under the guise of these two definitions, multiple tasks can be undertaken by the surgical robot or computer-assisted devices.
- Computer-assisted surgery is a term that should include most of the active functions of these devices. In some situations robots act autonomously and would be truly robotic, not computer-assisted interventions.
- Current systems are for the most part, in fact, either surgical assistants or computer-enhanced telemanipulators.

# C.  Current Clinical Applications

Robotic surgery encompasses a variety of different types of interaction that extend from the passive use of a robotic machine to computer-enhanced telemanipulators and even to truly robotic systems. The current state of computer-assisted surgery includes diagnostic and preoperative planning and image analysis, Simulation using patient specific information and data fusion, surgical navigation including surgical image overlay and fusion and surgical manipulation as a supervisory system or more commonly a remote telemanipulator system.

## 1. Image-Guided Robotic Systems

The various image-guided robots designed for targeting tissues and holding surgical instruments for biopsies and other relatively simple and linear uses exemplify the passive use of robots. The term "passive" implies that the surgeon provides the physical energy to manipulate the surgical tool. A system called PAKY, developed at Johns Hopkins

University for the percutaneous access of the kidney, has been found to offer an unquestionable improvement in needle placement accuracy and total procedure time, while reducing the radiation exposure to both patient and urologist. Another system has been designed to perform transperineal prostate biopsies under ultrasound guidance. A device compatible with magnetic resonance imaging techniques has been developed needle insertion manipulator for stereotactic neurosurgery. The **NeuroMate**™ (Integrated Surgical Systems, Sacramento, CA) is an image-guided, computer-controlled robotic system designed for stereotactic functional brain surgery.

## 2. Computer-Enhanced Robotic Telesurgery

The prefix *tele* in term "telesurgery" and "telemanipulator" implies distance between the surgeon and the patient. In this setting the surgeon sits at a dedicated workstation and uses either joysticks or more sophisticated devices to control the motion of the robotic arms at the bedside of the patient. The interposition of a computer allows for scaling of the surgeon's motions, while the presence of a camera attached to the robot by the use of dual imaging systems offers a true 3D view of the actions of the manipulators.

The **da Vinci** system (Intuitive Surgical, Sunnyvale, CA), is the only computer-enhanced robotic system with FDA approval that is currently available in the USA. This was the original clinical system offered first in the USA in 1999, and in 2010 had produced and placed over 1,700 devices throughout the world Fig. 16.1. In Canada, the Amadeus system (Titan Medical, Toronto, Ontario, CA) is in use. Elsewhere in the world other systems are being developed. The Amadeus system has received regulatory approval. Its clinical results and capabilities, including four arm mulitarticulated technology and instrumentation, are similar to da Vinci. Both devices include the remotely located control console and the surgical unit that holds and manipulates the instruments. The da Vinci instruments are capable of delivering 7 degrees of freedom of movement, while its cable-driven **EndoWrist** device adds another 3 degrees of freedom. The EndoWrist instruments allow for an impressively complete range of motion of the instrument tips, facilitating tissue dissection, optimal needle positioning, and direct suturing comparable to open surgery. Additionally, the **da Vinci** system incorporates a magnified 3D display of the operative field through the integration of the view offered by a two-channel endoscope. A primary feature, also, of this robotic system is the

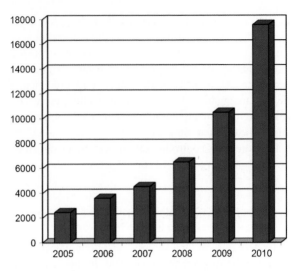

Fig. 16.1. Total procedures (*n*).

complete "immersion" of the surgeon to the endoscopic operative field without any external or operative cues, enabling for intuitive hand–eye coordination and superb depth perception. While the device is designated a telerobotic system, the distance separating the surgeon form the patient is still small. Remote applications and distant manipulation involve challenges that are not yet clinically relevant. A variety of research and study protocols has been completed and is underway to demonstrate such feasibility and identify barriers for future innovation.

## 3. True Robotic Surgery

True robotic surgery is accomplished with such advanced devices such as **ROBODOC** (Integrated Surgical Systems), designed for orthopedic surgery; this device can be programmed to perform primary or revision total hip or knee replacement. The task is facilitated by a preoperative planning workstation called **ORTHODOC** that simulates the surgery using the actual computed tomographic (CT) scan of the patient. Using the CT scans of the patient along with models of the virtual prosthesis, the surgeon is able to provide all the necessary preoperative data for the robotic surgery.

## 4. "Computer-Enhanced" Telesurgery: Operative Procedures

The clinical usefulness of computer-enhanced telesurgery is under intense development. Many applications have been utilized, and feasibility has been reported in a variety of clinical scenarios and operative techniques. The use by various specialties is diverse and encompasses many aspects of surgery (see Fig. 16.2).

### a. Cardiac Surgery

During the last 10 years the demand for a minimally invasive cardiac surgery has been met by the introduction of the beating heart surgery that eliminates the need for cardiopulmonary bypass and by decreasing the size of the incision so that some procedures can be performed through small incisions and limited thoracotomies. However, the development of a total endoscopic cardiac procedure proved extremely difficult, mainly owing to the inherent limitations of the laparoscopic technique in the microsurgical environment. The introduction of computer-enhanced robotic systems addressed many of the physical limitations of traditional

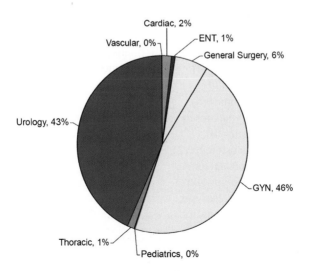

Fig. 16.2.  2010 Procedure mix by specialty.

endoscopic surgery in the microsurgical setting and allowed the performance of various procedures such as the following:

- Harvesting of the left internal thoracic artery.
- Total endoscopic coronary artery bypass grafting (TECABG).
- Mitral valve repair and replacement.
- Repair of atrial septal defects.

Current data demonstrates limited use of these applications in selected patients and disease states. In experienced centers there appears to be advantages over conventional approaches. The field of minimally invasive cardiac surgery continues to evolve rapidly so that many transthoracic or transcardiac procedures are done using endoluminal techniques. Thousands of cardiac surgical procedures have been performed worldwide.

## b. General Surgery

The feasibility of computer-enhanced robotic surgery (daVinci) in noncardiac procedures was reported in a study that described the initial clinical experience of four centers in the USA. The vast majority of the procedures were intra-abdominal, including the following:

- Various antireflux procedures (69).
- Cholecystectomies (36).
- Heller myotomies (26).
- Bowel resections (17).
- Donor nephrectomy (15).
- Left internal mammary artery mobilization (14).
- Gastric bypasses (7).
- Splenectomies (7).
- Adrenalectomies (6).
- Exploratory laparoscopies (3).
- Pyloroplasties (4).
- Gastrojejunostomies (2).
- Distal pancreatectomy.
- Duodenal polypectomy.
- Gastric mass resection.
- Lysis of adhesions.

The study concluded that the clinical results of robotic assisted surgery compared favorably with those of conventional laparoscopy with respect to mortality, complications, and length of stay.

Antireflux surgery has been extensively evaluated by Melvin et al. (2001) in a prospective trial comparing the results of computer-enhanced robotic fundoplication and traditional laparoscopic antireflux procedures. With 20 patients in each arm of the study, there was little difference in clinical outcomes. Operative times were longer with the robot, but decreased as experience was gained. The study concluded that computer-assisted laparoscopic antireflux surgery is safe, but at the current level of development, offered little advantage over standard laparoscopic approaches.

Certain procedures such as Heller myotomy may be improved with the use of robotic devices. This assumption is based on the fact that computer-enhanced robotic devices, through the features of visual magnification, motion scaling, and fine tremor reduction, drastically improve manual performance in the microsurgical setting. Further case series demonstrated that robotic surgery could reduce the incidence of intraoperative esophageal perforation utilizing this advanced technology.

Bariatric surgery has been shown to be feasible using robotic technology. A variety of case series have demonstrated the safety and effectiveness. Few have reported on cost-effectiveness in these high volume surgeries. It would appear that compared to hand sewn anastomosis, the robotic technology can be as effective and efficient, but compared to high volume centers that routinely use stapling techniques in procedures such as Roux en Y Gastric bypass, use of the robot allows similar outcomes with more time in the operating room and more costs. The use of the robot in placing an adjustable gastric band for the treatment of obesity has been similarly reported.

Other complex gastrointestinal procedures have been reported as well. Several case series from Asia have demonstrated the ability to perform extensive lymph node dissections in the setting of gastrectomy for cancer, in many centers this has emerged as the procedure of choice. Colon resections are often not significantly enhanced by robotic technology. This is in part due to the limitations of performing dissection in different quadrants of the abdomen. (i.e., mobilizing the splenic flexure and doing a sigmoid mobilization), necessitating varying the robotic set up during the case. This disadvantage is not seen in rectal resection and surgery limited to the pelvis. Reported data suggests that rectal resection can be more safely and efficiently performed using this technology when compared to standard laparoscopic techniques and even open surgery.

Endocrine surgery has also seen feasibility demonstrated by robotic surgical innovations. Adrenalectomy was initially identified as a feasible procedure using either a transabdominal or strictly a retroperitoneal approach. Both approaches can be enhanced by robotic technology allowing a minimally invasive approach to a diverse types and sizes of adrenal pathology. Surgical innovators identified problems, mostly cosmetic, in offering standard open surgical approaches to the thyroid and parathryoid glands, that could be addressed with robotic technology. Large series of patients from Korea have now been reported utilizing either a transaxillary approach or a transareolar approach to the thyroid or parathyroid glands, avoiding a cervical incision that, in some cultures, is seen as socially restricting.

## c. Urology

The feasibility of robotic assisted telesurgery initially in urologic laparoscopy lagged behind that of general surgery, However, modern data has demonstrated significant use, not only addressed in the prostate, but in fact a wide range of urologic procedures and urologic procedures. There are significant technical advantages over standard laparoscopy in complex procedures such as prostatectomy, specifically where space is limited such as a narrow male pelvis. Advanced procedures such as partial nephrectomy and pyeloplasty are now preferentially performed using telerobotic enhancement. The experience with these advanced urological procedures is increasing rapidly at many centers throughout the world.

## d. Gynecology

Gynecologic surgeons have embraced minimally invasive technology as they have with robotic assisted surgery. Feasibility has been demonstrated for almost all gynecologic procedures. Specific procedures that utilize the benefit of articulated instruments and motion scaling are recognized clear indications for robotic surgery. These include not only minor procedures (but technically demanding procedures) such as tubuloplasty but also more radical procedures especially oncologic procedures that require pelvic lymphadenectomy. Some published reports now suggest superiority of the computer enhanced procedures.

## e. Thoracic Surgery

Noncardiac thoracic surgery has been a target for robotic surgery since its inception. The ability to perform complex intrathoracic procedures without open thoracotomy and the associated disability and trauma from the in incision is significant. Approaches to the mediastinum with intrathoracic mobilization and anastamosis or resection provide an enhanced ability to the thoracic and gastrointestinal surgeon. Thymectomy and other tumor resections from a single sided approach may offer more benefit than pulmonary resection. Esophagectomy for selected reasons can be performed via thoracotomy; however, using robotic technology the transabdominal, transhiatal approach is made possible by angled scopes and mulitarticulated robotic technology and has been reported with generally good results.

# D.  Limitations

Current technology is somewhat limited by the lack of tactile feedback; this includes not only simple force feedback but also proprioception. The reason for these continued limitations is complex; however, measuring the forces, transmitting the data, and applying the forces correctly in a very short time frame remain difficult. Ongoing engineering and computational work continues in this arena in order to address this issue.

Apart from the technological limitations, a serious issue regarding the clinical use of these robotic systems has to do with the assessment of their outcomes. Since computer-enhanced telesurgery has become clinically relevant, there exist little high-quality data demonstrating a clear-cut superiority in the clinical results associated with its use. The lack of this data has not significantly reduced implementation; however, it is imperative that clinical, as well as financial data, continue to be accumulated and analyzed in order to best serve the health needs of the public. While the technical superiority of these systems in the areas of motion and optics in comparison with standard laparoscopic instruments is taken for granted, the limited objective data remains mildly problematic. The cost of these systems, both initial purchase price and maintenance, is significant and will likely be a large determinant in the extent of dissemination of robotic surgery.

Credentialing of current surgeons and resident training appear to gain significant value as the use of robotic surgery is anticipated to expand. Skill for the novice may be acquired more rapidly with computer-assisted surgery, as shown by Melvin et al. (2002), who found that skill performance on a standardized test with the robotic system remains superior to that with standard laparoscopic instrumentation, even after training. However, the true learning curve for such complex devices has not been well demonstrated, and the encountered difference may be eliminated for the experienced surgeon.

# E. Emerging Issues

The introduction of robotics to the field of minimally invasive surgery has affected the practice of medicine and surgery. It is certain that technologic advances will continue to enhance the ability to care for patients in the foreseeable future. Advances will be seen in the immediate future in further decreasing the trauma of surgical interventions. Assessment of the addition of these advances will have to continue in order for the medical and political community to most appropriately adopt these advances for the benefit of improving medical care throughout society.

A significant potential advantage of computer enhancement is the ability to increase the precision of surgery beyond that capable with the free hand. This would be most important in procedures requiring fine motor skills, high magnification, and microsurgical skills. Preliminary work with the existing devices has demonstrated the feasibility of using robotic devices for enhancement of open surgical procedures.

Merging imaging systems with computer-controlled operating systems may allow some significant benefits. This would potentially allow procedures to be performed without direct visualization. Another clear benefit would be the ability to simulate a patient-specific surgery and allow for preoperative planning and preoperative simulation to help reduce errors.

Continued technologic advances have allowed further miniaturization of various devices. Future devices will allow intracorporeal flexible instruments and perhaps complex therapeutic interventions via existing body orifices. Telerobotic control and information system integration will allow these advanced procedures and technology to improve patient care outcomes.

# F. Conclusion

The role of robotic surgery remains under development. However, it is certain that as technology advances, robotic technology will continue to change the patient–surgeon interface with the potential to improve patient outcomes.

# Selected References

Aiono S, Gilbert JM, Soin B, Finlay PA, Gordan A. Controlled trial of the introduction of a robotic camera assistant (EndoAssist) for laparoscopic cholecystectomy. Surg Endosc. 2002;16:1267–70.

Cadeddu JA, Stoianovici D, Chen RN, Moore RG, Kavoussi LR. Stereotactic mechanical percutaneous renal access. J Endourol. 1998;12:121–6.

Davies B. A review of robotics in surgery. Proc Inst Mech Eng. 2000;214(H):129–40.

Galvani CA, Gorodner MV, Moser F, Jacobsen G, Chretien C, Espat NJ, Donahue P, Horgan S. Robotically assisted laparoscopic transhiatal esophagectomy. Surg Endosc. 2008;22(4):1139–40.

Lavallee S, Brunie L, Mazier B, et al. Image guided operating robot: a clinical application in stereotactic surgery. In: Taylor R, et al., editors. Computer integrated surgery. Cambridge, MA: MIT Press; 1996;77–98.

Luketich JD, Fernardo HC, Buanaventura PO, Christie NA, Grondin SC, Schauer PR. Results of a randomized trial of HERMES-assisted vs non-HERMES-assisted laparoscopic antireflux surgery. Surg Endosc. 2002;16:1264–8.

Massamune K, Kobayashi E, Masutani Y, et al. Development of an MRI-compatible needle insertion manipulator for stereotactic neurosurgery. J Image Guid Surg. 1995;1:242–8.

Melvin WS, Dundon JM, Talamini MA, Horgan S. Computer enhanced robotic telesurgery reduces esophageal perforation during Heller myotomy. Surgery. 2005;138(4): 553–8; discussion 558–9.

Melvin WS, Needleman JB, Krause RK, Schneider C, Ellisson EC. Computer-enhanced vs. standard laparoscopic antireflux surgery. J Gastroint Surg. 2002;6:11–6.

Prasad SM, Ducko CT, Stephenson ER, Chambers CE, Ralph J. Prospective clinical trial of robotically assisted endoscopic coronary grafting with 1-year follow-up. Ann Surg. 2001;233(6):725–32.

Rovetta A, Sala R. Robotics and telerobotics applied to a prostate biopsy on a human patient. In: Proceedings of the second international symposium on medical robotics and computer–assisted surgery, Baltimore, 2000. p. 104.

Talamini M, Chapman W, Melvin S, Horgan S. A prospective analysis of 211 robotic assisted surgical procedures. Surg Endosc. 2002;16 Suppl 1:S205.

Weinstein GS, O'Malley Jr BW, Cohen MA, Quon H. Transoral robotic surgery for advanced oropharyngeal carcinoma. Arch Otolaryngol Head Neck Surg. 2010;136(11): 1079–85.

Weissenbacher A, Bodner J. Robotic surgery of the mediastinum. Thorac Surg Clin 2010;20(2):331–9.

Part II

# Diagnostic Laparoscopy and Biopsy

# 17. Emergency Laparoscopy

*Brian T. Valerian, M.D.*
*Steven C. Stain, M.D.*

## A. General Considerations

The entire peritoneal cavity can be visualized by the laparoscope, and diagnostic laparoscopy is an effective modality for determining pathology within the abdominal cavity. The decision to perform diagnostic laparoscopy is based on clinical judgment, weighing the sensitivities and specificities of other modalities [computed tomographic (CT) scan, ultrasound, diagnostic peritoneal lavage, mesenteric arteriography] versus the relative morbidity of minimally invasive laparoscopy. Although some centers have experience in performing laparoscopy in the emergency room or intensive care unit, most surgeons have reserved laparoscopy for the operating room. Once a surgical diagnosis has been made, laparoscopic therapeutic options are based upon the expertise of the surgeon. Equally important is the ability to exclude disease processes requiring surgical intervention, sparing the patient the potential morbidity of a negative laparotomy.

The **indications for emergency laparoscopy** can be grouped into those related to abdominal pain of uncertain etiology and those related to trauma resulting in intra-abdominal injury (Table 17.1). The therapies for individual conditions once identified are described elsewhere in this text.

## B. Abdominal Pain

1. The most common indication for emergent abdominal operation or diagnostic laparoscopy is **suspected appendicitis**. Laparoscopic appendectomy is part of the modern surgeon's

Table 17.1. Indications for emergency laparoscopy.

| Abdominal pain | • | Right lower quadrant pain (rule out gynecologic pathology) |
|---|---|---|
| | • | Right upper quadrant pain (rule out Fitz-Hugh–Curtis syndrome) |
| | • | Peritonitis |
| | • | Mesenteric ischemia |
| | • | Intra-abdominal abscess, not amenable to image-guided drainage |
| | • | Acalculous cholecystitis |
| | • | Small bowel obstruction |
| | • | Fever of unknown origin |
| | • | Gastrointestinal hemorrhage of unexplained etiology |
| | • | Acute complicated diverticulitis with peritonitis |
| Trauma | • | Blunt abdominal trauma |
| | • | Penetrating trauma |
| | | Exclude peritoneal penetration |
| | | Evaluate diaphragm |

armamentarium, and diagnostic laparoscopy provides an excellent opportunity to establish and treat the diagnosis of appendicitis, but it also can diagnose other pathology mimicking the signs and symptoms of appendicitis. This enthusiasm of diagnostic laparoscopy for suspected appendicitis, which can accurately establish a diagnosis, should be weighed against the accuracy of thin-section CT scanning.

2. Diagnostic laparoscopy may be most appropriate for women of childbearing age because this group has historically had the highest rates of negative appendectomy. In such patients, the differential diagnosis of appendicitis versus gynecologic pathology may be difficult, and laparoscopy can establish a precise diagnosis, and therapy if indicated. The gynecologist may be consulted preoperatively, or intraoperatively if necessary. The technique of laparoscopic appendectomy is described in Chap. 30. It is the policy of most surgeons to complete the appendectomy (if possible), even if alternate diagnoses are found at operation. Salpingitis is readily identified by visualization of inflamed fallopian tubes. A tubo-ovarian abscess may warrant gynecologic consultation. In women of reproductive age with right upper quadrant pain and negative radiologic studies, the diagnosis of Fitz-Hugh–Curtis syndrome should be entertained. Laparoscopy provides the opportunity to confirm the diagnosis and divide the perihepatic adhesions.

3.  Small bowel obstruction due to adhesions is generally diagnosed radiologically, but may be treated laparoscopically (Chap. 28). Preoperative CT scan may provide information about the location of the obstructing adhesion and direct the exploration.

4.  In certain patients with symptoms suggestive of peritonitis despite nondiagnostic radiologic studies, laparoscopy can accurately exclude surgical pathology, direct the placement of the appropriate surgical incision, or provide access for treatment (perforated duodenal ulcer, small bowel obstruction, Meckel's diverticulitis, etc.).

5.  Emergency laparoscopy may be indicated for certain critically ill patients in the intensive care unit, especially those with sepsis of unknown etiology, whose instability would make a trip to the CT scan suite or operating room hazardous. Diagnostic laparoscopy can exclude surgical pathology or identify ischemic bowel, acalculous cholecystitis, or perforated viscus as the source.

6.  Infrequently, diagnostic laparoscopy may be employed in patients with fever of unknown origin. In the patient presenting with vague abdominal signs and fever, especially if there is a history of foreign travel or recent immigration, the diagnosis of tuberculosis or brucellosis should be considered. Laparoscopy can assist with confirming these diagnoses.

7.  A patient suffering from Acute complicated diverticulitis with peritonitis may be considered for laparoscopic lavage and drain placement without resection in the acute setting. Several recent studies have demonstrated low morbidity and mortality, although this has not become the standard of care.

# C. Method of Diagnostic Laparoscopy for Abdominal Pain

Emergency diagnostic laparoscopy requires a skill set different from that for a therapeutic laparoscopy for a known diagnosis (e.g., appendicitis or cholecystitis). If no pathology is found, the surgeon must be confident that he or she was able to exclude pathology requiring definitive surgical treatment. One must feel comfortable exposing solid organs and manipulating bowel for a thorough exploration. **It should never be considered a failure to resort to laparotomy for complete exploration or definitive therapy**.

Although it is feasible to perform diagnostic laparoscopy in the intensive care unit or the emergency department, diagnostic laparoscopy is best performed in the operating room.

Several principles of technique facilitate the procedure.

1. Unless prior abdominal surgery suggests otherwise, insert the laparoscope at the umbilicus. In cases of abdominal distension, the open insertion of a Hasson cannula is safer.

2. Both a 30° laparoscope and a 0° laparoscope should be available. The 30° scope will be especially useful to "see around corners" and visually approach bowel or viscera from different angles for optimal maneuvering or dissection. A **10-mm laparoscope** provides better light and view, although a 5-mm scope may be adequate. Remember the important objective of complete exploration if the anticipated pathology is not readily identified.

3. Maximal working area is available when the surgeon stands on the side of the patient that is opposite the anticipated pathology. It may be advantageous to move from side to side if necessary to gain access to all four quadrants of the abdomen.

4. Two video monitors should be available, preferably mobile units, to locate the most favorable positions for the surgeon and assistant.

5. A second, or third, trocar will be necessary to manipulate, palpate, and move viscera for a thorough exploration. While 5-mm trocars are often adequate for laparoscopic instruments necessary for bowel manipulation, placement of 10-mm trocars may provide increased opportunity to relocate the laparoscope for improved visualization. Alternatively, a 5-mm laparoscope may be used for the alternate views.

6. If pathology is identified that requires a therapeutic intervention (e.g., appendectomy, patch of perforated ulcer), it can be performed by conversion to celiotomy, or laparoscopic treatment (refer to the appropriate chapter).

# D.  Laparoscopy for Trauma

The proper role of laparoscopy for injured patients is contingent upon the expertise of the surgeon, available instrumentation, and the diagnostic algorithm adopted for blunt or penetrating trauma. The established priorities provided by advanced trauma life support (airway, breathing, and circulation) must be adhered to.

Patients with **blunt abdominal trauma** and obvious indications for laparotomy (hypotension, increasing abdominal girth, and other signs of hemorrhage) should have open exploration. There are few indications for emergency diagnostic laparoscopy for blunt trauma. Focused abdominal sonography for trauma (FAST) scans are indicated for unstable patients, and CT scan provides reliable definition of solid viscus injury of stable patients after blunt trauma. Laparoscopy may be appropriate for patients with a "**seat belt sign**" in who suspicion of bowel injury exists. These patients have a 15–35% incidence of significant injury and warrant further investigation. Free abdominal fluid without solid organ injury may also warrant laparoscopy. A thorough diagnostic laparoscopy can identify bowel injury or exclude intra-abdominal pathology. Laparoscopy in head-injured patients should be performed with caution, as abdominal insufflation leads to increased intracranial pressure.

The evaluation of patients with **penetrating abdominal trauma** is evolving. Most centers perform laparotomy for all patients with gunshot wounds; however, laparoscopy can be utilized to reliably exclude peritoneal violation in patients with anterior or flank tangential injuries. Laparoscopic evaluation of posterior gunshot wounds (posterior to the midaxillary line) is not appropriate. The majority of stab wounds do not require therapeutic laparotomy. The diagnostic evaluations used most frequently for stable patients are observation by serial physical examinations, CT scan, or ultrasonography. The application of local wound exploration and diagnostic peritoneal lavage appears to be decreasing. Several centers have reported their experience with diagnostic laparoscopy for anterior abdominal stab wounds as a valuable tool to exclude peritoneal violation, and select patients for early discharge.

Laparoscopy has an important role for **thoracoabdominal stab wounds**, especially on the left, that may have violated the diaphragm. These patients have up to a 24% incidence of diaphragm injury, which may present years later with diaphragmatic hernia and intestinal strangulation. No other modality (short of abdominal exploration) can reliably exclude diaphragm injury. Isolated diaphragm injuries can be repaired laparoscopically or by open exploration.

# E. Method of Laparoscopy for Trauma

Hemodynamically unstable patients with abdominal injury require exploration. Emergency laparoscopy can be performed in the emergency room or operating room. Because trauma patients are assumed to have full stomachs, general endotracheal anesthesia in the operating room is preferred, and the surgical team should be prepared to convert to open laparotomy. The purpose of laparoscopy for trauma is to **exclude or confirm intra-abdominal injury**. Appropriate use of diagnostic laparoscopy for trauma may reduce the incidence of nontherapeutic celiotomies that may occur with diagnostic peritoneal lavage or CT scan.

Application of the modality in the diagnostic algorithm adopted requires consideration of the technical expertise of the surgeon, the available resources in the hospital, and the relative strengths and weaknesses of other diagnostic tests available.

For penetrating trauma, diagnostic laparoscopy can be used to exclude peritoneal violation or to diagnose enteric injury. CT scan provides better information about the severity of solid organ injury because the entire organ is imaged, whereas laparoscopy allows only a surface view. It may be difficult to adequately evaluate the entire spleen with laparoscopy owing to overlying omentum.

Some principles to guide the exploration are as follows:

1.   Position the patient supine, with a standard trauma prep, from clavicles to pelvis to allow for access for open exploration if necessary.
2.   Always review the chest X-ray prior to general anesthesia with positive pressure ventilation. Penetrating wounds to the chest may result in a pneumothorax, which can be **converted to a tension pneumothorax** from abdominal insufflation and a diaphragm injury. An occult pneumothorax (not recognized by chest X-ray) may also lead to a tension pneumothorax with positive pressure ventilation or peritoneal insufflation. Pneumothorax may be visible laparoscopically as a bellowing out (toward the abdomen) of the ipsilateral diaphragm.
3.   Generally, the laparoscope (10 mm) should be inserted through the umbilicus. Mobile monitors should be positioned opposite the surgeon and assistant. The operating room table should allow Trendelenburg, reverse Trendelenburg, and side-to-side tilting of the table.
4.   **Close any stab wound entrance site** (simple skin closure) to allow creation of the pneumoperitoneum. If no peritoneal injury is identified, one can assume that there has not been peritoneal violation and therefore no intra-abdominal injury.
5.   Peritoneal violation from a stab wound **does not mandate open exploration**. If peritoneal violation has occurred, complete exploration is necessary to exclude injury, and additional

Table 17.2. Grading system for hemoperitoneum observed at diagnostic laparoscopy.

- **Grade 0**: No blood is seen within the peritoneal cavity
- **Grade 1**: Small flecks of blood on the bowel or small amounts of blood in the paracolic gutters. Blood does not recur when aspirated. No bleeding sight is seen
- **Grade 2**: Blood is seen between loops of bowel and in the paracolic gutter. Blood recurs after aspiration
- **Grade 3**: Frank blood is aspirated from the Veress needle, or the intestines are noted to be floating on a pool of blood

trocars will be needed. Five-millimeter trocars will suffice, and utilizing atraumatic bowel graspers, the colon should be inspected and the small bowel should be run.

6. Diagnostic laparoscopy from a gunshot wound is generally performed to exclude peritoneal violation. Because the energy associated with ballistic injury, and the variability of the paths of bullets, peritoneal violation by a gunshot wound warrants open exploration.

7. In the case of blunt abdominal trauma, the bleeding can be characterized by a standard grading system (Table 17.2). Generally, grade 2 or 3 hemoperitoneum requires open laparotomy. Depending upon the mechanism of injury, the surgeon may choose to observe patients with grade 1 hemoperitoneum. Grade 0 is a normal examination.

The complications of laparoscopy for trauma include the complications of anesthesia and laparoscopy, but also some that are unique to the trauma patient.

1. Blunt trauma patients may have sustained closed head injury. It has been demonstrated that both pneumoperitoneum and reverse Trendelenburg position lead to increased intracranial pressure with potentially serious consequences.

2. Hypothermia may be exacerbated with insufflation of cold carbon dioxide gas, leading to worsening of acidosis.

3. Pneumothorax, from occult pulmonary injury or peritoneal insufflation through a diaphragm injury, may occur.

4. Physiologic changes, such as acidosis, cardiac depression, arrhythmias, and gas absorption causing subcutaneous emphysema, may have more profound consequences in the trauma patient.

# Selected References

Alamili M, Gogenur I, Rosenberg J. Acute complicated diverticulitis managed by laparoscopic lavage. Dis Colon Rectum. 2009;52:1345–9.

Bender JS, Talamini MA. Diagnostic laparoscopy in critically ill intensive care patients. Surg Endosc. 1992;6:302–4.

Berci G, Sackier JM, Paz-Partlow M. Emergency laparoscopy. Am J Surg. 1991;161: 355–60.

Chandler DF, Lane JS, Waxman KS. Seatbelt sign following trauma is associated with increased incidence of abdominal injury. Am Surg. 1997;63(10):885–8.

Chelly M, Major K, Spivak J, et al. The value of laparoscopy in management of abdominal trauma. Am Surg. 2003;69(11):957–60.

Decadt B, Sussman L, Lewis MPN, et al. Randomized clinical trial of early laparoscopy in the management of acute non-specific abdominal pain. Br J Surg. 1999;86(11):1383–6.

Eachempati SR, Barie PS. Minimally invasive and noninvasive diagnosis and therapy in critically ill and injured patients. Arch Surg. 1999;134(11):1189–96.

Forde KA, Treat MR. The role of peritoneoscopy (laparoscopy) in the evaluation of the acute abdomen in critically ill patients. Surg Endosc. 1992;6:219–21.

Halverson A, Buchanan R, Jacobs K, et al. Evaluation of mechanism of increased intracranial pressure with insufflation. Surg Endosc. 1998;12(3):266–9.

Kaban GK, Novitsky YW, Perugini RA, et al. Use of laparoscopy in evaluation and treatment of penetrating and blunt abdominal injuries. Surg Innov. 2008;15:26–31.

Murray JA, Demetriades D, Asensio JA, et al. Occult injuries to the diaphragm: prospective evaluation of laparoscopy in penetrating injuries to the left lower chest. J Am Coll Surg. 1998;187(6):626–30.

Paw P, Sackier JM. Complications of laparoscopy and thoracoscopy. J Intensive Care Med. 1994;9:290–304.

Sackier JM. Second-look laparoscopy in the management of acute mesentery ischemia. Br J Surg. 1994;81:1546.

Schob OM, Allen DC, Benzel E, et al. A comparison of the pathophysiologic effects of carbon dioxide, nitrous oxide, and helium pneumoperitoneum on intracranial pressure. Am J Surg. 1996;172(3):248–53.

Simon RJ, Rabin J, Kuhls D. Impact of increased use of laparoscopy on negative laparotomy rates after penetrating trauma. J Trauma. 2002;53(2):297–302.

Sosa JL, Sims D, Martin L, Zeppa R. Laparoscopic evaluation of tangential abdominal gunshot wounds. Arch Surg. 1992;127:109–10.

Zantut LF, Ivatury RR, Smith RS, et al. Diagnostic and therapeutic laparoscopy for penetrating abdominal trauma: a multicenter experience. J Trauma. 1997;42:825–9.

# 18. Elective Diagnostic Laparoscopy and Cancer Staging

*Michael D. Honaker, M.D.*
*Frederick L. Greene, M.D., F.A.C.S.*

## A. Diagnostic Laparoscopy

The laparoscope has become an important tool in the diagnosis of benign and malignant conditions in the abdominal cavity. Laparoscopy should be utilized in conjunction with conventional imaging techniques such as computed tomography (CT), transcutaneous ultrasound, magnetic resonance imaging (MRI), positron emission tomography (PET), and other radiologic and nuclear medicine studies to differentiate between benign and malignant processes as well as to assess the potential metastatic disease in the abdominal cavity. Diagnostic and staging laparoscopy can also be performed just prior to a planned definitive operation. This will eliminate a separate trip to the operating room for a diagnostic/staging laparoscopy. The laparoscope may also be used to identify the underlying cause of unexplained ascites as well as identify the cause of unexplained abdominal and pelvic pain.

## 1. Indications for Elective Diagnostic Laparoscopy

Patients with underlying malignancy may have either primary or metastatic malignant disease within the abdomen. Common indications for laparoscopic evaluation include carcinoma of the esophagus, stomach, pancreas, and colorectum as part of a complete preoperative assessment (Table 18.1). Frequently, melanoma of the trunk or extremities may metastasize to the small bowel, causing unexplained bleeding or chronic intermittent small bowel obstruction. A patient with these

N.J. Soper and C.E.H. Scott-Conner (eds.), *The SAGES Manual: Volume 1 Basic Laparoscopy and Endoscopy*, DOI 10.1007/978-1-4614-2344-7_18,
© Springer Science+Business Media, LLC 2012

Table 18.1. Indications for laparoscopic staging of abdominal tumors.

| |
|---|
| • Preoperative assessment prior to major extirpation |
| • Documentation of hepatic or nodal involvement |
| • Confirmation of imaging studies |
| • Full assessment of ascitic fluid |
| • Borderline resectable tumors after pre-op imaging |

Table 18.2. Techniques utilized during diagnostic or staging laparoscopy.

| |
|---|
| • Full abdominal and pelvic evaluation |
| • Division of gastrohepatic omentum |
| • Biopsy using cupped forceps or core needle |
| • Abdominal lavage for cytologic study |
| • Retrieval of ascitic fluid for cytology and culture |
| • Identification and removal of enlarged lymph nodes |
| • Laparoscopic ultrasound |

findings may benefit from a laparoscopic examination. Other indications for laparoscopic staging include the full assessment of patients with Hodgkin lymphoma to plan appropriate chemotherapy and/or radiation therapy and to further evaluate the patient with borderline respectable disease on preoperative imaging.

The laparoscope may be utilized for general inspection of the abdominal cavity and as a method of obtaining tissue from solid organs such as liver or lymph nodes (Table 18.2). Imaging studies give only indirect evidence of underlying disease and, therefore, the laparoscope may be used for directed biopsy, obtaining cytologic specimens along with peritoneal lavage, or fine-needle aspiration techniques. In some parts of the world, infectious diseases (such as tuberculosis or parasitic infestation) causing abdominal problems may be more prevalent than cancer, and laparoscopic examination assists in the differential diagnosis of these entities. Diagnostic laparoscopy is also beneficial for patients with chronic abdominal pain who have had limited abdominal procedures in the past. This is especially true in women who have undergone hysterectomy and who have chronic pelvic pain. The identification and lysis of adhesions may be beneficial in this group.

## 2. Technique of Elective Diagnostic Laparoscopy

After appropriate preoperative evaluation, diagnostic laparoscopy is usually performed under general anesthesia. Diagnostic laparoscopy may be performed in the operating room (most common) or in a treatment area equipped for administration of anesthesia and with full resuscitative support. A proper table that allows the patient to be placed in both full Trendelenburg and reverse Trendelenburg positions during examination is essential. Appropriate time should be taken for a full examination of the upper and lower abdomen. This generally requires creating a pneumoperitoneum using carbon dioxide at 10–12 mmHg.

A 10-mm laparoscope is preferred utilizing both 0° and 30° cameras for full visualization. Place the laparoscope through a midline infraumbilical trocar site using a 10/11-mm trocar sleeve. Depending on the area to be examined, place one or two additional 5-mm trocars in each upper quadrant. These will be used for grasping forceps, palpating probes, and biopsy forceps.

Biopsy may be performed with cupped forceps passed through either a 5- or 10-mm trocar sleeve. Alternatively, cutting biopsy needles may be used to obtain liver or nodal tissue (Fig. 18.1). Needle biopsy may be performed percutaneously under laparoscopic guidance, or the biopsy needle may be passed through one of the 5-mm trocar sheaths. When a cupped forceps is used, it is important to perform biopsy cleanly without crushing tissue, since this might reduce the opportunity for pathologic review.

Specific areas of biopsy depend on the nature of the lesion and the tumor undergoing staging, and several malignancies will be discussed individually in the sections that follow. For example, in patients with lower esophageal and gastric cancer, the liver must be closely inspected and biopsies should be performed on any lesions on the surface of the liver. In addition, the gastrohepatic and gastrocolic omental areas may be divided to allow for evaluation of nodal tissue in these areas. Lymph nodes should be removed intact, if possible, to achieve better histologic identification. In assessing the patient with pancreatic cancer, the duodenum may be mobilized by means of Kocher maneuver allowing for biopsies of retroduodenal and other node-bearing areas.

Divide the gastrocolic omentum and inspect the superior pancreatic area for evidence of local or regional pancreatic cancer. Perform abdominal lavage with 500 mL of saline to obtain fluid for cytologic investigation. Angle the operating table into various positions to allow for the

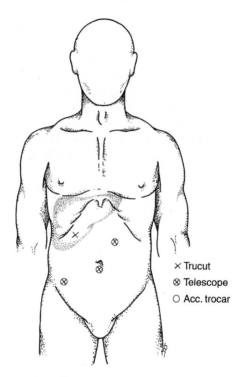

× Trucut
⊗ Telescope
○ Acc. trocar

Fig. 18.1.  Trocar and needle placement for liver biopsy. The biopsy needle may be passed through a trocar or percutaneously through the abdominal wall.

disbursement of the lavage fluid. Aspirate all of the fluid and send it to the cytology laboratory to be centrifuged and evaluated for malignant cells. Staging for pancreatic cancer prior to the planning of a Whipple procedure should be a separate event to allow for the assessment of cytology results and any biopsy specimens taken during the procedure, as positive peritoneal cytology is classified as stage IV disease. The laparoscope may not completely aid in the examination of the retropancreatic region especially in the region of the superior mesenteric artery and vein. Additional techniques specifically utilizing intraoperative laparoscopic ultrasound may aid in this assessment.

# B.  Esophageal Carcinoma (Squamous and Adenocarcinoma)

Historically, squamous cell carcinoma accounted for the majority of esophageal cancers. However, recently adenocarcinoma has dramatically increased to the point that now the two occur in almost equal frequencies. Adenocarcinoma is associated with Barrett's esophagus, which is related to reflux esophagitis. The classic approach to esophageal cancer management has been esophagectomy with reconstruction using either the stomach or the colon as an interposed organ. Because of the recent advances in esophageal cancer management using chemotherapy and radiation, neoadjuvant as well as postoperative adjuvant therapy may be important in many of these patients. Nodal involvement in carcinoma of the esophagus occurs in the mediastinum as well as in the celiac region and may be advanced even when imaging studies fail to show nodal disease. Fifty to sixty percent of patients present with locally advanced or metastatic disease. Careful assessment of the liver as well as the celiac axis can identify occult nodes in these regions or small metastases that have not been apparent on preoperative imaging studies. These patients, although amenable to palliation, will not benefit from major extirpative surgery, as there has been reported close to 50% morbidity with surgical treatment of esophageal cancer alone. Diagnostic laparoscopy can help exclude those patients in which a major operation would not be beneficial. In these cases radiation with placement of expandable stents may give appropriate treatment and support quality of life.

The technique of laparoscopy for the assessment of esophageal cancer utilizes three ports: an umbilical port for the laparoscope and two accessory ports, one in each subcostal region.

1.  Begin the assessment of the abdomen by placing the patient in steep Trendelenburg position and inspecting the pelvic peritoneum, looking for small peritoneal metastases.
2.  Next, place the operating table in a neutral position. Rotate it sequentially to the right and left decubitus positions (commonly termed "airplaning" the table) and look for ascites. Aspirate any fluid and send it for cytology.
3.  Next, inspect the liver. The reverse Trendelenburg position, with the left side down, assists by allowing the liver to drop down out of the subdiaphragmatic space. Look at all visible surfaces of the liver, using an angled (45°) laparoscope to facilitate inspection. Carefully assess the liver for any unusual

adhesions or plaques, which may initially appear benign yet harbor small metastases. Perform a biopsy on any suspicious areas with cup forceps or cutting needle.

4. Biopsy any lesions seen on the peritoneum or omentum with cupped forceps. As bleeding may occur, always have electro-cautery available when performing diagnostic laparoscopy.

5. Examine the anterior wall of the stomach and the region of the esophageal hiatus (Fig. 18.2). Place the table in reverse Trendelenburg position and use a 30° laparoscope.

6. Divide the gastrohepatic omentum to search for lymph nodes in the region of the subhepatic space and the lesser curvature of the stomach extending up to the esophageal hiatus. Lymph nodes in the region of the left gastric and celiac vessels may be inspected by this technique. Pass the laparoscope into the lesser sac for full identification (Fig. 18.3). If positive nodes are found, place metal clips to facilitate planning of radiation therapy, if appropriate.

## C. Gastric Cancer

Although the approach to cancer of the stomach is generally resection, whether it be for cure or palliation, laparoscopic evaluation may be important in patients who present with advanced disease or in patients that have questionable resectability after preoperative imaging. The main advantage of laparoscopic evaluation is to identify those patients with peritoneal metastases that were missed by conventional imaging, which can occur in up to 30% of patients. In this setting laparoscopy can select those patients who would not benefit from laparotomy. It also allows for sampling of involved lymph nodes and liver metastases. During staging, laparoscopy, a feeding jejunostomy tube can be placed for enteral feeding should it be needed. The assessment of the patient with gastric cancer is similar to that noted is esophageal cancer, and many of the same maneuvers are involved.

Recently, sentinel node techniques have been advocated for the enhancement of staging in gastric cancer. There may be additional roles for staging laparoscopy in this disease, as recognition of the nodal drainage patterns in gastric cancer is increased by radionuclide and vital staining.

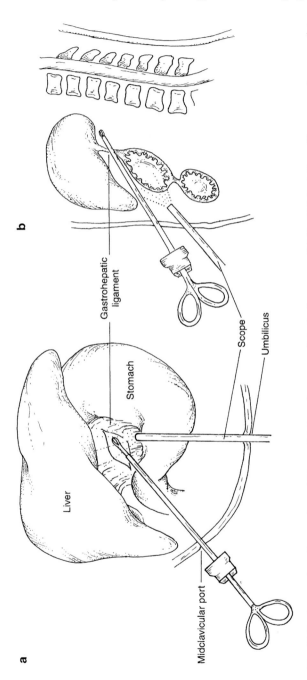

Fig. 18.2. Approach to the esophageal hiatus. (**a**) Anterior approach to the lesser sac. (**b**) Sagittal depiction of laparoscopic approach to the lesser sac.

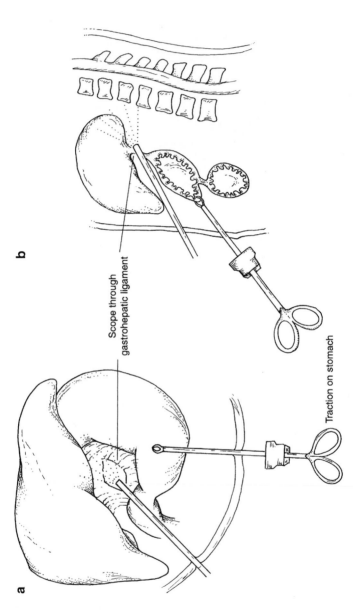

Fig. 18.3. Laparoscope switched to right upper quadrant portal and passed into lesser sac through opening in avascular portion of gastrohepatic omentum. Traction on the stomach facilitates this maneuver. (**a**) Anterior approach to the lesser sac. (**b**) Sagittal depiction of laparoscopic approach to the lesser sac.

# D. Tumors of the Liver (Primary and Metastatic)

Laparoscopic assessment of primary hepatic tumors is ideal because many of these tumors involve the surface of the liver. The recent application of laparoscopic ultrasound has aided in the identification of tumors deep to Glisson's capsule. Although metastatic disease of the liver is the most common indication for laparoscopic assessment, given the worldwide incidence of hepatocellular cancer and the increase in hepatic tumors associated with chronic hepatitis, evaluation of hepatocellular cancer is becoming increasingly more important. Staging laparoscopy in this setting also helps to categorize the severity of cirrhosis and the amount of liver that will remain if resection is undertaken. Traditional imaging studies may underestimate involvement of the liver, and this becomes critically important when hepatic resection is being considered.

1. A three-trocar technique is used for hepatic assessment, with an umbilical trocar for the laparoscope, and accessory ports in the left and right upper quadrants. Peritoneal attachments to the liver may need division based on the anatomical findings in the specific patient (Fig. 18.4).
2. Hepatic lesions may have a variety of colors including white, gray, or yellow, and may be nodular or have a depressed center

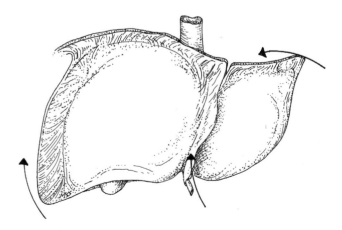

Fig. 18.4. Schematic of peritoneal attachments of liver, which may need to be divided for full assessment of the hepatic surface. Generally, this is not required, but the laparoscopist should be aware of the regional anatomy.

forming a "moon crater" or a "volcano" appearance. These lesions may also have increased vascularity, giving a hyperemic appearance.

3.  Biopsy techniques may involve either the use of cutting needles or cup forceps. Electrocautery should be immediately available to achieve hemostasis. If a bleeding vessel is noted, it is generally just below the liver capsule and can be handled easily by combining pressure with the cautery tip at the time of applying cauterization.

4.  In patients with hepatocellular cancer, diffuse lesions in both lobes of the liver as well as extrahepatic disease are obvious contraindications to primary resection. These patients may also have associated cirrhosis as a manifestation of chronic alcohol ingestion or hepatitis. Laparoscopy is important in the identification of the cirrhotic liver and the severity of the cirrhosis, which may also be a major contraindication to further resection.

# E.  Pancreatic Carcinoma

With peripancreatic cancers, surgery remains the only treatment that offers a potential cure. However, in pancreatic cancer the majority of patients present with unresectable and metastatic disease excluding them from surgical resection with an overall 5-year survival of less than 5%. Patient presentation depends upon the location and stage of the disease. Most tumors are found in the pancreatic head resulting in obstructive jaundice. However, there is a wide range of presenting symptoms from common symptoms such as vague abdominal pain and nausea to the infrequent symptoms of obstruction and GI bleeding. Staging laparoscopy is used to identify metastatic disease in patients with locally advanced tumors and in circumstances where radiological imaging did not show unresectable disease. One third of patients will have radiologically occult metastases or unresectable disease that was not seen on preoperative imaging.

Peritoneal cytology may also be performed during staging laparoscopy. A patient with positive cytology has stage IV disease according to the AJCC TNM staging system. Up to 10% of patients thought to have resectable disease will have positive peritoneal cytology. The role for laparoscopic staging and peritoneal cytology in all patients is unclear and currently a topic of debate, but advanced disease will be revealed when imaging studies show disease limited to the pancreas. For this reason, allow adequate time after performing laparoscopy to obtain and evaluate results (that is, do not schedule laparoscopy under the same anesthesia as the planned definitive surgery).

1. The goals of laparoscopic evaluation in pancreatic cancer are to assess peripancreatic nodes as well as remote sites that may harbor metastases.

2. Perform direct inspection of the pancreas by dividing the gastrocolic and gastrohepatic omental areas and by inserting the laparoscope into the lesser sac. Needle aspiration or biopsy of peripancreatic masses may be accomplished in this manner if a tissue diagnosis has not previously been obtained.

3. Pancreatitis and the development of adhesions in this area may render inspection of the lesser sac difficult. Gentle dissection of these adhesions by means of electrocautery may allow for excellent inspection of the pancreatic body and tail with opportunity for laparoscopically guided biopsy in a large number of patients.

4. The major purpose of laparoscopy is to look for superficial peritoneal and hepatic masses that have not been identified by conventional imaging studies. Using a combination of laparoscopy and CT or MRI of the abdomen, at least 90% of unresectable tumors can be identified, which benefits a large group of patients without the need for exploratory laparotomy.

5. Cytologic investigation of peritoneal washings should be performed if results of other examinations are negative. Carcinoma cells may be obtained from the free peritoneal cavity even when the peritoneum itself is grossly free of metastatic implants. Positive cytology indicates metastatic (M1) disease.

# F. Laparoscopic Ultrasound in Cancer Staging

Laparoscopic cancer staging should include routine adjunctive laparoscopic ultrasound (LUS), which assists in identifying small lesions and directing biopsies. LUS examination uses either linear array or sector scan probes with rigid or flexible tips in frequencies ranging from 5 to 10 MHz. Color Doppler imaging may be available to discern venous or arterial blood flow. These probes allow high-resolution imaging of the liver, bile ducts, pancreas, abdominal vessels, and lymph nodes. Overall, the application of LUS in cancer staging increases the accuracy by approximately 5–25% in patients evaluated.

This section gives specific techniques for various anatomic regions and should be considered complementary to the previous sections (which deal with specific malignancies).

1. **Liver**. Generally three trocars are used, including a 10/11-mm trocar in the right upper quadrant, an umbilical port for the laparoscope, and a left upper quadrant port (Fig. 18.5). Pass a flexible or rigid ultrasound probe over the right liver, medial segment of the left liver, and lateral segment of the left liver to identify lesions in the hepatic parenchyma. The anterior and posterior surfaces may be scanned easily without mobilization of the liver.

   a. Contact between the ultrasound probe and the liver surface may be improved by lowering the pressure setting on the

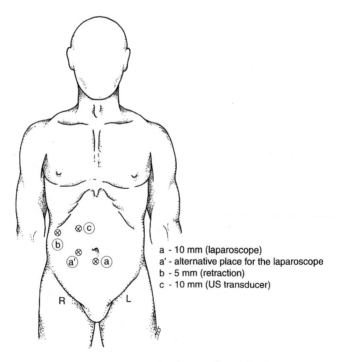

a - 10 mm (laparoscope)
a' - alternative place for the laparoscope
b - 5 mm (retraction)
c - 10 mm (US transducer)

Fig. 18.5. Trocar sites for laparoscopic ultrasound examination.

insufflator and allowing the pneumoperitoneum to partially collapse.

b. Identify hemangiomas and differentiate these from metastatic lesions by their compressibility, elicited either by contact with the ultrasound probe directly or by palpation with an instrument. Small hemangiomas are usually hyperechoic.

c. Small liver metastases are usually hypoechoic compared with normal liver parenchyma or isoechoic with a hypoechoic halo. Biopsy suspicious lesions with a cutting needle or biopsy forceps. Lesions as small as 3 mm may be identified by LUS.

2. **Biliary tract** (see also Chap. 20, Laparoscopic Cholecystectomy)

a. Image the intrahepatic bile ducts, the bifurcation, and the proximal common bile duct by placing the probe on the anterior surface of segment IV of the liver. Use the umbilical and subcostal trocars alternately to obtain longitudinal and transverse scans. Bile duct dilatation, inflammatory bile duct thickening, and localized bile duct tumors of 1 cm or less may be seen.

b. Image the gallbladder either through the liver or by placing the probe on the gallbladder itself.

c. Tumors of the bifurcation or the proximal common bile duct are usually isoechoic in comparison to liver parenchyma. In some patients the falciform ligament prevents the appropriate application of the laparoscopic ultrasound probe during the evaluation of tumors of the left hepatic duct and surrounding area. This may be resolved by scanning segment IV as well as segments II and III to the left of the falciform ligament.

3. **Pancreas and periampullary region**

a. Visualize the pancreas, pancreatic duct, and common bile duct by placing the LUS probe on the stomach and duodenum. Tumors in this region are best imaged through the left and right subcostal trocars, which produce transverse or oblique sections of the pancreas.

b. The portal venous system may also be imaged with LUS. The superior mesenteric vein is best evaluated from the left subcostal trocar, while the more obliquely oriented portal vein is best imaged from the right subcostal trocar. Vessels of the low-pressure portal system are easily compressed by the ultrasound probe, falsely implying stenosis when in fact the vessel is normal. Tumor infiltration into the portal vein is characterized by loss of the hyperechoic interface between the vessel lumen and the tumor.

c.  Adenocarcinomas of the pancreas as well as small cholangiocarcinomas and carcinomas of the papilla of Vater (approximately 1 cm) may be seen as a hypoechoic mass in comparison to normal pancreas. In contrast, neuroendocrine tumors of the pancreas and duodenal wall show higher echogenicity than adenocarcinomas.

d.  Differentiation between pancreatic inflammation and tumor may be quite important. Generally, inflamed pancreatic tissue is hypoechoic compared to normal pancreatic parenchyma.

4. **Lymph nodes**. LUS is an ideal technique for evaluating nodes without performing a formal node dissection. Ultrasound features suggesting benign nodes include a hyperechoic center, which represents hilar fat within the lymph node. If the image is more rounded and more hypoechoic with a loss of the hyperechoic center, metastasis must be assumed. There is overlap on occasion between benign and malignant features of nodes on ultrasound exam. Enlargement of lymph nodes by itself is not a characteristic of either benign or malignant lesions.

a.  Nodes in the hepatoduodenal ligament and celiac axis are best seen through the left lobe of the liver or by direct approximation of the LUS probe directly on the hepatoduodenal ligament or celiac axis. Localization of these nodes will then allow for laparoscopic biopsy. This is especially helpful in the preoperative staging of gastric carcinoma, or during staging laparoscopy for Hodgkin lymphoma.

b.  Tumors of the gastric cardia or distal esophagus have an isoechoic appearance on LUS. Nodal involvement especially in the celiac and lesser curve areas is apparent on LUS.

## Selected References

Angst E, Hiatt JR, Gloor B, et al. Laparoscopic surgery for cancer: a systematic review and a way forward. J Am Coll Surg. 2010;211:412–23.

Conlon KC, Dougherty E, Klimstra DS, et al. The value of minimal access surgery in the staging of patients with potentially resectable peripancreatic malignancy. Ann Surg. 1996;223:134–40.

Edge SB, Byrd DR, Compton CC, Fritz AG, Greene FL, Trotti A. AJCC cancer staging manual. 7th ed. New York: Springer; 2010.

Feld RI, Liu J-B, Nazarian L. Laparoscopic liver sonography: preliminary experience in liver metastases compared with CT portography. J Ultrasound Med. 1996;15:289–95.

Gaujoux S, Allen PJ. Role of staging laparoscopy in peri-pancreatic and hepatobiliary malignancy. World J Gastrointest Surg. 2010;2:283–90.

Greene FL. Laparoscopy in malignant disease. Surg Clin North Am. 1992;72:1125–37.

Greene FL, Heniford BT. Minimally invasive cancer management. 2nd ed. New York: Springer; 2010.

Greene FL, Rosin RD. Minimal access surgical oncology. Oxford: Radcliffe Medical; 1995.

Hidalgo M. Pancreatic cancer. N Engl J Med. 2010;362:1605–17.

Hohenberger P, Conlon K. Staging laparoscopy. Berlin: Springer; 2002.

Hunerbein M, Rau B, Schlag PM. Laparoscopy and laparoscopic ultrasound for staging of upper gastrointestinal tumours. Eur J Surg Oncol. 1995;21:50–4.

John TG, Greig JD, Crosbie JL, et al. Superior staging of liver tumors with laparoscopy and laparoscopic ultrasound. Ann Surg. 1994;220:711–9.

John TG, Greig JD, Carter DC, Garden OJ. Carcinoma of the pancreatic head and periampullary region: tumor staging with laparoscopy and laparoscopic ultrasonography. Ann Surg. 1995;221:156–64.

Johnstone P, Rohde DC, Swartz SE, et al. Port site recurrences after laparoscopic and thoracoscopic procedures in malignancy. J Clin Oncol. 1996;14:1950–6.

Mahadevan D, Sudirman A, Kandasami P, Ramesh G. Laparoscopic staging in gastric cancer: an essential step in its management. J Minim Access Surg. 2010;6:111–3.

Mayo SC, Austin DF, Sheppard BC. Evolving preoperative evaluation of patients with pancreatic cancer: does laparoscopy have a role in the current era? J Am Coll Surg. 2009;208:87.

National Comprehensive Cancer Network. http://www.nccn.org. Accessed 15 Dec 2010.

Pratt BL, Greene FL. Role of laparoscopy in the staging of malignant disease. Surg Clin North Am. 2000;80:1111–26.

Ramshaw BJ. Laparoscopic surgery for cancer patients. CA Cancer J Clin. 1997;47:327–50.

Ravikumar TS. Laparoscopic staging and intraoperative ultrasonography for liver tumor management. Surg Oncol Clin N Am. 1996;5:271–82.

Warshaw AL, Tepper J, Shipley W. Laparoscopy in the staging and planning of therapy for pancreatic cancer. Am J Surg. 1986;151:76–80.

Watt I, Stewart I, Anderson D, et al. Laparoscopy, ultrasound, and computed tomography in cancer of the esophagus and gastric cardia: a prospective comparison for detecting intra-abdominal metastases. Br J Surg. 1989;76:1036–9.

Yoon HH, Lowe VJ, Cassivi SD, Romero Y. The role of FDG-PET and staging laparoscopy in the management of patients with cancer of the esophagus or gastroesophageal junction. Gastroenterol Clin N Am. 2009;38:105–20.

# 19. Lymph Node Biopsy, Dissection, and Staging Laparoscopy

*Lee L. Swanstrom, M.D., F.A.C.S.*

## A. Indications

Laparotomy is commonly used to perform biopsies on nodal tissue, to perform therapeutic lymphadenectomies, and to perform palliative gastrointestinal bypasses. Image-guided percutaneous biopsy is a less traumatic but significantly less accurate alterative. Most recently, laparoscopy and thoracoscopy has been shown to be an accurate, less invasive staging method and, in some cases, a procedure to allow extended lymphadenectomies for improved survival. The role of surgical node biopsy is rapidly evolving as introduction of new imaging modalities such as positron emission tomography scans and endoscopic ultrasonography become more widely available and increasingly accurate as staging tools. New evidence indicates that there may be a survival benefit from both a more aggressive policy of en bloc lymphadenectomy and the use of laparoscopy vs open procedures. Some practitioners are using a surgical robot for dissections. To date, this has not been shown to be better than laparoscopic/thoracoscopic dissections and is not currently cost-effective but may be eventually. In the future, techniques such as natural orifice transluminal endoscopic surgery (NOTES) may offer a new paradigm of even less invasive local resection and node biopsies. Current **indications** for the use of laparoscopy for intra-abdominal node dissections or biopsies are listed in Table 19.1.

## B. Patient Preparation, Positioning, and Setup

Informed consent for all procedures should include not only a discussion of the procedure, its risks, and alternatives but also further treatment options for various scenarios. Patient and surgeon should reach

N.J. Soper and C.E.H. Scott-Conner (eds.), *The SAGES Manual: Volume 1 Basic Laparoscopy and Endoscopy*, DOI 10.1007/978-1-4614-2344-7_19, © Springer Science+Business Media, LLC 2012

Table 19.1. Tumor sites for which laparoscopic lymph node biopsy or dissection has been reported, grouped by purpose of laparoscopic intervention.

| Purpose of intervention | Tumor site |
| --- | --- |
| Staging (including sentinel node biopsy) | Ovary |
| | Uterine cervix |
| | Endometrium |
| | Prostate |
| | Bladder |
| | Testis (including germ cell) |
| | Hodgkin lymphoma[a] |
| | Esophagus |
| | colorectal |
| Determination of resectability for cure | Esophagus |
| | Stomach |
| | Pancreas |
| | Hepatobiliary |
| | Unknown retroperitoneal masses |
| Therapeutic lymph node dissection | Colon[b] |
| | Stomach[b] |
| | Esophagus[b] |
| | Nonseminomatous testicular |
| | Uterine cervix or endometrium |

[a] Also see Chap. 18 for more details on staging laparoscopy for Hodgkin lymphoma
[b] As part of resection

consensus on how to proceed with surgical cancer treatment depending on possible findings of the laparoscopic staging procedure. This allows the surgeon to proceed with an orderly plan of treatment that is consistent with the patient's wishes (e.g., to perform a formal resection under the same anesthesia, to attempt palliation, or to do nothing further) all depending on the intraoperative findings.

The details of preparation depend upon the anticipated site of dissection, duration of surgery, and associated pathology. Here are some general guidelines.

1. Place a **Foley catheter** for iliac node dissection, mediastinal explorations, pelvic dissection, or long cases.
2. Retrogastric biopsy or other upper abdominal procedures require an orogastric tube.

3.  Formal bowel preparation is advisable for para-aortic lymph node dissection as both the transabdominal and the retroperitoneal approaches involve extensive colon manipulation.

4.  Patients with malignancy are at high risk for deep-vein thrombosis (DVT), and the effects of position and pneumoperitoneum may contribute to intraoperative venous stasis. **Anti-DVT prophylaxis** is extremely important.

5.  A single dose of **antibiotics** is given immediately preoperatively, usually a first-generation cephalosporin.

6.  Patient position and monitor setup in the operating room varies for these cases.

    a.  Position the patient supine with the legs spread on a "split-leg" OR table for **upper abdominal node biopsies/dissections, transhiatal dissections, or Hodgkin staging** (Fig. 19.1). A restraining belt is not feasible so footrests and care with securing the legs is necessary. Arms can be tucked or secured to arm boards at less than a 90° angle. A bracket for a liver retractor holder should be attached to the bed before draping.

    b.  **Para-aortic dissections** can also be done in this position (with the arms tucked), but are more commonly done through a retroperitoneal approach with the patient positioned in the lateral decubitus position (Fig. 19.2). This position requires a beanbag with the patient positioned over the table break to allow lateral flexion. Attention to padding of the axilla, arms, and legs is critical to prevent neuropraxia. The monitors should be placed at the head and foot of the table.

    c.  For **iliac and low pelvic node dissection** the patient lies supine with both arms tucked (Fig. 19.3).

    d.  Laparoscopic staging procedures for **gynecologic and urologic malignancies** are often done in full lithotomy position, to allow access to the urethra or vagina for biopsy, hysterectomy, placement of a uterine elevator or endoscopy (hysteroscopy, cystoscopy, or sigmoidoscopy). The laparoscopic monitors are placed at the patient's feet.

    e.  Robotic and NOTES procedures require additional and complex equipment sets, but the concepts of patient positioning are the same.

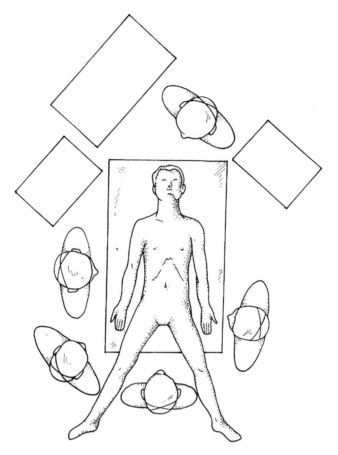

Fig. 19.1. Room setup and patient position for upper abdominal node dissection.

## C. Access Ports and Equipment for Laparoscopic Node Biopsy or Dissection

Simple biopsy can often be performed with three ports (two 5 mm and one 10 mm), but more formal retroperitoneal node dissections may require up to six ports (three 10 mm and three 5 mm). Recent developments in "mini-laparoscopy," utilizing scopes, ports, and instruments between 1.5 and 3 mm in diameter, have permitted even less invasive access for at least staging and diagnosis. Placement obviously varies according to the area

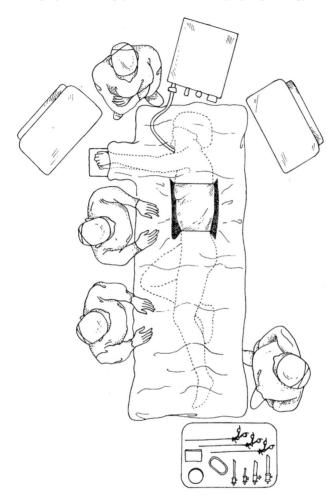

Fig. 19.2. Room setup and patient position for retroperitoneal para-aortic node biopsy.

being sampled. Finally, single incision laparoscopic surgery (multiple instruments via one incision) is gaining traction for many abdominal procedures and has been described for some oncologic resections including node dissections. This requires specialized ports with multiple lumens and often special endoscopes and instruments (curved or steerable).

Instruments that are typically needed for standard laparoscopy are listed in Table 19.2.

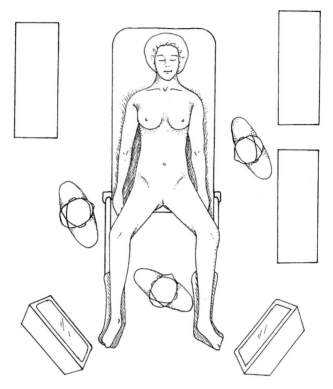

Fig. 19.3.   Room setup and patient position for iliac node dissection.

Table 19.2.   Instruments for laparoscopic node biopsy and dissection.

| | |
|---|---|
| Angled laparoscope (3–10 mm) | 5- or 10-mm endoclip applier |
| Atraumatic graspers (Glassman) | Specimen retrieval sac |
| Maryland dissector | Ultrasonically activated scissors[a] |
| | Bipolar sealing devices[a] |
| Laparoscopic ultrasound probe | Dissecting balloons[a] |
| Endoscopic Metzenbaum scissor | Needle holders[a] |

[a] Not needed in all cases

# D.  Technique of Retrogastric Dissections

Retrogastric dissection for esophageal cancer staging or in conjunction with gastrectomy is approached much the same as for a laparoscopic antireflux procedure.

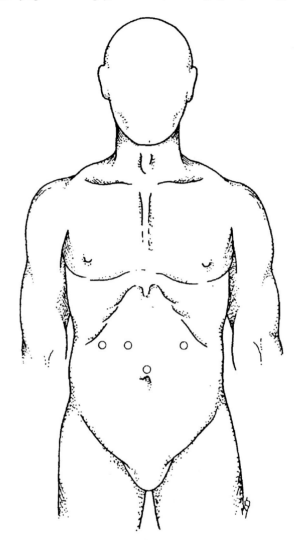

Fig. 19.4. Trocar placement for upper abdominal dissection.

1. Position the patient on a split leg table with arms out on arm boards, as previously noted (Fig. 38.1) and in reverse Trendelenburg position.
2. Place the initial trocar 3 cm above the umbilicus in the midline, the second (10-mm) trocar in the left midclavicular line, and the third (5-mm) in the right midclavicular line (Fig. 19.4).

3.  Use a **25- to 50° angled laparoscope** to carefully perform a complete peritoneoscopy, which should include inspection of the pelvic cul-de-sac, Morrison's pouch, and the diaphragm. This is done to rule out any carcinomatosis that may obviate a more extended procedure.

4.  Next, use **laparoscopic ultrasound** to assess the liver, porta hepatic, celiac, and retrogastric nodes. Any nodes identified as enlarged should be targeted for biopsy.

5.  If no adenopathy is noted, or the findings are equivocal, open the avascular portion of the gastrohepatic omentum and retract the lesser curvature of the stomach to the patient's left. This gives good access to the **celiac nodes** at the base of the patient's right crus. It also allows access to the head of the pancreas and the nodal tissue overlying this area as well as those immediately superior to the portal vein (Fig. 19.5).

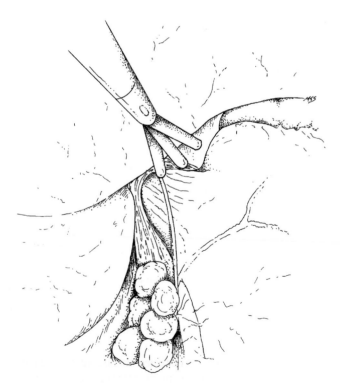

Fig. 19.5.  Exposure of the celiac nodes.

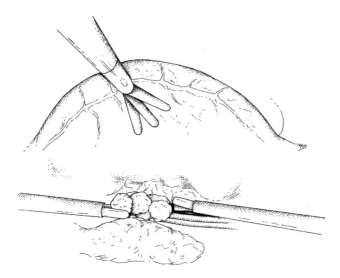

Fig. 19.6. Retrogastric nodes exposed.

6.   Grasp the selected node(s) with an atraumatic grasper, and coagulate lymphatics and small feeding vessels with electrocautery, bipolar sealers or ultrasonic scissors.

7.   Access the **retrogastric nodes** by dividing the gastrocolic omentum and entering the lesser sac behind the stomach. Take care when dividing the gastrocolic omentum to avoid injuring the gastroepiploic vasculature (Fig. 19.6).

8.   Inside the lesser sac, divide the avascular adhesions between stomach and pancreas and use an atraumatic liver retractor to elevate the stomach. This retractor is best held by a table-mounted retractor holding system.

9.   Node-bearing tissue also lies along the superior border of the splenic vein and pancreas and adjacent to the superior mesenteric vein and artery.

10.   For simple staging, grasp and excise isolated nodes. Sentinel node techniques, now standard in breast surgery, are being investigated for GI cancers as well and may well be an ideal minimally invasive procedure in the future (see "Selected References").

11.   For more extended therapeutic dissections, the paraceliac and porta hepatic nodes are usually dissected as one contiguous mass.

12.   Node tissue between the superior mesenteric vein and splenic hilum is next removed in continuity.

13. The nodal tissue is placed in a specimen bag and removed through a trocar site (which may be enlarged if necessary).
14. A closed suction drain should be left in the field when an extensive node dissection is performed. This may control any postoperative lymphatic leakage. No drain is needed for simple biopsy.

# E. Staging for Hodgkin Disease

Surgical staging of Hodgkin lymphoma is seldom performed anymore. When it is done, it is ideally performed laparoscopically. It typically involves biopsy of multiple node-bearing areas and solid organ tissue. This indication has enjoyed some renewed interest with the ability to do it laparoscopically because it yields greater sensitivity and specificity than is possible with imaging techniques while minimizing patient morbidity and length of hospital stay. Chapter 18 contains additional information about Hodgkin staging. The discussion here focuses on the specific techniques of lymph node biopsy which is applicable to all GI, urologic, or Gyn cancers.

1. Position the patient supine with legs spread.
2. Five trocars are used (three 5-mm trocars and two 10-mm trocars).
3. Perform laparoscopic ultrasonography to identify any obvious retroperitoneal masses (Fig. 19.7).
4. Perform a biopsy on any grossly (or ultrasonographically) visible nodes or peritoneal lesions.
5. Obtain mesenteric nodes.
   a. Gently elevate the midjejunum with atraumatic graspers and use sharp and blunt dissection to dissect out mesenteric nodes, which are usually visible under the visceral peritoneum.
   b. The ultrasonic coagulating shears are useful for control of the lymphatic and vascular supply to the nodes.
   c. Single nodes can be withdrawn through the 10-mm port, labeled, and fixed in formalin for pathologic assessment. One node from each area should also be sent fresh to allow touch-prep slides to be made.
   d. Obtain nodes from the transverse colon mesentery in the same way. The omentum should be swept into the upper

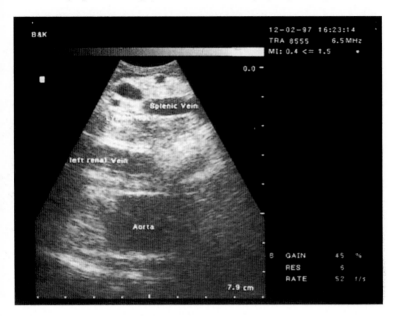

Fig. 19.7. Ultrasonic image of retroperitoneal nodes.

abdomen while the transverse colon is being elevated to allow mesenteric node sampling.

6. Access para-aortic nodes by carrying the dissection down to the root of the mesentery adjacent to the ligament of Treitz.
7. A wedge liver biopsy is performed (see Chap. 18).
8. Finally, a laparoscopic splenectomy is performed (see Volume II Chap. 26).

## F. Para-aortic Node Dissections

A formal para-aortic node dissection is usually indicated for staging or therapy of endometrial or cervical carcinomas, or as a treatment for early stage germ cell tumors of the testicle. A formal dissection is best approached with retroperitonoscopy.

1. Place the patient in the **lateral decubitus position** on a beanbag with the midabdomen positioned over the table break.
2. **Flex the table** so that the lateral abdominal musculature is stretched taut.

3.  **Take care to prevent nerve injury** An axillary roll must be carefully positioned, the uppermost arm supported, and abundant padding placed between the flexed legs.

4.  **Gain access** by a direct cut down to the preperitoneal plane in the midclavicular line 2–3 cm lateral to the umbilicus. Use blunt finger dissection to establish the working space. Introduce a dissecting balloon (Origin MedSystems, Menlo Park, CA) and advance it posteriorly. Insufflate between 800 and 1,600 mL into the balloon (with the scope in place to observe the resulting dissection). Stop the dissection when the aorta is visualized (Fig. 19.8).

5.  Use insufflation at 10–15 mmHg to maintain the created space and insert **additional ports** (5 and 10 mm) under direct vision. Additional dissection can be done to allow full access to the aorta between the hypogastric takeoff and the renal artery.

6.  **Node sampling** is done throughout the entire area, with the nodes either removed individually or placed in a tissue bag, which is removed at the end of the procedure.

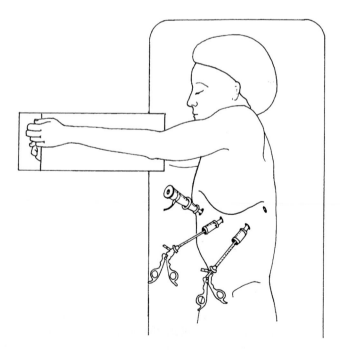

Fig. 19.8.  Trocar placement for retroperitoneal aortic node dissection.

7. Take care to **avoid injury** to the lumbar sympathetics, anterior spinal nerve roots, and ureters.

8. While efforts are made to remove most of the nodes on the ipsilateral side of the tumor, it is also wise to **cross the midline** and sample nodes from the contralateral side.

9. For therapeutic dissections, take the nodes **in continuity** as much as possible. This may be combined with an ipsilateral iliac node dissection.

10. **No drains** are placed, and at the conclusion of the procedure the retroperitoneum is allowed to deinsufflate, the trocars are withdrawn, and fascias are closed for the larger port sites.

# G. Iliac Dissection

Iliac dissection can be performed either transabdominally or properitoneally. There is no clear-cut advantage of one approach over the other. Dissection is usually bilateral for prostate, cervical, or vulvar cancers, and unilateral (ipsilateral) for other malignancies confined to one side of the patient.

1. Room setup is the same for both approaches, with a single monitor at the foot of the bed.

2. Place the patient supine with arms tucked at the side.

3. The surgeon stands on the side opposite the initial dissection (Fig. 19.3).

4. Three ports are used for both approaches (two 10 mm and one 5 mm).

5. Place the laparoscope through a trocar in the subumbilical site.

6. For the **transperitoneal approach**, the trocars are placed as shown in Figure 19.9.

    a. Incise the peritoneum overlying the iliac artery in a longitudinal fashion and dissect the edges of the peritoneum back medially and laterally.

    b. The lymphatic tissue lies medial to the iliac artery and vein and within the obturator fossa (Fig. 19.10).

    c. Dissect out the nodal tissues in continuity, beginning at the femoral ring and working from top to bottom.

    d. Take care not to injure the obturator nerve, which marks the posterior boundary of the obturator fossa. A minimum of electrocautery should be used in this area.

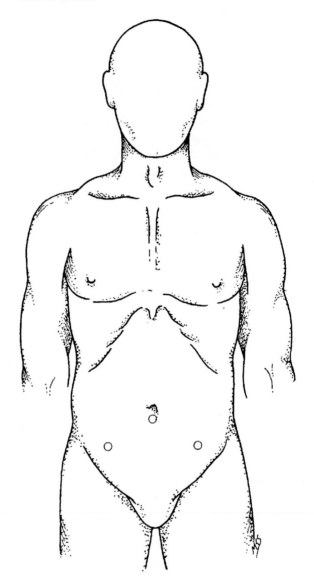

Fig. 19.9.   Trocar placement for transperitoneal iliac node dissection.

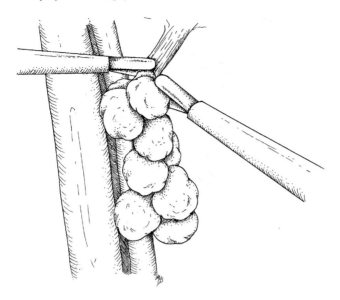

Fig. 19.10. Exposure of iliac nodes.

    e.   Continue the dissection to the iliac bifurcation. Frozen section is usually obtained when doing nodes for prostate cancer, and if positive, there is no need to perform the contralateral node dissection.

    f.   There is debate about closing the resulting peritoneal defect. If left open, there is a risk of bowel adhesions to this area. If closed, a lymphocele could form potentially, compromising the iliac vein. If the peritoneum is closed, a closed suction drain may be advisable.

7.   The preperitoneal approach utilizes the same technique used for a totally extraperitoneal hernia repair (see Chap. 32).

    a.   Enter the preperitoneal space via an infraumbilical port.

    b.   Create the initial entry into the preperitoneal space by finger dissection.

    c.   Pass a dissecting balloon or trocar into the space. If a dissecting balloon is not used, the pressure of insufflation can be turned up (20 mmHg) and the preperitoneum space dissected bluntly using the laparoscope.

    d.   When this space is developed, additional trocars may be placed along the abdominal midline (Fig. 19.11). The same

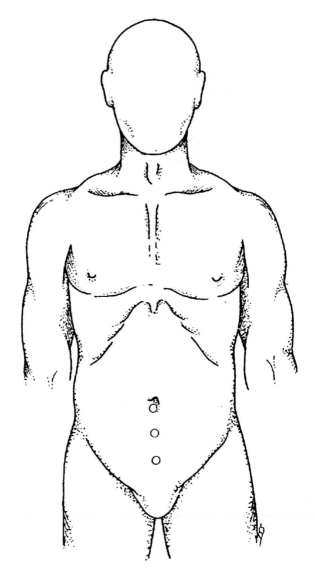

Fig. 19.11.  Trocar placement for preperitoneal node biopsy.

dissection as the transabdominal approach is then performed. A drain is not usually placed, but the patient should be counseled to watch closely for extremity swelling.

# H. Novel Techniques

Evolution, even of surgical procedures, never stops. Several new techniques to further minimize access trauma are currently in early phases of investigation. These include single port laparoscopic procedures, continued work on sentinel node biopsy for GI malignancy and even incisionless surgery via natural orifices.

a.  Single incision procedures are known by a multitude of names SILS (single incision laparoscopic surgery), SPS (single port Surgery), LESS (laparoscopic entry via single site), etc. These approaches which typically create a single larger skin incision through which multiple ports or a single multichannel device are inserted have particularly found favor with urologic radical resections as the access is essentially through the specimen retrieval site. The true benefits of this single incision approach have yet to be documented and there are particular concerns with the possibility of increased wound complications and the possibility of increased operative complications due to compromised ergonomics.

b.  Sentinel node approaches continue to evolve and are increasingly explored in the GI cancer field. There have been papers recently showing the accuracy of sentinel node detection for both colon cancer and gastric cancer. Early esophageal cancer may be another place for sentinel node staging due to the high incidence of node positivity for even early cancer. The future of early cancer in the GI tract may well be one of early endoscopic full thickness excision with local harvesting of the sentinel node through the defect and subsequent endoscopic closure.

c.  NOTES or natural orifice transluminal endoscopic surgery, once again seeks to avoid the trauma and complications of skin incisions by using flexible endoscopy to gain access to the chest, abdomen or retroperitoneum through the mouth, vagina or rectum. Of particular interest to our current subject is transoral mediastinal access and transrectal or vaginal retroperitoneal access.

These difficult to reach areas may be accessible with flexible scopes allowing harvesting or even dissection of lymph nodes. To date, NOTES is mostly experimental or limited to fairly basic surgical procedures, but lab work has been done on paraesophageal node harvest and retroperitoneal node dissections.

# I.  Complications

1.  **Diffuse bleeding from a peritoneal biopsy site**
    a.  **Cause and prevention**. Cancer patients frequently bleed from simple biopsies because of hypocoagulability (from decreased platelet counts, anti-inflammatory medications, clotting factor depletion, etc.) or portal hypertension secondary to hepatic or extrahepatic tumor involvement. Obtain a coagulation panel before surgery and correct any abnormalities. Look for clinical signs of portal hypertension (ascites, spider veins, history of variceal gastrointestinal bleeds, etc.) during preoperative assessment; this may represent a relative contraindication for the surgery.
    b.  **Recognition and treatment. Bleeding from a biopsy site** is usually recognized at the time of biopsy and should be treated by judicious electrocautery. If this fails, a thrombogenic material can be inserted and pressure applied for 5–10 min. If bleeding continues, an endoscopically placed figure-of-eight suture tied intracorporally will almost always control the bleeding. Rarely, an extended node dissection will result in diffuse bleeding over a wide area. The laparoscopic argon beam coagulator can be useful in these circumstances.

    Always check the security of hemostasis by lowering the insufflation pressure to less than 10 mmHg at the end of the procedure. In spite of this, delayed bleeding can occur and postoperative lymph node dissection patients should be carefully watched for the first 24 h for signs of bleeding (tachycardia, increasing pain, dropping hematocrit, flank discoloration from a retroperitoneal bleed). Treatment of delayed bleed depends on the hemodynamic stability of the patient. Stable patients with mild symptoms may require fluids and/or blood, check of coagulation factors, and administration of appropriate factors if indicated. Unstable patients should be returned to the operating room without delay for a laparoscopic or open exploration.

2. **Bleeding from a liver biopsy**
   a. **Cause and prevention**. Cancer patients are at increased risk of bleeding. Patients with severe coagulopathy or known portal hypertension who have to have a liver biopsy should have blood products given before surgery to correct anemia and normalize coagulation indices. Maximal medical treatment (diuretics) should also be undertaken to control ascites.

   b. **Recognition and treatment**. Bleeding from the site of a liver biopsy is hard to miss. Needle biopsy site bleeding is almost always controllable with cautery. Oozing is controlled with a monopolar device set on a high pure coagulating setting. This allows arcing of the current and prevents the resulting eschar from pulling away with the probe. High-pressure bleeds require a lower setting and direct contact of the probe to apply pressure and heat simultaneously. Recalcitrant bleeding may require 15–20 min of direct pressure, argon beam coagulation, or injection of fibrin glue into the needle tract.

   Bleeding from the exposed surface of a wedge resection should be controlled with a woven oxidized cellulose material and pressure. If this fails, the argon beam coagulator is useful.

3. **Chylous ascites**
   a. **Cause and prevention**. Rarely, disruption of major lymphatic channels can lead to a massive lymphatic leak and chylous ascites. Clip or ligate large lymph ducts before division, and perform all extended dissections with ultrasonic coagulating shears or electrocautery.

   b. **Recognition and treatment**. Sometimes division of a major lymph channel is recognized at the time of the dissection when milky chyle appears. Identify the ends of the duct and ligate, cauterize, or clip it. Chylous ascites may present many weeks after the surgery with increasing abdominal distention and discomfort (rarely pain). Treatment almost always involves reexploration, identification of the severed duct, and ligation.

4. **Lymphocele**
    a. **Cause and prevention**. Minor lymphatic leaks within the peritoneal cavity are seldom a problem because of the absorptive capacity of the peritoneum. When a leak occurs within a confined retroperitoneal space, a lymphocele may result. Lymphoceles may be asymptomatic, or they may present with pain or unilateral extremity swelling. They can occasionally obstruct venous outflow and have even been implicated in major venous thrombosis. It may be prudent to leave a temporary drain in the preperitoneum if it is closed or to leave this space open to the peritoneal cavity.
    b. **Recognition and treatment**. Ipsilateral extremity swelling, a palpable mass, and diffuse back pain are signs of a possible lymphocele. Ultrasound is the test of choice to make the diagnosis. Treatment usually requires operative intervention via a laparotomy or laparoscopy, with the goal of opening the retroperitoneum, controlling obvious lymph leaks, and either draining the space with closed suction drains or leaving it open to the peritoneal cavity. Percutaneous drainage is seldom more than a temporizing maneuver and could lead to secondary infection. A lymphangiogram may be needed for the rare patient with a persistent leak.

5. **Port site tumor implantation** There have been reports of tumor implantation in the retrieval port site after dissections for malignancies. Prevention of such occurrences depends on meticulous technique (avoiding node disruption) and use of a tough, impermeable specimen retrieval bags or wound protector.

# Selected References

Cahill RA, Perretta S, Forgione A, Leroy J, Dallemagne B, Marescaux J. Multimedia article. Combined sentinel node biopsy and localized sigmoid resection entirely by natural orifice transluminal endoscopic surgery: a new challenge to the old paradigm. Dis Colon Rectum. 2009;52(4):725.

Casaccia M, Torelli P, Cavaliere D, Panaro F, Nardi I, Rossi E, Spriano M, Bacigalupo A, Gentile R, Valente U. Laparoscopic lymph node biopsy in intra-abdominal lymphoma: high diagnostic accuracy achieved with a minimally invasive procedure. Surg Laparosc Endosc Percutan Tech. 2007;17(3):175–8.

Childers JM, Balserak JC, Kent J, Surwit E. Laparoscopic staging of Hodgkin's lymphoma. J Laparoendosc Surg. 1993;3(5):495–9.

Cho WY, Kim YJ, Cho JY, Bok GH, Jin SY, Lee TH, Kim HG, Kim JO, Lee JS. Hybrid natural orifice transluminal endoscopic surgery: endoscopic full-thickness resection of early gastric cancer and laparoscopic regional lymph node dissection–14 human cases. Endoscopy. 2011;43(2):134–9.

Das S. Laparoscopic staging pelvic lymphadenectomy: extraperitoneal approach. Semin Surg Oncol. 1996;12(2):134–8.

Du J, Zheng J, Li Y, Li J, Ji G, Dong G, Yang Z, Wang W, Gao Z. Laparoscopy-assisted total gastrectomy with extended lymph node resection for advanced gastric cancer—reports of 82 cases. Hepatogastroenterology. 2010;57(104):1589–94.

Ehrlich PF, Friedman DL, Schwartz CL, Children Oncology Group Hodgkin Lymphoma Study Section. Monitoring diagnostic accuracy and complications. A report from the Children's Oncology Group Hodgkin lymphoma study. J Pediatr Surg. 2007;42(5): 788–91.

Fanning J, Hossler C. Laparoscopic conversion rate for uterine cancer surgical staging. Obstet Gynecol. 2010;116(6):1354–7.

Gallotta V, Fanfani F, Rossitto C, Vizzielli G, Testa A, Scambia G, Fagotti A. A randomized study comparing the use of the Ligaclip with bipolar energy to prevent lymphocele during laparoscopic pelvic lymphadenectomy for gynecologic cancer. Am J Obstet Gynecol. 2010;203(5):483.e1–6.

Guzzo TJ, Gonzalgo ML, Allaf ME. Laparoscopic retroperitoneal lymph node dissection with therapeutic intent in men with clinical stage I nonseminomatous germ cell tumors. J Endourol. 2010;24(11):1759–63.

Holub Z, Jabor A, Kliment L, Lukac J, Voracek J. Laparoscopic lymph node dissection using ultrasonically activated shears: comparison with electrosurgery. J Laparoendosc Adv Surg Tech A. 2002;12(3):175–80.

Katai H, Sasako M, Fukuda H, Nakamura K, Hiki N, Saka M, Yamaue H, Yoshikawa T, Kojima K, JCOG Gastric Cancer Surgical Study Group. Safety and feasibility of laparoscopy-assisted distal gastrectomy with suprapancreatic nodal dissection for clinical stage I gastric cancer: a multicenter phase II trial (JCOG 0703). Gastric Cancer. 2010;13(4):238–44.

Kawahara H, Watanabe K, Ushigome T, Noaki R, Kobayashi S, Yanaga K. Laparoscopy-assisted lateral pelvic lymph node dissection for advanced rectal cancer. Hepatogastroenterology. 2010;57(102–103):1136–8.

Kitagawa Y, Ohgami M, Fujii H, et al. Laparoscopic detection of sentinel lymph nodes in gastrointestinal cancer: a novel and minimally invasive approach. Ann Surg Oncol. 2001;8(9 Suppl):86S–9.

Konishi T, Kuroyanagi H, Oya M, Ueno M, Fujimoto Y, Akiyoshi T, Yoshimatsu H, Watanabe T, Yamaguchi T, Muto T. Lateral lymph node dissection with preoperative chemoradiation for locally advanced lower rectal cancer through a laparoscopic approach. Surg Endosc. 2011;25:2358–9.

Levy RM, Wizorek J, Shende M, Luketich JD. Laparoscopic and thoracoscopic esophagectomy. Adv Surg. 2010;44:101–16.

Li GX, Zhang C, Yu J, Wang YN, Hu YF. A new order of D2 lymphadenectomy in laparoscopic gastrectomy for cancer: live anatomy-based dissection. Minim Invasive Ther Allied Technol. 2010;19(6):355–63.

Park do J, Kim HH, Park YS, Lee HS, Lee WW, Lee HJ, Yang HK. Simultaneous indocyanine green and (99m)Tc-antimony sulfur colloid-guided laparoscopic sentinel basin dissection for gastric cancer. Ann Surg Oncol. 2011;18(1):160–5.

Schwartz MJ, Kavoussi LR. Controversial technology: the Chunnel and the laparoscopic retroperitoneal lymph node dissection (RPLND). BJU Int. 2010;106(7):950–9. doi:10.1111/j.1464-410X.2010.09659.x.

Shao P, Meng X, Li J, Lv Q, Zhang W, Xu Z, Yin C. Laparoscopic extended pelvic lymph node dissection during radical cystectomy: technique and clinical outcomes. BJU Int. 2010;108:124–8. doi: 10.1111/j.1464-410X.2010.09774.x.

Smith BR, Chang KJ, Lee JG, Nguyen NT. Staging accuracy of endoscopic ultrasound based on pathologic analysis after minimally invasive esophagectomy. Am Surg. 2010;76(11):1228–31.

Spirtos NM, Eisenkop SM, Schlaerth JB, Ballon SC. Laparoscopic radical hysterectomy (type III) with aortic and pelvic lymphadenectomy in patients with stage I cervical cancer: surgical morbidity and intermediate follow-up. Am J Obstet Gynecol. 2002; 187(2):340–8.

Touijer K, Fuenzalida RP, Rabbani F, Paparel P, Nogueira L, Cronin AM, Fine SW, Guillonneau B. Extending the indications and anatomical limits of pelvic lymph node dissection for prostate cancer: improved staging or increased morbidity? BJU Int. 2010;108:372–7. doi: 10.1111/j.1464-410X.2010.09877.x.

Turner BG, Gee DW, Cizginer S, Kim MC, Mino-Kenudson M, Sylla P, Brugge WR, Rattner DW. Endoscopic transesophageal mediastinal lymph node dissection and en bloc resection by using mediastinal and thoracic approaches (with video). Gastrointest Endosc. 2010;72(4):831–5.

Vasiley SA, McGonigle KF. Extraperitoneal laparoscopic para-aortic lymph node dissection. Gynecol Oncol. 1996;61(3):315–20.

# Part III
# Laparoscopic Cholecystectomy and Common Duct Exploration

# 20. Laparoscopic Cholecystectomy

*Pradeep Pallati, M.B.B.S.*
*Dmitry Oleynikov, M.D.*

## A. Indications

1. **Cholelithiasis.**
   a. **Asymptomatic cholelithiasis:**
      Asymptomatic cholelithiasis in itself is not an indication for prophylactic cholecystectomy in the general population, except in patients on chronic immunosuppression. Presence of a porcelain gallbladder, along with gallstones, is generally considered to be an indication for cholecystectomy due to the increased risk of carcinoma.
   b. **Symptomatic cholelithiasis:**
      Biliary colic and cholecystitis are relieved with laparoscopic cholecystectomy. Nonspecific symptoms such as nausea, bloating, indigestion, and flatulence are sometimes benefited by cholecystectomy.
   c. **Complicated cholelithiasis:**
      In patients with **gall stone pancreatiti**s, cholecystectomy should be performed close to discharge during the index hospitalization. **Choledocholithiasis with cholangitis**—Laparoscopic cholecystectomy is performed after the cholangitis has resolved. The common duct must be cleared of stones—generally this will have been done by ERCP as part of initial treatment; if not, laparoscopic Common Bile Duct Exploration can be performed at the time of cholecystectomy.
2. **Conditions unrelated to gallstone disease**
   a. **Acute acalculous cholecystitis**—Although laparoscopic cholecystectomy may be performed, percutaneous cholecystostomy is the management option of choice for critically ill patients.

N.J. Soper and C.E.H. Scott-Conner (eds.), *The SAGES Manual: Volume 1 Basic Laparoscopy and Endoscopy*, DOI 10.1007/978-1-4614-2344-7_20,
© Springer Science+Business Media, LLC 2012

b. **Gallbladder dyskinesia**—presenting with episodes of Right Upper Quadrant pain but no evidence of chole lithiasis and decreased ejection fraction on Hepatobiliary IminoDiacetic Acid (HIDA) scan. Although good prospective trials are lacking, there is retrospective data stating that cholecystectomy relieves symptoms in a significant number of patients.

c. **Polyps, cholesterolosis, and adenomyomatosis**—polyps larger than 1 cm in size are an indication for laparoscopic cholecystectomy. Smaller polyps may be treated by close observation. Patients with cholesterolosis and adenomyomatosis should be operated on if they have classic symptoms of biliary colic.

3. **Absolute Contraindications** for laparoscopic cholecystectomy are now very limited, as the advances in laparoscopic equipment have made it possible to perform the surgery in most patients. Relative contraindications include patients with major upper abdominal surgery, history of ascites, and coagulopathy.

# B.  Patient Position

1. Operating table should have the capability to allow fluoroscopy and to place the patient in steep reverse Trendelenburg position.
2. Position the patient supine with both arms tucked.
3. Place one monitor at the head of the patient at the level of the eye (Fig. 20.1). This way, both the surgeon and the assistant view the same monitor and good coordination is obtained.
4. Stomach is emptied with an orogastric tube, and a Foley catheter may be placed, based on the expected difficulties in the case.

# C.  Trocar Placement

1. Typically, we use four trocars (Fig. 20.2).
   a. Supraumbilical or infraumbilical 11-mm optical entry trocar. The exact location is based on the relative location of the umbilicus.
   b. Epigastric 11-mm trocar is placed based on the liver edge.

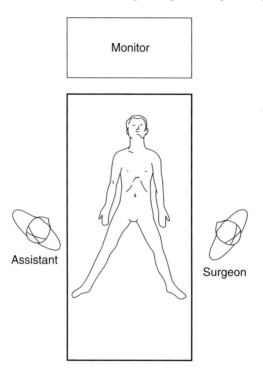

Fig. 20.1. Operating room setup.

    c.    Two additional 5-mm trocars laterally on the right side, one in midclavicular line and another in anterior axillary line.

2.    Initial access is obtained with the use of a Veress needle near the umbilicus.

    a.    Access can be modified if patient has had previous abdominal operations and if any difficulties arise.

3.    We use an optical access trocar, placed under vision near the umbilicus. Perform general laparoscopy and check the entry site of the Veress needle.

4.    Under laparoscopic guidance, place an epigastric port. We routinely place an 11-mm dilating trocar in this location, in order to be able to pass a large clip applicator.

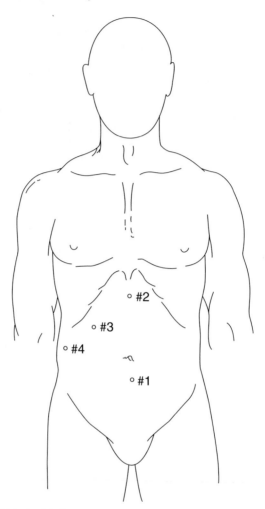

Fig. 20.2. Usual trocar sites.

5. Place two additional 5-mm trocars along the right costal margin. We usually place these trocars after identifying the liver edge and the location of the epigastric trocar. Placing the midclavicular trocar closer to epigastrium helps with the two-handed technique, while placement closer to the lateral-most trocar helps in teaching mode.

# D.  Identification of Calot's Triangle (Critical View of Safety)

1. Place the patient in reverse Trendelenburg position with right side up.
2. Dissect down any adhesions of the omentum to the gallbladder, using blunt graspers from the epigastric port site.
3. A locking grasper placed through the lateral-most trocar holds the fundus and retracts superiorly, to the right and over the liver edge.
4. Another locking grasper placed through the midclavicular port site holds the infundibulum, and retracts laterally and to the right to separate the cystic duct away from the common bile duct.
5. Next gently strip the peritoneal covering of the gallbladder obscuring Calot's triangle with the use of either blunt graspers or short bursts of electrocautery.
6. Identify the node of Calot in this location and gently separate it from the gallbladder.
7. Retraction of the infundibulum of the gallbladder to the left at this point reveals the posterior peritoneal lining, which needs to be dissected too.
8. Once the entire peritoneal lining is taken down, gently dissect the fatty tissue overlying the infundibulum, cystic duct, and cystic artery with blunt instruments.
9. Taking the peritoneal covering superiorly helps expose the cystic plate as well, and delineates the critical view of safety.
10. "Critical View of Safety" is achieved when only two structures are entering the gallbladder, and the lower part of the cystic plate is clearly visualized (Fig. 20.3).
11. Intraoperative cholangiogram can be performed at any point prior to dividing the duct, in the case of unclear anatomy or the need to rule out common bile duct stone, as explained in the following chapters.
12. Apply clips on the cystic duct at this time, with one clip very close to the infundibulum and two clips towards the common bile duct (CBD). Take care to avoid placement of the clips too close to CBD to prevent injury. Similarly, divide the cystic artery between the clips either before or after division of the cystic duct.

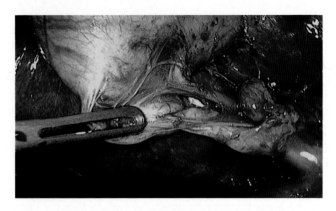

Fig. 20.3.   Critical view of safety with lymph node of Calot dissected down.

# E.  Removal of Gallbladder

1.   Use L-hook electrocautery to remove the gallbladder from the liver bed. Take care to dissect in the loose adventitial plane, with adequate traction from the grasper holding the infundibulum.

2.   After a while, the gallbladder will need to be flipped over the liver edge to clearly identify the posterior peritoneal lining close to the fundus.

3.   Before completely removing the gallbladder, make a final observation of the liver bed as well as the cystic structures, to confirm hemostasis.

4.   If the gallbladder is not severely inflamed or perforated, it can be extracted through the umbilical port site by holding the region of the cystic duct with a large grasper.

5.   In other cases, the gallbladder is placed in an endoscopic retrieval bag and extracted through the umbilical port site. Some surgeons extract the gallbladder from the epigastric port site.

# F. Difficult Situations

## 1. Difficult Fundus Retraction

a. If the gallbladder wall is severely inflamed with a thick wall and unable to grasp well, two things can help.

    i. Aspiration of bile from the gallbladder, with a long laparoscopic needle placed through one of the trocars, or a Veress needle placed though a separate incision.

    ii. If the problem is not fluid, but a large stone or contracted gallbladder, the lateral-most trocar can be upsized to a 10 mm dilating trocar, and a large claw forceps can be used to hold the gallbladder efficiently and retract well.

## 2. Inflamed and Indurated Calot's Triangle

a. In these circumstances, persistence with gentle dissection usually yields.

b. A suction irrigator can be used bluntly to delineate the structures. Use electrocautery judiciously to prevent inadvertent damage to ductal structures.

c. Liberal use of intraoperative cholangiogram in these difficult cases is very useful to avoid any injuries.

d. If the gallbladder is severely contracted and adherent to the liver bed, dissection closer to the gallbladder, even if this requires leaving the posterior wall of the gallbladder in place, is good judgment. The alternative of trying to completely remove the back wall of the gallbladder usually results in severe bleeding from the liver, and sometimes bile leaks.

## 3. Fundus First Approach

a. The fundus first technique is indicated when the triangle of Calot cannot be easily visualized, due to dense inflammation and foreshortening of the cystic duct. This procedure should be performed by experienced surgeons as the technical considerations are much more difficult.

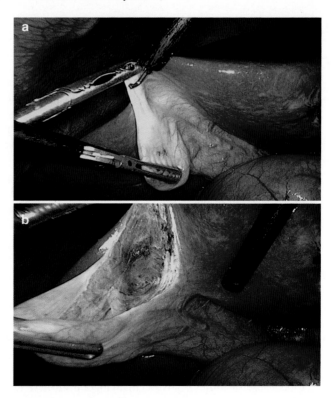

Fig. 20.4. Fundus first technique.

b.  The port placement is similar to traditional cholecystectomy
    techniques, but the assistant's job is to grab the gallbladder just
    as it meets the uppermost portion of the liver bed.
c.  In the second step, the surgeon grabs next to the assistant's
    placement on the gallbladder side and uses electrocautery to
    incise the peritoneum around the gallbladder (Fig. 20.4).
d.  Cautery is then used to carefully separate the gallbladder away
    from the liver bed, with the assistant maintaining traction on the
    gallbladder bed and remaining peritoneum. The gallbladder is
    circumferentially dissected, with the surgeon staying close to
    the gallbladder while doing the dissection circumferentially.
    Blunt dissection, as well as using a suction irrigation, may be
    necessary at this point, as this is likely an ongoing acute inflam-
    matory process and the plane may be obscured.

e. As the gallbladder is approached inferiorly, the first structure that should be identified is the cystic artery. This structure needs to be carefully dissected and divided using clips. The dissection then continues along the infundibulum of the gallbladder until no structure, other than the cystic duct, remains. This is identical to the technique used in open cholecystectomy, but needs to be carefully adhered to, as tactile sensation is not available to the laparoscopic surgeon.

f. Once the cystic duct is completely skeletonized and the cystic artery taken, the cystic duct can be traversed with clips, or in the event of thickening and inflammation, the use of an Endoloop device. The gallbladder is then removed in the standard fashion, and intraoperative cholangiogram can be helpful if anatomy needs to be further delineated.

# Acknowledgment

This chapter was contributed by Karen Deveney in the previous edition.

# Selected References

Strasberg SM, Brunt LM. Rationale and use of the critical view of safety in laparoscopic cholecystectomy. J Am Coll Surg. 2010;211(1):132–8.

Way LW, Stewart L, Gantert W, Liu K, Lee CM, Whang K, Hunter JG. Causes and prevention of laparoscopic bile duct injuries: analysis of 252 cases from a human factors and cognitive psychology perspective. Ann Surg. 2003;237(4):460–9.

# 21. Laparoscopic Cholecystectomy: Avoiding Complications

*Jessemae Welsh, M.D.*
*Joseph J. Cullen, M.D., F.A.C.S.*

## A. Introduction

Laparoscopic cholecystectomy has become the operation of choice for gallstone disease, and the incidence of complications is low. Major complications occurring during surgery or in the immediate postoperative period include hemorrhage, common bile duct injury, bile leak, iatrogenic gallbladder perforation, bowel injury, and retained bile duct stone. Risk factors leading to increased complications include acute or chronic cholecystitis, a wide and short cystic duct, previous upper abdominal surgery, obesity, anatomic variation, cirrhosis, cholecystoenteric fistula, cholangiocarcinoma, and surgeon experience. Knowledge of these common complications and risk factors may aid in prevention or early recognition of problems that may occur.

## B. Hemorrhage

### 1. Cause and Prevention

Bleeding during laparoscopic cholecystectomy can vary from inconsequential oozing to major hemorrhage.

   a.  Bleeding can occur at a trocar insertion site and blood may drip into the operative field. Obtain hemostasis in the skin before placing a trocar and avoid any obvious vessels during insertion.
   b.  Blunt dissection of adhesions from the gallbladder and liver can result in bleeding from vessels in the omentum. Cautious

use of electrocautery when dividing omental adhesions prior to applying traction on the gallbladder can be helpful in preventing this type of bleeding.

c.  Dissection in the triangle of Calot can result in sudden and often pulsatile bleeding. This may be due to an inadvertent, tangential injury to the cystic artery which can be controlled with application of clips between the source of bleeding and the artery's origin. Careful and meticulous dissection in this area with accurate identification of the cystic artery and subsequent application of clips can often avoid this complication.

d.  One of the more difficult sources of bleeding is from the gallbladder fossa. This is more frequent in the setting of acute cholecystitis. If bleeding occurs in the area between the posterior wall of the inflamed gallbladder and liver bed, it should be controlled immediately rather than waiting until the entire operative field is obscured.

## 2. Recognition and Management

a.  Trocar site bleeding typically either drips from the abdominal wall or runs down instruments to drip into the operative site. There are several strategies for dealing with this kind of bleeding. Identify and gain temporary control by angling the trocar against the abdominal wall; when the trocar is pressed against the region of the bleeding, it may slow or stop. Injecting epinephrine solution (1:10,000) in the vicinity of the bleeding site may stop the bleeding. If disposable trocars are being used, screwing in the anchoring device may compress and stop the bleeding. Finally, a suture ligature may be advanced through the abdominal wall, into the peritoneal cavity, and back out again, thus encompassing the bleeding site. Remember to reinspect the area for hemostasis at the conclusion of the case. Remove the trocar under laparoscopic visual control and watch for recurrence of bleeding.

b.  When significant, unexpected bleeding occurs in the triangle of Calot, do not apply clips blindly. Indiscriminate application of clips in this area may injure the right hepatic artery, right hepatic duct, or common bile duct. If bleeding obscures the laparoscope, remove it and clean the lens. Do not hesitate to insert an additional trocar in the midline between the epigastric and umbilical ports, to provide an extra port for manipulation. Gently pushing the gallbladder against Calot's triangle by manipulating the fundic and infundibular graspers may provide temporary hemostasis while the situation is assessed and additional trocars inserted. Irrigate and aspirate aggressively to determine the exact source of bleeding. Grasp and elevate the bleeding vessel and perform any needed additional dissection around the area. Apply clips after precise isolation of the bleeding vessel. The surgeon should have a low threshold for performing a laparotomy if bleeding continues or worsens.

c.  Bleeding from the gallbladder fossa can usually be controlled by judicious use of electrocautery. If the cautery tip tends to dig into the liver, apply the metal tip of a suction irrigator to the liver and cauterize on the suction tip instead. Multiple, small areas of bleeding in this area can be controlled by application of oxidized cellulose or topical collagen hemostatic agents.

# C. Problems Related to Gallbladder Anatomy

## 1. Cause and Prevention

a.  The tensely inflamed gallbladder often proves difficult to grasp and hold. Preliminary needle decompression is sometimes helpful. Stabilize the fundus of the gallbladder and pass a large-gauge needle percutaneously into the part of the gallbladder closest to the anterior abdominal wall. Connect the needle to suction and aspirate the contents. Close the hole with a grasping forceps or a pretied suture ligature. Some laparoscopic forceps have been designed specifically for retracting an inflamed and edematous gallbladder. An endoscopic Babcock clamp may also prove useful. Other techniques include suture placement in the gallbladder fundus for additional retraction. If the extent of inflammation makes the anatomy unclear, consider dissection in an antegrade fashion, fundus first. If anatomy still remains unclear, the surgeon should have a low threshold for conversion to an open procedure. In cases of difficult anatomy, laparoscopic subtotal cholecystectomy has been described and demonstrated to be safe in recent small retrospective series.

b.   Perforation of the gallbladder still occurs frequently in the setting of acute cholecystitis. Perforation during dissection can lead to contamination of the peritoneal cavity with potentially infected bile and gallstones. Tears in the gallbladder wall can also lead to further disruption of the wall, making subsequent dissection difficult. Needle decompression of a distended, tense gallbladder, as mentioned above, may also help minimize contamination.

c.   Gallbladders containing large stones or those with a thickened wall may also be difficult to remove from the abdominal cavity.

d.   Occult carcinoma of the gallbladder, although rare, is occasionally found in the setting of long-standing chronic cholecystitis. Trocar site recurrence has been reported when laparoscopic cholecystectomy was performed in this setting. If gallbladder carcinoma is suspected, pathologic examination may be requested specifically analyzing the gallbladder mucosa with frozen section examination of any suspicious areas. The incidence of gallbladder carcinoma is increased in elderly patients with chronic cholecystitis and those with calcifications within the wall of the gallbladder. If preoperative ultrasound is suspicious, or the patient has a calcified gallbladder, open cholecystectomy may be considered.

## 2. Recognition and Management

a.   When acute cholecystitis is encountered, partially decompress the tense, distended gallbladder by aspirating its contents through the fundus. Occlude the aspiration site by applying a grasping forceps over the opening or a pretied laparoscopic suture.

b.   If disruption of the wall has occurred with spillage, copious irrigation and suctioning can remove the majority of stones and bile, while larger stones may be placed in a laparoscopic tissue pouch and removed. Placement of closed suction catheters may be indicated for extensive bile spillage. These drainage catheters can be introduced through a lateral port. The tip of the catheter is then held in place in the subhepatic space while the cannula is removed.

c.   Gallbladders containing large stones may be placed in a retrieval bag to avoid spillage of stones if the gallbladder tears during attempted removal. Alternatively, the neck of the gallbladder may be pulled partially out of the abdomen and the stones within the gallbladder crushed and removed piecemeal. Gallbladders with thickened walls should be placed in a retrieval bag prior to removal. On rare occasion an occult carcinoma of the gallbladder will be found, and this method minimizes contamination of the trocar site. Finally, enlarging the skin and fascial incisions at the extraction site will usually suffice in completing the removal of the gallbladder from the abdomen. If the adjacent rectus muscles are not incised, enlarging the incision will add minimal additional postoperative pain or cosmetic defects.

d.  Carcinoma of the gallbladder is best recognized and dealt with at the time of the original operation. The surgeon should maintain a high index of suspicion and request frozen section examination in doubtful cases. If carcinoma of the gallbladder is identified, consider conversion to open surgery, with excision of the gallbladder bed, regional lymphadenectomy (depending upon depth of penetration), and excision of trocar sites. Implantation of carcinoma of the gallbladder has been reported to occur as rapidly as 1 week after laparoscopic cholecystectomy and is not limited to the trocar used for specimen removal.

# D.  Postoperative Bile Leakage

1.  **Cause and prevention**. Postoperative bile leaks or collections may be the result of common duct or right hepatic duct injury, cystic duct stump leakage, or injury to an accessory bile duct. Severely edematous tissues from acute cholecystitis may result in failure of standard clips to completely occlude the cystic duct, resulting in postoperative bile leak. Similarly, a short and wide cystic duct may make application of clips difficult. When dissection of the gallbladder is difficult in the setting of acute cholecystitis or when there is significant bile spillage, place a closed suction drain. This may prevent bile collections due to minor leaks from the liver bed or aid in controlling cystic duct stump leaks.

2.  **Recognition and management**. Recognition of conditions that predispose to bile leaks can help in management and avoidance of complications. If the cystic duct appears edematous and inflamed, both surgical clips and pretied laparoscopic sutures may be used to securely occlude the cystic duct. Endoscopic staplers are another option. Bile leakage from small accessory ducts in the gallbladder may not be recognized at the time of laparoscopic cholecystectomy but may be the source of a postoperative bile leak. These accessory ducts should be suspected if the gallbladder fills with contrast during intraoperative cholangiography despite occlusion of the junction of the gallbladder and cystic duct. When this filling is noted at operation, these ducts should be recognized and clipped, ligated, or coagulated. Placement of closed suction drains is also recommended in this situation. When a collection is suspected, an ultrasound or computed tomography scan of the abdomen with subsequent percutaneous drainage may establish the diagnosis and initiate treatment.

If a bile collection occurs, the biliary tree should be investigated by radionuclide scan and endoscopic retrograde cholangiopancreatography (ERCP). ERCP is useful in both the diagnosis and treatment. Cholangiography often demonstrates extravasation from the cystic duct stump. When a leak is noted, treatment consists of decreasing the pressure of the common bile duct by placing a nasobiliary drain or transpapillary stent, or by, endoscopic sphincterotomy. All these methods decrease the pressure in the duct and allow rapid closure in cases of both cystic duct stump leaks and accessory bile duct leaks. Early investigation of bile leaks with ERCP also allows prompt diagnosis of bile duct injury, facilitating early repair and increasing the chance of long-term success.

# E.  Bile Duct Injury

1.  Cause and prevention. Injury to the ductal system usually occurs during the dissection at the triangle of Calot while exposing the cystic duct. Cephalad traction will often cause the cystic duct to lie parallel with the common bile duct, allowing the common

duct to be mistaken for the cystic duct. To prevent this from happening, the infundibulum of the gallbladder should be retracted laterally to fully expose the cystic duct and gallbladder from the common duct.

Excessive retraction of the gallbladder when the clips are applied to the proximal cystic duct may result in trapping a portion of the common duct in the clips which can be avoided by leaving a longer cystic duct remnant. Dissecting the cystic duct from the infundibulum of the gallbladder downward, incising the medial and lateral peritoneal attachments of the infundibulum to the liver, while removing all connective tissue and fat to clearly expose the junction of the cystic duct with the gallbladder allows identification of these structures. Avoid excessive use of electrocautery in the triangle of Calot, which may lead to late injury and strictures to the ductal system. Intraoperative cholangiography may outline the biliary anatomy and likely facilitates intraoperative detection of bile duct injuries, but does not prevent major ductal injuries.

2.  **Recognition and management**. Major injuries to the ductal system may be noted with continued dissection as bile leaks into the operative field, or later, when the patient presents with jaundice or an intra-abdominal bile collection.

    When such injuries are recognized at operation, conversion to laparotomy is advised. If a significant portion of the ductal system has been excised, reconstruction with a hepaticojejunostomy is indicated. When only a small choledochotomy has been made, reconstruction over a T-tube may be attempted. A clean transection without tissue loss may require a ductal anastomosis over a T-tube. Patients with injury to the biliary system recognized several days later need cholangiography to adequately define the injury. If cholangiography reveals total occlusion or transection of the ductal system, immediate operative repair, usually by hepaticojejunostomy, is indicated. Repair of injured bile ducts should be done only by individuals with extensive experience in biliary surgery, preferentially in a tertiary center, to optimize outcomes. Injuries to the lateral wall of the common duct may be treated with external drainage of any intra-abdominal collections and biliary stenting.

# Selected References

Duca S, Bala O, Al-Hajjar N, et al. Laparoscopic cholecystectomy: incidents and complications. A retrospective analysis of 9542 consecutive laparoscopic operations. HPB.
2003;5(3):152–8.

Khan MH, Howard TJ, Fogel EL, et al. Frequency of biliary complications after laparoscopic cholecystectomy detected by ERCP: experience at a large tertiary referral
center. Gastrointest Endosc. 2007;65(2):247–52.

Rosenberg J, Bisgaard T. The difficult gallbladder: technical tips for laparoscopic cholecystectomy. Surg Laparosc Endosc Percutan Tech. 2000;10(4):249–52.

Singhai T, Balakrishnan S, Hussain A, et al. Laparoscopic subtotal cholecystectomy: initial
experience with laparoscopic management of difficult cholecystitis. Surgeon.
2009;7(5):263–8.

# 22. Cholangiography*

*Rahul Gupta, M.B.B.S., M.S., D.N.B.*
*Daniel B. Jones, M.D., M.S.*
*Mark P. Callery, M.D.*

## A. Introduction

Cholangiography is a special imaging procedure for outlining the major bile ducts by direct instillation of radiopaque contrast material. Mirrizi reported the first static portable operative cholangiogram in 1931. Berci and Steckell introduced portable C-arm fluoroscopy in 1970s. Since then multiple modalities such as ERCP, MRCP, and laparoscopic ultrasound have been developed for assessment of CBD, which complement operative cholangiography.

Operative cholangiography is mainly undertaken to delineate the biliary anatomy and to evaluate the common bile duct for filling defects, obstruction (pathologic or iatrogenic), or contrast extravasation indicative of injury.

## B. Routine Intraoperative Cholangiography Versus Selective Operative Cholangiography

Cholangiography may be performed routinely (in virtually every case) or selectively. This section summarizes arguments on each side of the debate although SAGES Guidelines state that intraoperative cholangiography diminishes the risk of bile duct injury, when used routinely.

---

*This chapter was contributed by George Berci, MD in the previous edition.

N.J. Soper and C.E.H. Scott-Conner (eds.), *The SAGES Manual: Volume 1 Basic Laparoscopy and Endoscopy*, DOI 10.1007/978-1-4614-2344-7_22, © Springer Science+Business Media, LLC 2012

## 1. Benefits of Routine Cholangiography

Benefits of routine cholangiography have been detailed by Berci, G in the second edition of SAGES Manual. These include the following:

a.   Defining biliary anatomy and recognition of anomalies and thus decreasing the incidence of common bile duct injury. The argument also states that it is impossible to predict who is at higher risk of CBD injury and thus making IOC safer practice.

b.   Discovery of common bile duct injuries allows intraoperative repair and potentially superior outcomes.

c.   Diagnosis missed CBD stones allow the surgeon to manage these stones intraoperatively.

d.   Eliminates the need for preoperative ERCP.

The diversity of anomalies and intraoperative hazards that may be detected by Routine IOC is shown in Figs. 22.1–22.4.

## 2. Selective Cholangiography

Selective cholangiography is performed for a specific indication as appreciated in the pre and perioperative period (Table 22.1).

Several studies have shown benefits from this approach, including the following:

a.   The incidence of missed stones is relatively small (4%), and only a small percentage (15%) of these will be clinically relevant in the postoperative period.

b.   Reduction of expense and operative time associated with routine intraoperative cholangiography given large number of cholecystectomies performed in a year.

c.   Intraoperative cholangiography does not prevent CBD injuries but merely facilitates early detection of these injuries.

d.   False positive results lead to negative duct explorations. Misinterpretation of cholangiogram can be limited by direct communication with the radiologist.

e.   Common bile duct exploration by laparoscopic or open choledochotomy is a more morbid procedure than ERCP for CBD stones. The management of T tube which is left in situ compounds postoperative morbidity. The inflammation surrounding the T tube renders any reoperative procedure exponentially more difficult as compared to ERCP and stone extraction.

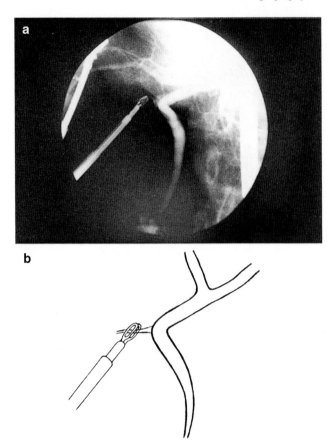

Fig. 22.1. (**a**) Slight traction on the cholangiograsper can tent the common duct, especially if the cystic duct is very short. In the two-dimensional view seen on the monitor, the common duct may be misinterpreted as the cystic duct and transected. The length of the cholangiograsper jaws is 10 mm. (**b**) Schematic diagram of cholangiogram seen in (**a**). It is very important to recognize the short cystic duct.

f.  Hartmann's pouch–cystic duct junction dissection (Gallbladder down) as compared to cystic duct–CBD confluence (Calot's triangle focused dissection) ameliorates the necessity to identify anatomical variations in the biliary system.

g.  Laparoscopic ultrasound of CBD and MRCP have remarkable sensitivity and specificity in diagnosing CBD stones. Routine availability and reduction in expense are expected to change the dynamics of intraoperative cholangiogram.

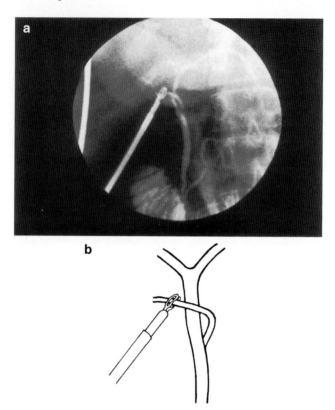

Fig. 22.2. (**a**) Very close spiral drainage of cystic duct into the common duct. (**b**) Schematic diagram of cholangiogram.

## C.  Techniques of Performing Intraoperative Cholangiography

Intraoperative cholangiography is most commonly performed by cannulating the cystic duct. When this is difficult or impossible, it may be possible to obtain a cholangiogram by instilling contrast directly into the gallbladder. Both techniques are described here.

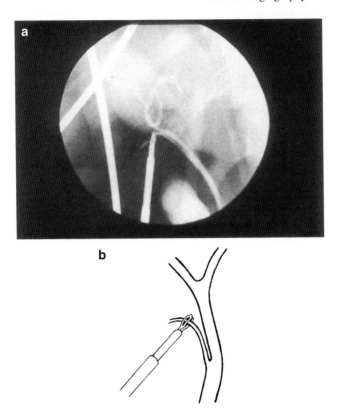

Fig. 22.3. (**a**) Close parallel run of cystic duct and common duct. Note how close the cholangiograsper jaw is to the common hepatic duct. (**b**) Schematic diagram of cholangiogram. The cholangiograsper jaw is 10 mm long; this gives some hint of distances and proximities.

## 1. Cystic Duct Cholangiography (Fig. 22.5)

### a. Selection of Catheter or Instrumentation

The final selection is typically made after the cystic duct has been dissected and isolated.

- Balloon tipped catheter—helpful if the duct is transected and in dilating the duct for manipulation and choledochoscopy.
- Taut Catheter (Taut Inc., Geneva, IL).
- Stiff Ureteral catheter.
- Curved tip catheter—Kaplan arrow cholangiogram catheter.

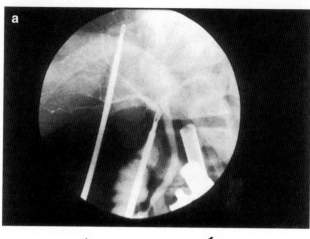

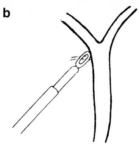

Fig. 22.4. (**a**) Dangerously short cystic duct draining directly into right hepatic duct. (**b**) Schematic drawing of cholangiogram.

Table 22.1. Indications of selective intraoperative cholangiography

| Preoperative indications | History | • Acholic stools |
|---|---|---|
| | | • Icterus |
| | | • Pancreatitis |
| | | • Cholangitis |
| | Ultrasound | • Dilated common bile duct |
| | Biochemical | • Elevated bilirubin |
| | | • Elevated alkaline phosphatase |
| | Anatomy which precludes ERCP | • Previous surgery—RYGB |
| | | • Duodenal diverticulum |
| Intraoperative indications | • Dilated bile duct | • Cystic duct >5 mm |
| | • Stones or sludge in cystic or bile duct | • Common duct >10 mm |
| | • Unclear anatomy | |
| | • Suspected bile duct injury | |

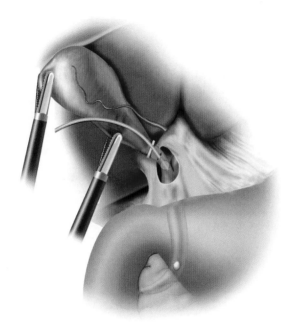

Fig. 22.5. Cartoon showing intraoperative cholangiogram using a balloon tipped catheter. Illustration reprinted with permission from Atlas of Minimally Invasive Surgery, Jones et al. Cine-Med © 2006.

- Butterfly needle (wings clipped)—may be utilized for common duct cholangiogram or blind stick cholangiogram. It is beneficial in extremely difficult cases with frozen Calot triangles, severely contracted gallbladder and in suspected Mirrizi syndrome (Cholecystocholedochal fistula).
- Infant feeding tube.
- Kumar's clamp (Nashville surgical instruments, Springfield, TN) for Cholecystocholangiogram.
- Olsen Cholangiogram fixation clamp (Karl Storz Endoscopy, Culver city, CA) (Figs. 22.6 and 22.7).

## b. Abdominal Access Selection

Select the port site with the most direct access to the cystic duct. This is also vital for choledochoscopy and Dormia basket stone extraction. The site can be used for placement of T tube and is helpful in percutaneous retrieval of stones in the postoperative period.

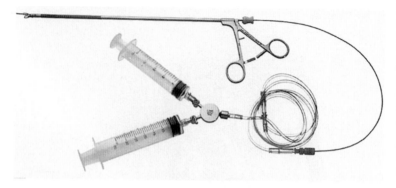

Fig. 22.6. Cholangiograsper with 4-Fr ureteral catheter inserted, extension tubing, Y-shaped adapter, and two syringes of different sizes (Karl Storz, Endoscopy-America, Culver City, CA).

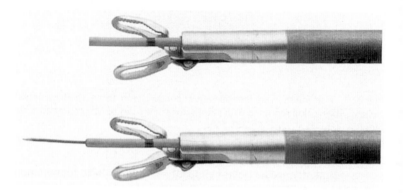

Fig. 22.7. Cholangiograsper seen in close-up with protruding ureteral catheter (*top*). In case of difficult introduction, a guide wire is advanced and introduced into the cystic duct, followed by the catheter (*bottom*).

A Separate incision may be required at times to provide most undeviating access. The best location will generally be subcostal, in the midclavicular line.

### c. Cystic Duct Dissection, Isolation, and Cannulation

Meticulously dissect Hartmann's pouch and the cystic duct junction. It is essential to visualize the cystic duct entry into the gallbladder. Place a clip or ligature at the junction of cystic duct and gallbladder.

Select a cholangiocatheter (4 or 5 Fr, depending on the size of cystic duct). Connect the catheter through a Y or a three-way stop cock system to saline and contrast. It is convenient to add a short length of extension IV tubing. This augments one's flexibility during the contrast injection/imaging.

Make a small incision on the anterolateral aspect of cystic duct and milk the duct retrograde with the help of flat grasper to unclog any sludge or small stones. Clear flow of bile indicates unobstructed passage into the common duct.

Insert the cholangiography grasper with catheter into the peritoneal cavity. Arranging the system in a way that the catheter protrudes only about 1 cm from the grasper aids in controlling the tip for insertion. Mild counter traction will help negotiate the catheter although excessive counter traction may occlude the lumen and make it more difficult. Slide the cholangiograsper coaxially over the catheter to ensure a tight seal. Saline may be injected to confirm an airtight seal. Do not introduce more than 1–2 cm of the catheter into the cystic duct. The aim is to instill the dye into the cystic duct and then follow its progress through the CBD. If too much catheter is inserted, the cystic duct–common duct junction will not be well visualized. Remove all radiopaque objects from the field.

### d. Contrast Selection and Dilution

Contrast medium diluted to a concentration of 45% gives optimum results. Concentrated contrast demonstrates the anatomy better but may shield small calculi within the densely radiopaque dye column, while diluted contrast displays the reverse.

### e. Operating Table Position and Fluoroscopy Equipment

A tube potential of 100–110 kV provides the best images for cholangiogram.

Fluoroscopy delivers real-time imaging for surgeons to evaluate for CBD abnormalities. The functional flow is visible and study may be repeated conveniently. Cholangiograms are conducted with the patient in 15° Trendelenberg (allows for superior filling of proximal ducts) and depressing the right side (avoid overlap of cholangiographic images with the vertebrae).

### f. Injection of Contrast

Ensure exclusion of all air bubbles from the system. Flushing saline through the catheter and then retrograde into the contrast syringe by obstructing forward flow should ensure a bubble free system.

A check image is performed to center the field and to confirm unobstructed images. In a normal caliber system, 10–15 ml of contrast is adequate.

g. Interpretation

Inspect the films (or fluoroscopic image) for the following:

   i.   The length of cystic duct and location of its junction with the CBD.
   ii.  The size of the CBD.
   iii. The presence of intraluminal filling defects.
   iv.  Free flow of contrast into the duodenum.
   v.   Anatomy of the extra hepatic and intrahepatic biliary tree. The cholangiogram should confirm drainage of all segments of liver. Non filling of a particular segment or sector should raise a red flag as to potential variation in drainage of that segment.

h. Drugs Influencing Sphincter of Oddi Function

   i.   Morphine causes spasm of sphincter of Oddi (SO) in a complex manner not completely understood at present. In a study in human subjects Morphine was administered in four successive doses of 2.5, 2.5, 5, and 10 µg/kg IV at 5-min intervals. Morphine in subanalgesic doses increased the frequency of SO phasic pressure waves to a maximum of 10–12/min, caused the phasic waves to occur simultaneously along the sphincter segment, increased phasic wave amplitude from 72 to 136 mmHg, and increased SO basal pressure from 10 to 29 mmHg ($p$ less than 0.05). The response is directly proportional to the amount of drug administered. Morphine administration improves filling and delineation of proximal ducts and is more pronounced in patients with floppy sphincter of Oddi.
   ii.  Glucagon is a smooth muscle relaxant and has an intense hypotonic action, counteracts spasm of sphincter of Oddi, and decreases the resistance of biliary tree. It has a consistent and rapid onset of action, the effect of short duration, and there are relatively few side effects. This makes it potentially useful in every type of cholangiographic examination. The standard dose is 1 mg of 0.1% glucagon hydrochloride. Forward flow is augmented by glucagon, and this clarifies the visualization of obstructing lesions in the distal system.

## 2. Modification of Technique Under Special Circumstances

### a. Inability to Cannulate the Cystic Duct

   i. **Spiral valves of Heister**

      Inability to cannulate the cystic duct can be overcome by passing the guide wire and then threading the catheter over the guide wire. Alternatively, infuse saline while inserting to distend the duct.

   ii. **Cystic duct obstruction due to pathology or impacted stone**. In such a situation, alternate methods of common bile duct evaluation should be considered.

Direct needle access to CBD using percutaneous spinal needle or butterfly needle.

Intraoperative ultrasound (see Chap. 23).

### b. Flaccid Sphincter

During operative cholangiography, the proximal biliary system must fill retrograde, and a flaccid sphincter may allow too rapid passage of dye into the duodenum. Placing the patient in Trendelenberg position or injection of morphine may help. Alternatively after evaluation of the distal system a blunt occlusive grasper may be used to delineate the proximal system.

### c. Abnormal Appearance of the Sphincter

Use the magnification function to observe the sphincter in greater detail (be sufficiently familiar with the equipment to do this!) and observe the sphincter for 5 or 10 s. By watching for sphincter motion a "pseudo-calculus" may disappear (Fig. 22.8).

### d. Rounded Lucency: Bubble Versus Stone

Inject contrast and then withdraw the plunger to create vacuum. Air bubbles tend to move back and forth synchronously as compared to stones, which are generally impacted. Air bubbles tend to be spherical in contrast to stones, which rarely have a perfect outline.

Alternately flush the CBD with saline for contrast to wash out and then repeat the procedure.

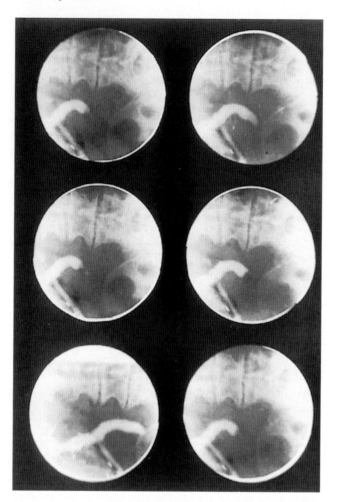

Fig. 22.8. Sphincter function during the opening and closing cycles. The thumb-print configuration shown in middle figures can easily be misinterpreted as a stone. By observing the sphincter for a few seconds longer, one can easily see the opening and closing of the sphincter and interpret the image correct.

e. Overfilled System

Too much contrast on the film creates difficulties in interpretation. Wash out the duct with warm saline (to avoid sphincter spasm) and then do another cholangiogram (Fig. 22.9).

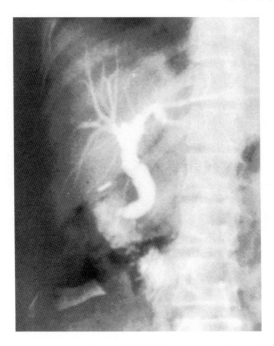

Fig. 22.9. The ductal system is overfilled with contrast and no early filling stage is seen. The cystic duct drainage into the common duct is obscured by excess contrast.

## f. Danger Signs

The surgeon should be able to recognize certain radiographic danger signs, which might warrant immediate exploration:

    i.    Contrast material is seen in the distal CBD below the cystic duct but contrast extravasation is observed above this site. This may indicate a transection of the common hepatic duct (Fig. 22.10).

    ii.   The distal duct is well filled with contrast, but there is no filling of the proximal system. If these images do not change with repeated injection and with maneuvers described previously, there may be an obstructing clip on the common hepatic duct. It may be visible on fluoroscopy. (Fig. 22.11).

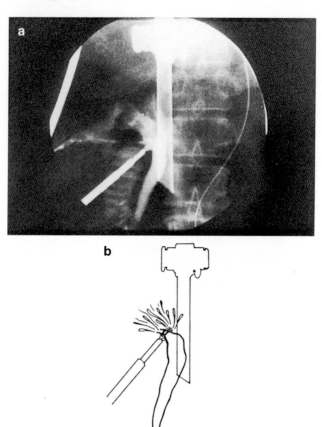

Fig. 22.10. (**a**) The distal duct is well seen, but there is obvious extravasation of dye proximal. The duct was found to be transected. (**b**) Schematic diagram of cholangiogram.

## 3. Cholecystocholangiogram (Fig. 22.12)

When it is not possible to access the cystic or common duct for any of the techniques described above, it may still be possible to produce a cholangiogram by injecting contrast directly into the gallbladder. Place the patient in Trendelenberg position and right side down to prevent the gallbladder from falling medially and to prevent overlap of the biliary tree and vertebrae shadows. Introduce a 5 mm atraumatic long grasper

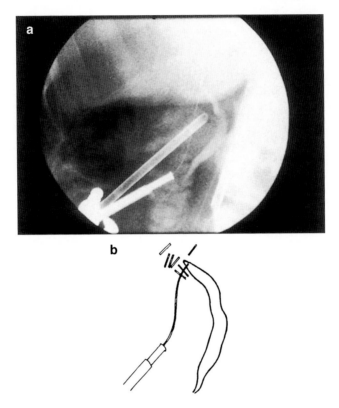

Fig. 22.11. (a) Distal duct is visible, but no contrast material is seen in the proximal duct. If the proximal duct cannot be filled with contrast, consider conversion to open procedure. (b) Schematic diagram of cholangiogram.

and clamp the gallbladder just above the infundibulum. Stick the gall bladder with Veress needle or cholangiogram catheter. A larger volume of contrast is required to perform cholangiogram, and it may be necessary to dissect the gallbladder from hepatic bed in order to elevate the gall bladder for absolute occlusion.

The advantages of this technique include defining the anatomy before Calot's triangle dissection. Disadvantages include higher failure rate due to obstructed cystic duct or scarred valves of Heister.

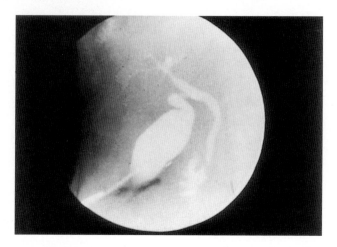

Fig. 22.12. Cholecystocholangiogram. In the difficult case, direct puncture of the gallbladder with contrast injection can display the anatomy. In this example, the cystic duct drains directly into the common hepatic duct.

# D.  Complications of Intraoperative Cholangiography

1.   The process of dissecting around the ducts or introducing the catheter may produce a common bile duct injury.
2.   Injection of contrast under pressure induces biliovenous reflux, which may precipitate a septic response in an infected system.
3.   Pancreatitis, although rare, has been reported.
4.   Allergic reaction to contrast.

## Selected References

Berci G, Steckell R. Modern radiology in the operating room. Arch Surg. 1973;161: 355–60.

Berci G. Laparoscopic cholecystectomy: cholangiography. In: Scott-Connor CEH, editor. The SAGES manual, fundamentals of laparoscopy, thoracosopy and GI endoscopy. 2nd ed. New York: Springer; 2006. p. 145–64.

Birth M, Carroll BJ, Delinikolas K, et al. Recognition of laparoscopic bile duct injuries by intraoperative ultrasonography. Surg Endosc. 1996;10:794–7.

Flum DR, Dellinger EP, Cheadle A, et al. Intraoperative cholangiography and risk of common bile duct injury during cholecystectomy. JAMA. 2003;289:1639–44.

Helm JF, Venu RP, Geenen JE, Hogan WJ, Dodds WJ, Toouli J, et al. Effects of morphine on the human sphincter of oddi. Gut. 1988;29(10):1402–7.

Holzman MD, Holcomb GW, Frexes-steed M, Richards WO. An alternative technique for laparoscopic cholangiography. Surg Endosc. 1994;8:927–30.

Jones DB, Dunnegan DL, Soper NJ. Results of a change to routine fluorocholangiography during laparoscopic cholecystectomy. Surgery. 1995;118(4):693–702.

Jones DB, Maithel S, Schneider B. Atlas of minimally invasive surgery. CT: Cine Med Publishing; 2006.

Ludwig K, Bernhardt J, Steffen H, Lorenz D. Contribution of intraoperative cholangiography to incidence and outcome of common bile duct injuries during laparoscopic cholecystectomy. Surg Endosc. 2002;16:1098–104.

Lundstrom B, Rydh A, Wickman G. Experimental evaluation of tube potential and contrast medium concentration for cholangiography. Acta Radiol Diagn (Stockh). 1976;17(3): 353–60.

Machi J, Tateishi T, Oishi AJ, et al. Laparoscopic ultrasonography versus operative cholangiography during laparoscopic cholecystectomy: review of the literature and a comparison with open intraoperative ultrasonography. J Am Coll Surg. 1999;188:360–7.

Metcalfe MS, Ong T, Bruening MH, et al. Is laparoscopic intraoperative cholangiogram a matter of routine? Am J Surg. 2004;187:475–81.

Mirrizi PL. Operative cholangiography. Surg Gynecol Obstet. 1937;65:702–10.

Overby DW, Apelgren KN, Richardson W. SAGES guidelines for the clinical application of laparoscopic biliary tract surgery. Surg Endosc. 2010;24:2368–86.

Ponsky PL. Laparoscopic biliary surgery: will we ever learn. Surg Endosc. 2010;24:2367.

Snow LL, Weinstein LS, Hannon JK, Lane DR. Evaluation of operative cholangiography in 2043 patients undergoing laparoscopic cholecystectomy. A case for selective operative cholangiogram. Surg Endosc. 2001;15(1):14–20.

Soper NJ, Brunt LM. The case for routine operative cholangiography during laparoscopic cholecystectomy. Surg Clin North Am. 1994;74:953–9.

Soper NJ. Intraoperative detection: intraoperative cholangiography vs. intraoperative ultrasonography. J Gastrointest Surg. 2000;4:334–5.

Way LW, Stewart L, Gantert W, et al. Causes and prevention of laparoscopic bile duct injuries: analysis of 252 cases from a human factors and cognitive psychology perspective. Ann Surg. 2003;237:460–9.

Z'Graggen K, Wehrli H, Metzger A, et al. Complications of laparoscopic cholecystectomy in Switzerland. A prospective 3-year study of 10,174 patients. Swiss Association of Laparoscopic and Thoracoscopic Surgery. Surg Endosc. 1998;12:1303–10.

# 23. Laparoscopic Ultrasound of the Biliary Tree

*Michael Lalla, M.D.*
*Maurice E. Arregui, M.D.*

## A. Introduction

Laparoscopic ultrasound (LUS) is a safe, effective, sensitive, and specific technique for detecting stones in the common bile duct (CBD) during laparoscopic cholecystectomy. It is quicker to perform than cholangiography and is a non-invasive method of preventing and determining CBD injury. It can also be useful in other circumstances such as evaluating unexpected anatomy or masses during laparoscopic cholecystectomy, and in the laparoscopic staging of pancreatic cancer, cholangiocarcinoma or other malignancies. This chapter demonstrates a technique for LUS and teaches the reader how to identify the common duct and surrounding structures aided by color Doppler. We give examples of pathology found in the biliary tree and surrounding structures (lymph nodes, pancreas, liver, etc.) which may be encountered during LUS of the biliary tree.

## B. Indications for LUS in Cholecystectomy

1. Detecting choledocholithiasis
2. Detecting bile duct injury
3. Difficult or ambiguous anatomy
4. Unsuspected mass

N.J. Soper and C.E.H. Scott-Conner (eds.), *The SAGES Manual: Volume 1 Basic Laparoscopy and Endoscopy*, DOI 10.1007/978-1-4614-2344-7_23,
© Springer Science+Business Media, LLC 2012

# C.  Equipment

High-frequency probes in the 7- to 10-MHz range using solid state linear array transducers are optimal. The probes are available in the 3–7.5 and 5–10 MHz ranges. Initially, there is a steep learning curve to be overcome as LUS is operator dependent. Color Doppler is helpful—though not required—to differentiate the CBD from the other structures especially for the novice. It largely becomes superfluous for the experienced sonographer.

# D.  Technique

1.  Dissect the cystic duct.
2.  Ligate or clip the cystic duct before performing LUS but do not transect until after LUS.
3.  Check the probe to determine the orientation of the image on the ultrasound screen and compare it to the position of the laparoscopic probe such that cephalad on the probe is on the left of the screen and caudad is on right, or if the probe is in the transverse position, the right side of the patient should be on the left of the screen as if looking at a CT.
4.  Pass a 5-mm laparoscope through a right upper quadrant port and use it to visualize placement of the ultrasound probe (passed through the 10-mm umbilical port).
5.  Place the probe on segment 4B of the liver (Fig. 23.1). Visualize the gallbladder to look at wall thickness and for stones or masses. Obtain a longitudinal view of the biliary tree and portal structures (Fig. 23.2). Rotate the probe or move it left to right in order to delineate the branches of the hepatic duct and the portal vein. Use higher frequencies to delineate the structures closer to the probe, and lower frequencies for deeper structures. Manipulate contrast and gain to improve the image quality.
6.  Place the probe on the porta hepatis with the tip in the liver hilum (Fig. 23.3). You should be able to identify the majority of structures on Figure 23.4 through this view. Stones may be seen in the cystic duct or CBD as a hyperechoic mass with an acoustic shadow—an artifact seen in ultrasound imaging in which an intensely hyperechogenic line appears at the surface of structures which block the passage of sound waves. The shadow is

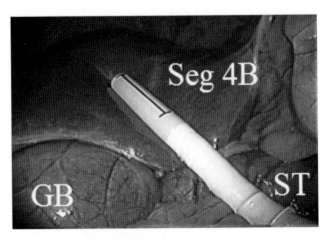

Fig. 23.1. Laparoscopic ultrasound probe on segment 4B of the liver (Seg 4B) with the gallbladder (GB) and stomach (ST) in view.

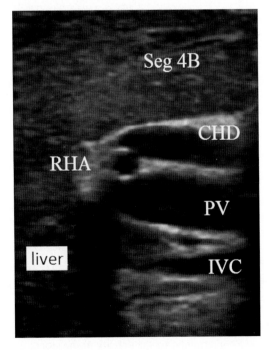

Fig. 23.2. Ultrasound image shows the liver, common hepatic duct (CHD), right hepatic artery (RHA), portal vein (PV), and Inferior vena cava (IVC).

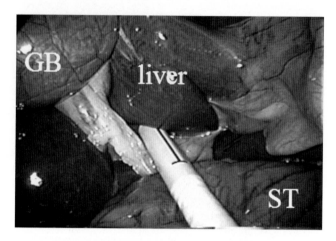

Fig. 23.3. Laparoscopic ultrasound probe on porta hepatis with stomach (ST) and gallbladder (GB) visualized.

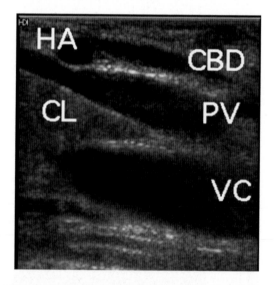

Fig. 23.4. Ultrasound view from porta hepatis with common bile duct (CBD), hepatic artery (HA), portal vein (PV), inferior vena cava (VC), and caudate lobe of the liver (CL).

cast by the stone and the degree of reflection of the ultrasound waves is determined by the density of the stone; the greater the density, the more intense the shadow formed (Fig. 23.5). For the novice sonographer, color Doppler can assist in identifying

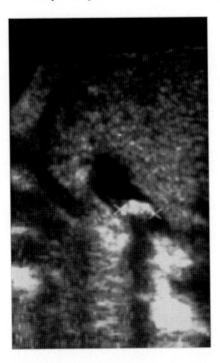

Fig. 23.5.  Hyperechoic stone in the common bile duct.

the bile ducts. There is no flow in the biliary system, while flow
will be seen in the portal vein and hepatic artery. Flow is seen as
either a blue or red color with red depicting flow towards the
transducer and blue away from the transducer. The cystic duct
common duct junction can be identified (Figs. 23.6 and 23.7),
but the key is to be able to follow the CBD from the confluence
of the right and left hepatic ducts to the ampulla to ensure that
the CBD is intact and that there are no CBD stones.

7.   The probe can then be manipulated to give a transverse view
     (Fig. 23.8) at the liver hilum. Here, the traditional "Mickey
     Mouse" view is seen with the CBD as the right ear, the hepatic
     artery as the left ear and the portal vein as the face. Follow the
     common duct from the hilum down to the Papilla using the
     transverse view (Fig. 23.9). Use the duodenum as an acoustic
     window to visualize the CBD as is traverses behind the duode-
     num and into the pancreas (Fig. 23.10). The distal CBD is the
     most common area to find stones.

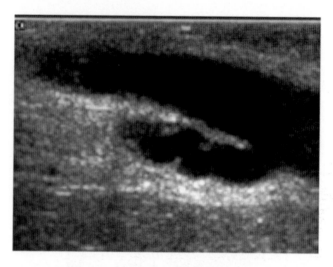

Fig. 23.6. Common hepatic duct, common bile duct, and cystic duct confluence.

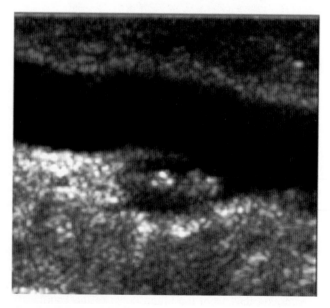

Fig. 23.7. Common hepatic duct, common bile duct, and cystic duct confluence with stones and sludge in the cystic duct.

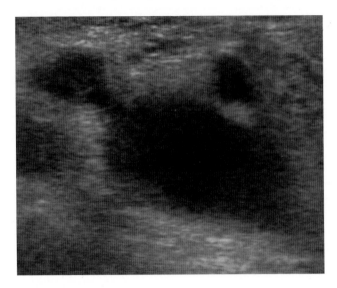

Fig. 23.8. "Mickey mouse" view: the common bile duct as the right ear, the hepatic artery as the left ear and the portal vein as the face.

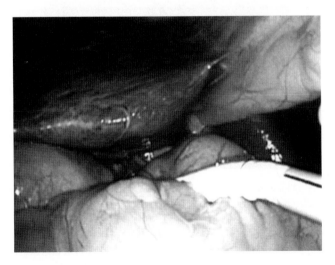

Fig. 23.9. Laparoscopic ultrasound probe on the duodenum using it as an acoustic window to show a transverse view of the porta on the ultrasound screen. The probe is depicted here between the omentum and the duodenum.

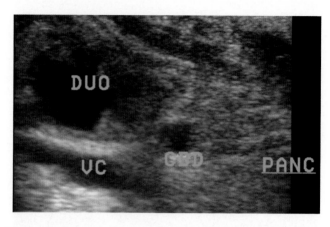

Fig. 23.10. Duodenal acoustic window shows duodenum (duo), common bile duct (CBD), pancreas (panc), and inferior vena cava (VC).

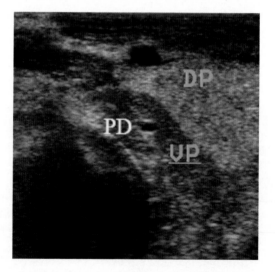

Fig. 23.11. Duodenal acoustic window shows pancreatic duct (PD), ventral pancreas (VP), and dorsal pancreas (DP).

8.  The head of the pancreas, pancreatic duct, ventral and dorsal pancreas may be visualized (Fig. 23.11). The ability to visualize these structures depends on the use of the duodenum as an acoustic window and the amount of fat in the surrounding tissue since fat

causes acoustic impedance. Acoustic impedance is the absorption of sound waves preventing penetration and visualization. The duodenum does not have a lot of fat and can be compressed lightly to remove any air allowing penetration of the ultrasound waves to the underlying ducts. The CBD can be followed transversely until it joins the pancreatic duct near or at the ampulla.

# E. Benefits

1. LUS has only the one-time cost of the ultrasound machine and probe. There is no requirement for a radiologist, technician, lead shields, or special operative table as with fluoroscopy.
2. There is no radiation.
3. Although user dependent, it may be used on "normal" anatomy to gain experience and as such allows for the identification of abnormal anatomy. Malignancy can be detected in the asymptomatic patient in surrounding structures such as the pancreas and liver.
4. There is virtually no contraindication to ultrasound.
5. Most bile duct injuries are caused by imprecise dissection and poor visualization of the anatomy. Simultaneous comparison of the laparoscopic and ultrasound images allows better mental imagery of the biliary ductal system and more precise localization of the CBD, thereby preventing injury. LUS may be performed even before dissection has taken place and may be repeated with reproducible images in real time if there is any doubt—aiding dissection in especially difficult patients. The structures can also be viewed from many different planes. After the dissected duct is ligated or clipped, LUS can be performed again to ensure that the CBD is not the ligated duct, thereby preventing transection of the CBD. Intraoperative cholangiogram (IOC) can investigate if the CBD has been clipped or damaged but cannot help prevent this from happening.
6. There is no risk of cystic duct or common duct injury during LUS, since the duct is not incised as in an IOC. The cystic duct common duct junction can be seen in 94% of patients.
7. LUS is as reliable as IOC in detecting choledocholithiasis.
8. In experienced hands, minimal intraoperative time is used.
9. LUS can be performed on patients with contrast allergies.

# F. Limitations

1.  The LUS probe is not available at all institutions.
2.  Results are user dependant. There is a steep learning curve.
3.  Air in the duodenum, a fatty pancreas or inflammatory tissue in acute cholecystitis can impede transmission of the sound waves thus impeding visualization of the CBD. Hence, an acoustic window through the bowel may be needed to see the ampulla, pancreas, and distal CBD. Right upper quadrant adhesions can impede the movement of the probe and render certain probe positions difficult to obtain.
4.  Incomplete visualization of the distal CBD is the major cause of false negative results. Fat causes acoustic impedence and identifying the distal CBD may be difficult in the obese. Artifacts (reverberation, mirror image) may prevent clear images. Reverberation occurs when the ultrasound wave reflects back and forth between a structure and the transducer. It is seen as "rings" or a "comet tail" behind the structure. A mirror image is caused by reflection of the ultrasound wave by a highly reflective surface (e.g., diaphragm) causing a mirror image across the reflective surface. If the diaphragm is the surface, the image of the liver will be seen across both sides of the diaphragm (which will appear intensely hyperechoic (white) on the screen). Small CBDs and the distal CBD are not always seen clearly.
5.  Calcifications in the pancreas in patients with a history of pancreatitis may cause false positive results for bile duct stones.
6.  IOC gives an excellent radiographic view of biliary anatomy and can be used to verify choledocholithiasis seen on LUS. IOC can also identify bile leaks which may not be seen with LUS.

# G. Pregnancy

LUS involves no radiation and in pregnancy is an effective tool in determining choledocholithiasis and the need for further intervention.

# H. Other Pathology

During LUS of the biliary tree, abnormalities can be discovered in the gallbladder, liver, pancreas and surrounding tissues. Normal common anatomical variants can be visualized to aid in operative planning (Fig. 23.12). The bile ducts and gallbladder may show stones or thickening, and polyps can be seen emanating from the gallbladder wall (Figs. 23.13–23.18) The liver may have cysts, tumors or metastasis (Figs. 23.19–23.24). The pancreas as well may have cysts or tumors, and stents can be visualized when placed in the ducts (Figs. 23.25 and 23.26). Enlarged lymph nodes can be seen (Fig. 23.27).

# I. Adopting LUS in General Surgery

Surgeons should try to master both LUS and intraoperative ultrasound initially then perform both IOC and LUS in order to validate their findings before replacing the use of IOC with LUS. Performing LUS on

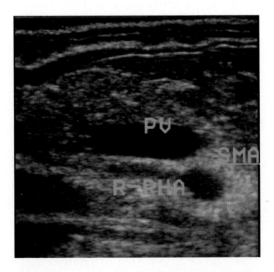

Fig. 23.12. Image of a replaced right hepatic artery (R-RHA) coming off the superior mesenteric artery (SMA) with portal vein (PV) visualized.

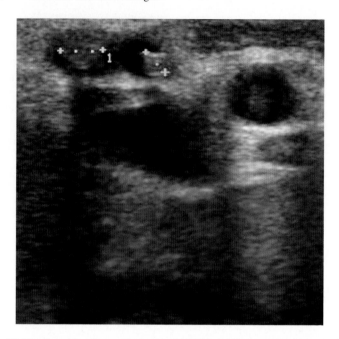

Fig. 23.13. Stone in the cystic duct and another in the common hepatic duct before the confluence to form the common bile duct seen in transverse view over the porta hepatis.

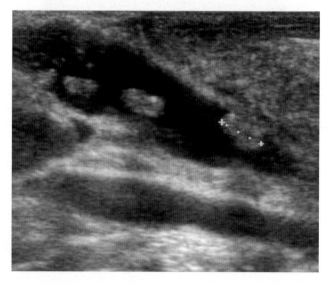

Fig. 23.14. Multiple stones in the common bile duct.

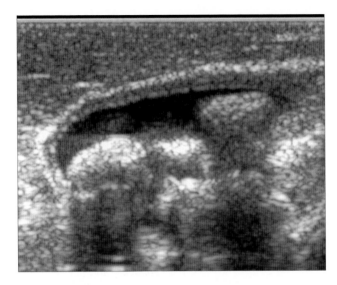

Fig. 23.15. Multiple stones with hyperechoic surface and posterior shadowing are seen in the gallbladder.

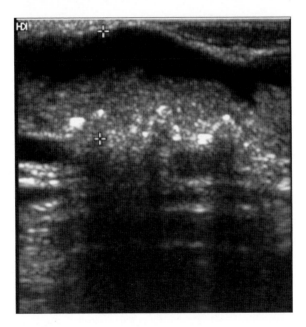

Fig. 23.16. Thickened common bile duct with stones and sludge within the common bile duct.

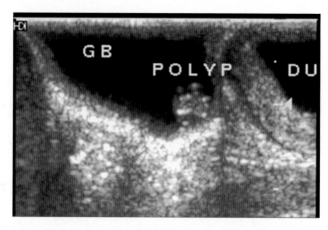

Fig. 23.17. Normal appearing gallbladder wall with polyp in the gallbladder. Duodenum (DU).

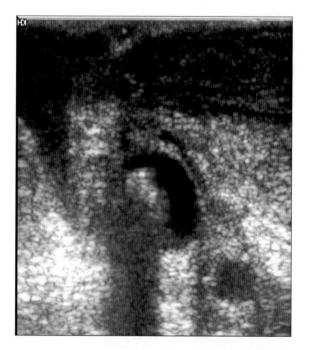

Fig. 23.18. Stone found at the ampulla of vater with dilated common bile duct.

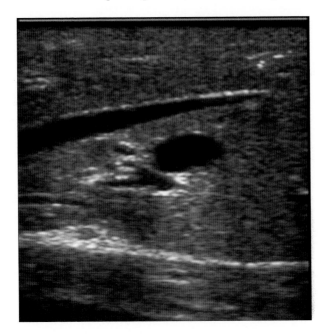

Fig. 23.19.  Benign simple liver cyst.

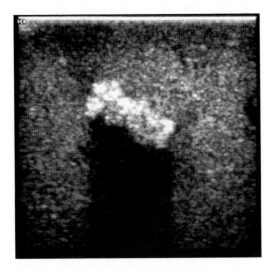

Fig. 23.20.  Calcified colorectal liver metastasis with intense posterior shadowing.

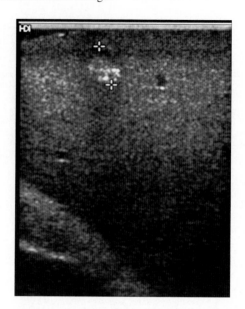

Fig. 23.21.  Hyperechoic liver metastasis.

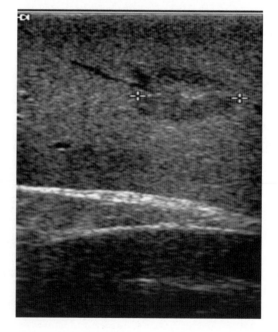

Fig. 23.22.  Hypoechoic liver metastasis.

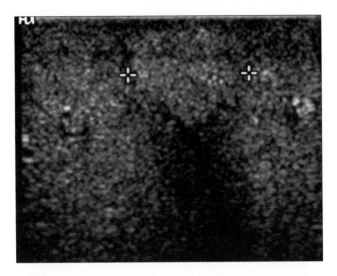

Fig. 23.23.   Isoechoic liver metastasis.

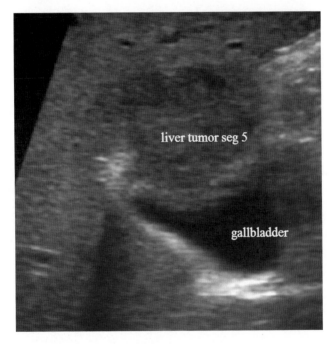

Fig. 23.24.  Hepatocellular adenoma tumor seen in Segment 5 above the gallbladder.

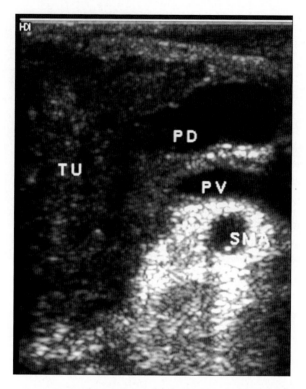

Fig. 23.25.  Dilated pancreatic duct (PD) caused by tumor (TU) in the pancreatic head with portal vein (PV) and superior mesenteric artery (SMA) visualized.

patients with low risk of choledocholithiasis with normal anatomy allows the novice to identify normal anatomy. This makes it easier to identify abnormal anatomy or identify the anatomy in difficult dissections. A novice with sonography should be able to identify the anatomy after 50–100 cases of LUS. For surgeons with sonographic experience this number lies between 25 and 50.

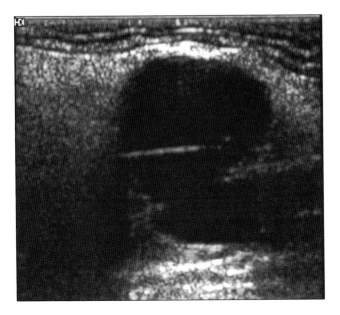

Fig. 23.26.  Pancreatic cyst incidentally found on routine cholecystectomy.

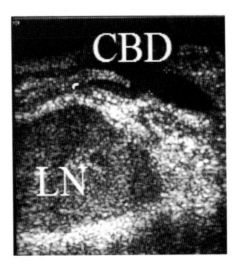

Fig. 23.27.  Enlarged periportal lymph node (LN) next to the common bile duct (CBD).

b.    Reverse Trendelenburg position and rotation to a slight left lateral decubitus position are often helpful in displaying the porta hepatis; this consideration is more important for LCDE than for laparoscopic cholecystectomy because it provides better visualization and access to the cystic duct–common duct junction.

## 2. Equipment Needed

a.    Use standard instrumentation for laparoscopic cholecystectomy including forceps, scissors, dissecting instruments, cholangiographic accessories, and a fluoroscope.

b.    Specialized tools and drugs are usually needed to perform CBD exploration (Table 24.3).

Table 24.3.  Instruments, drugs, and supplies that may be needed for LCDE.

The following equipment may be required for ductal exploration:

1.  Glucagon, 1–2 mg (given IV by the anesthetist)
2.  Balloon-tipped catheters (4 Fr preferred over 3 Fr and 5 Fr)
3.  Segura type baskets (4-wire, flat, straight in-line configuration)
4.  0.035 in. diameter long guide-wire
5.  Mechanical "over-the-wire" dilators (7–12 Fr)
6.  High pressure "over-the-wire" pneumatic dilator
7.  IV tubing (for saline instillation through the choledochoscope)
8.  Atraumatic grasping forceps (for choledochoscope manipulation)
9.  Flexible choledochoscope with light source ($\leq 3$ mm outside diameter, with $\geq 1.1$ mm working channel preferred)
10. Second camera
11. Second monitor (or second viewing area on the primary laparoscopic monitor)
12. Video switcher (for simultaneous same monitor display of choledochoscopic and laparoscopic images)
13. Waterpik™
14. Electrohydraulic lithotripter
15. Absorbable suture (polyglycolic acid suture, 4–0 or 5–0 size)
16. T-Tube (transductal) or C-Tube (transcystic)
17. Stent (straight, 7 Fr or 10 Fr)
18. Sphincterotome (for antegrade sphincterotomy)

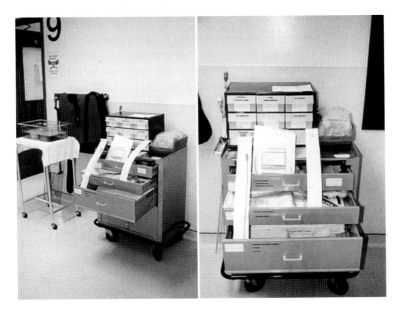

Fig. 24.1. Laparoscopic common bile duct exploration cart.

## 3. Equipment Placement

a. Keep the equipment in a central location, preferably on a separate movable cart near the operating room where the case is being performed (Fig. 24.1).

b. Place the specific items required for a particular case on a separate sterile Mayo stand, located to the right of the surgeon, near the patient's left shoulder (Fig. 24.2).

# C. Trocar Positioning and Choice of Laparoscope and Choledochoscope

1. Place laparoscopic ports in the standard *American* configuration.

a. Place a 10-mm port at the umbilicus.

b. Place 5-mm ports under direct laparoscopic vision in the

epigastrium just to right of the midline, in the right mid-clavicular line, and in the right anterior axillary line.

c.   The author uses the last port mentioned only for LCDE; the three other ports have been routinely used for laparoscopic cholecystectomy for over 20 years—>5,000 cases, without the need for the fourth port.

d.   The most lateral port is used to displace the gallbladder toward the right hemidiaphragm. This exposes the porta hepatis and elevates the CBD from the posterior structures, aiding considerably visualization of the cystic duct–common duct junction.

e.   The choledochoscope is inserted through the midclavicular port, and is guided into the cystic duct with forceps introduced through the medial epigastric port.

f.   Note: If LCDE is contemplated preoperatively, place the epigastric port slightly more inferiorly than for LC alone. Otherwise, suture closure of the choledochotomy may be awkward (suturing backward).

2.   The author prefers a **0°, 10 mm laparoscope** for visualization, but some other authors favor a 30°, 10-mm laparoscope. The angled scope is especially useful in obese patients where the

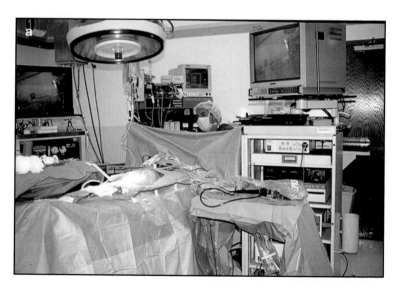

Fig. 24.2.  Separate sterile Mayo stand for common duct exploration equipment. (**a**) room setup; (**b**) graphic depiction of room setup from aerial view.

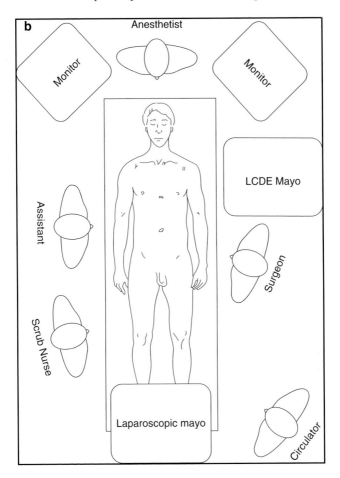

Fig. 24.2. (continued)

mesenteric and omental adipose tissue obscures visualization of the porta hepatis.

3.  There are many vendors who supply flexible choledochoscopes.

    a.  Generally, reusable scopes perform better than disposable scopes. However, reusable scopes are very expensive and very fragile and easily damaged by "heavy" or "harsh" manipulation.

    b.  Become facile with the gentle maneuvers required for manipulation of the scope.

    c.  Use atraumatic instruments if the choledochoscope requires grasping or manipulation for any internal positioning.

## D. Preparation for LCDE

1.  Generally, LCDE is performed in laparoscopic cholecystec-
    tomy cases when CBD abnormalities are found. Retract the
    gallbladder appropriately and expose the cystic duct in the usual
    fashion.
2.  Perform intraoperative imaging of the ductal system.
    a.  The surgeon should be facile with his or her favorite method:
        percutaneous cholangiography, portal cholangiography, or
        intraoperative ultrasonography.
    b.  Fluoroscopic imaging is the gold standard for intraopera-
        tive radiological evaluation because it is faster than other
        methods, more detailed, and allows the surgeon interact
        with the images in real time, i.e., he can scan the ductal
        system by moving the C-arm while injecting contrast mate-
        rial (Fig. 24.3).
3.  Dissection of the porta hepatis is usually carried out more thor-
    oughly in preparation for laparoscopic duct exploration than it
    is for routine laparoscopic cholecystectomy when abnormal
    cholangiograms are obtained.
    a.  In general, the dissection of the triangle of Calot should be
        approached from lateral to the neck of the gallbladder and
        carried toward the cystic duct–common duct junction as the
        anatomy is further defined.
    b.  Access to the cystic duct–common duct junction or the
        anterior surface of the common duct itself is often neces-
        sary for ductal exploration.
    c.  Use the cholangiogram as a guide to the anatomy in this
        sometimes-tedious dissection.
4.  Determine whether the transcystic approach or the choledo-
    chotomy approach will be suitable for LCDE.

## E. Techniques for LCDE

The techniques discussed below may be used with either access route,
although there is usually less morbidity with the transcystic approach.

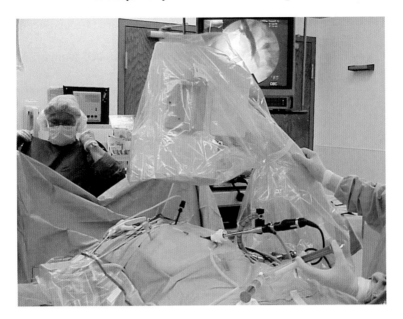

Fig. 24.3. Fluoroscopic imaging of the bile ducts.

## 1. Irrigation Techniques

When very small stones (≤2 mm diameter), sludge, or sphincter spasm is suspected to be responsible for lack of flow of contrast into the duodenum, transcystic flushing of the duct with saline or contrast material is occasionally successful in clearing the duct.

a. Intravenous glucagon (1–2 mg) administered by the anesthetist may relax the sphincter of Oddi and improve the success rate.

b. Monitor the progress, or lack thereof, fluoroscopically.

c. Surgeons should not expect this method to be successful in clearing stones 4 mm and larger from the duct.

## 2. Balloon Techniques

Fogarty™ type, low pressure, balloon-tipped catheters are sometimes useful in clearing the ductal system of stones or debris.
For Distal Stones:

a. A long 4-Fr sized catheter is inserted into the 14-gauge sleeve used for percutaneous cholangiography.

b. The insertion site for the sleeve is usually located 3 cm medial to the midclavicular port.

c. Guide the catheter through the cystic duct into the common duct with forceps introduced through the medial epigastric port.

d. Advance the balloon catheter all the way into the duodenum, at which point the 10 cm mark on the catheter will have just entered the cystic duct.

e. Inflate the balloon and withdraw the catheter slightly. Confirm the location of the papilla by observing movement of the duodenum as the catheter is moved.

f. Deflate the balloon, withdraw it an additional centimeter, and reinflate.

g. Withdraw the catheter until the balloon exits the cystic duct orifice.

h. Repeat this maneuver until no debris or stones exit from the cystic duct orifice.

This method appears to be most useful in delivering small debris or stones and in cases where it is combined with glucagon administration. In the latter, it may actually facilitate migration of small stones (<2 mm) into the duodenum. (This balloon technique may also be used through a choledochotomy if the surgeon has chosen that access route. In that case, even larger stones may be delivered through the choledochotomy with retraction on the balloon).

For Proximal Stones:

a. Use a 3-Fr Fogarty™ catheter for intrahepatic stones.

b. Insert the catheter through the cystic duct or a choledochotomy as in a., b., and c. above.

c. Advance the catheter past the stone.

d. Inflate the balloon and withdraw the catheter until it exits the cystic duct or the choledochotomy.

e. If these maneuvers result in displacement of the stone into the distal duct, follow the steps for removal of distal stones indicated above.

## 3. Basket Techniques

Basket stone retrieval methods may be used in cases where unsuspected stones are encountered (i.e., when the duct exploration equipment is not already prepared) while the nursing team is preparing the choledo-choscope. They are also useful in somewhat rare cases in which the patient's CBD is of such small diameter (<5 mm) that choledochoscope passage would be difficult or hazardous.

There are three primary methods of basket stone retrieval: under fluoroscopic control, under choledochoscopic control, or freely without either visual monitoring method.

a.  In the **fluoroscopic method**, insert the basket through a 14 gauge sleeve, (an IV sheath), placed 3 cm medial to the mid-clavicular port.

   i.  Advance the basket through the cystic duct into the CBD with forceps inserted through the medial epigastric port.

   ii.  Under fluoroscopic guidance identify and capture the stone in the contrast-filled CBD.

   iii.  If too much contrast has drained from the ductal system after completion of the cholangiograms, it may need to be instilled again with the cholangiocatheter. This cumbersome and time-consuming step is one of the disadvantages of this method.

   iv.  Another disadvantage of this method is the increased radiation exposure for the patient and the team during stone capture.

   v.  In addition, it is often difficult or impossible to manipulate the forceps controlling the basket while the C-arm is in place because the fluoroscope impedes movement of the forceps introduced through the medial epigastric port (Fig. 24.4).

b.  When the basket is used in conjunction with the **choledocho-scope**, insert it through the working channel of the scope.

   i.  Capture the stone is under direct vision.

   ii.  Remove the entire ensemble from the cystic duct and deposit the stone on the omentum.

   iii.  Remove the stone through the medial epigastric or other 10 mm port.

c.  Baskets may also be used without fluoroscopic or choledocho-scopic guidance. This is an advanced technique and should be used by the novice only with great caution.

   i.  Introduce the basket through the 14 gauge sleeve and guide it through the cystic duct into the common duct.

   ii.  Open the basket as soon the tip of the basket passes from the cystic duct into the CBD.

iii. Advance it to the distal portion of the duct with forceps introduced through the medial epigastric port. This minimizes the risk of accidental perforation of the duct by the basket tip and accidental capture of the papilla. In both instances, it is the rounded 1 cm diameter contour of the deployed basket that prevents excessive pressure from being applied by the basket tip and provides increased resistance when the papilla is reached, thereby preventing easy passage into the duodenum.

iv. After the basket has reached the distal duct, withdraw it proximally as the basket is closed. Incomplete closure of the basket handle usually signals stone capture.

v. The basket may have to be passed back and forth in the duct several times before the stone is captured.

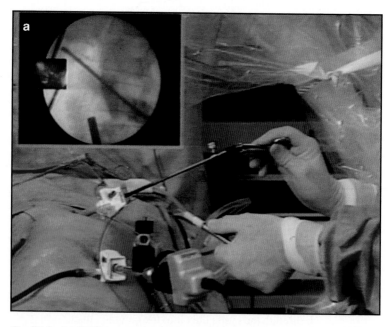

Fig. 24.4. (**a, b**) Fluoroscopic-guided basket manipulation for retrieval of common bile duct stones.

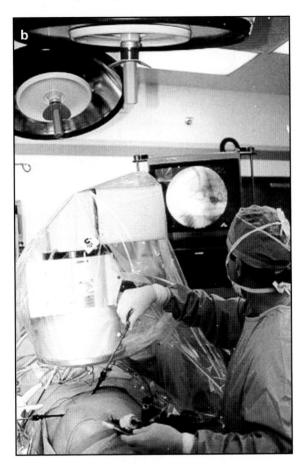

Fig. 24.4. (continued)

## 4. Choledochoscopic Techniques

Capturing stones under direct vision has always given the surgeon the greatest sense of safety and accuracy.

a.  While the surgeon may choose to look directly into the chole-dochoscope, attaching a camera to the choledochoscope to display the image on a video monitor facilitates choledochoscopy. This either requires a third monitor, replacement of the image on the "slave" or secondary monitor, or preferentially,

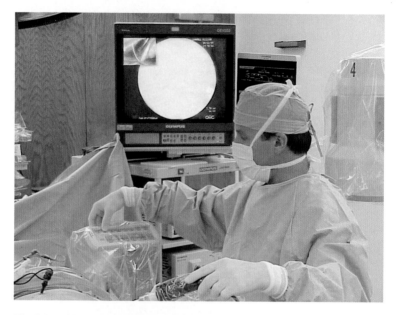

Fig. 24.5. Multiplexing video signals with a video switcher.

use of a video switcher to incorporate the image onto the same monitors used for the laparoscopic camera image.

    i.   The video switcher should reside on one of the monitor towers for easy manipulation. In some integrated systems, the switching controls are located on a sterile touch pad controlled by the surgeon. The display of both images on one monitor allows the surgeon to simultaneously engage the controls of the choledochoscope and externally manipulate the scope with atraumatic forceps (Fig. 24.5).

  b.   Smaller-diameter (<3 mm) flexible scopes facilitate transcystic choledochoscopy. Nevertheless, even when using such small scopes, the cystic duct may need to be dilated in order to allow passage of the scope.

    i.   Adequate dilatation is usually possible if the initial cystic duct diameter is greater than 2.5 mm, and unlikely if it is not.

    ii.  Dilatation may be carried out with either mechanical over-the-wire graduated dilators or pneumatic over-the-wire dilators. The former are found in most urology departments and are inexpensive.

       (a) Insert a guide-wire through the midclavicular port through the cystic duct and into the common duct.

(b) Guide a series of successively larger dilators over the guide-wire through the midclavicular port into the cystic duct and common duct, using forceps inserted through the medial epigastric port. Because these dilators exert a shearing type force, exercise great care to avoid disruption of the cystic duct–common duct junction.

(c) In general, **if the duct will not initially accept a 9-Fr** dilator easily, then adequate dilatation to the requisite 12 Fr is unlikely.

iii. High pressure balloon-tipped catheters may be used to dilate the cystic duct.

(a) Insert a guide-wire through the midclavicular port through the cystic duct and into the common duct.

(b) Advance the catheter is over the guide-wire.

(c) Position the balloon catheter in the cystic duct.

(d) Inflation of the balloon distends the duct with radially directed force, and might be safer than the graduated dilators. Still, both the pressure on the balloon and cystic duct changes must be closely observed to avoid injury. This is a more expensive way to dilate the cystic duct.

iv. Insert the choledochoscope is through the midclavicular port and guide it into the cystic duct with atraumatic forceps inserted through the medial epigastric port. Some authors have suggested the use of a semiflexible sleeve, inserted through the midclavicular port into the cystic duct, as a guide for the choledochoscope. In the author's experience, this impedes some of the manipulations necessary for adequate choledochoscopic intervention.

v. Control the scope both at its insertion site on the abdominal wall and with the controls on the head of the choledochoscope. This allows rotational movements of the shaft of the scope and deflection movements of the scope tip.

vi. Advance the scope into the common duct and locate the stone(s) (Fig. 24.6).

(a) Capture the most proximal stone first to avoid difficulty in removing it from the duct (i.e., do not try to drag it past other stones).

(b) Insert the basket through the working channel of the scope and advance it to the stone under direct choledochoscopic vision.

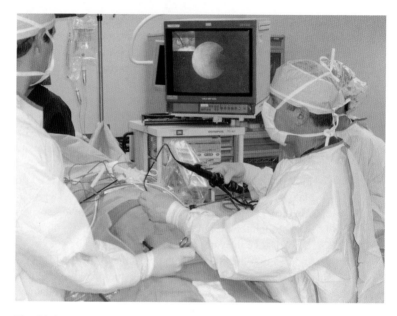

Fig. 24.6.  Transcystic choledochoscopy.

(c) Advance the closed basket beyond the stone. Open the basket and pull back, capturing the stone within the basket. Sometimes, the basket must be "jiggled" back and forth to capture the stone. Close the basket firmly but gently around the stone to secure and not crush the stone.

(d) Remove the entire ensemble through the cystic duct and deposit the stone temporarily on the omentum.

(e) Remove the stone with forceps inserted through the medial epigastric port.

vii. Balloon techniques may be combined with choledochoscopic techniques in order to retrieve hepatic duct stones and stones that defy capture with a basket.

(a) Pass the catheter through the 14-gauge sleeve in the abdominal wall into the ductal system adjacent to the scope, since the working channel of the scope is too small to admit it.

(b) Advance the catheter beyond the stone under direct vision.

(c) Inflate the balloon distal to the stone and withdraw the catheter enough to impact the stone against the scope.

(d) Remove the entire ensemble through the duct. Combined use of these techniques requires either a large diameter cystic duct or a choledochotomy approach.

(e) In the unlikely event that stones are displaced into the common hepatic duct during balloon manipulations, flush them back down into the distal system again by altering the position of the table, or retrieve them by passing the balloon catheter proximally. In the author's experience, this is a rare event and in no case have other measures been necessary to retrieve common hepatic duct stones.

## 5.  Lithotripsy

The primary indication for intraoperative lithotripsy continues to be an impacted stone that defies less aggressive removal techniques. Intraoperative electrohydraulic or laser lithotripsy techniques have been used sporadically since the introduction of LCDE. Laser lithotripters are far too expensive to encourage widespread implementation; electrohydraulic lithotripters (EHL)—previously found in many urology departments—are much less expensive, and consequently have been used somewhat more frequently. EHL devices must be used with great caution because they may cause unwanted ductal damage if the tip of the EHL probe is not accurately applied to the stone. However, with careful, direct visualization and application of EHL energy to the stone surface, stones may be safely fragmented without undue risk.

The unfortunate reality at this time (2011) is that in many hospitals, including the author's institution, EHL devices have been removed for unknown reasons—although it may be related to urologists' preferences. This leaves the surgeon with few options regarding impacted stones— biliary bypass or ERCP + S (endoscopic retrograde cholangiopancreatography and sphincterotomy).

## 6.  Intraoperative Sphincterotomy

Laparoscopic antegrade sphincterotomy was first described by DePaula and coworkers in Brazil in 1993.

a.  In this method, a sphincterotome is passed through the working channel of the choledochoscope and through the sphincter.
b.  Monitor the cutting action of the device by simultaneous side-viewing endoscopy of the duodenum.
c.  Alternatively, pass the sphincterotome through the side-viewing scope, rather than through the choledochoscope.
d.  While these techniques achieve excellent results as a drainage procedure, they are logistically quite difficult to accomplish.
    i.   More equipment and an additional endoscopic team must be present in an already crowded operating theater.
    ii.  It is more difficult to pass the ERCP scope and perform sphincterotomy with the patient supine (rather than in the typical semiprone position).
    iii. Laparoscopic visualization is hampered by excessive air insufflation during the endoscopy and ERCP+S.
    iv.  For all these reasons, laparoscopic antegrade and retrograde sphincterotomy have not gained widespread acceptance.
e.  An alternative, when stones cannot be removed using the methods detailed above, is to pass a guide-wire or cystic duct tube (C-Tube) through the cystic duct and advance it into the duodenum. This assists in postprocedure ERCP and sphincterotomy.

# 7. Drainage Procedures

Biliary bypass procedures may be indicated in patients with an impacted distal stone, a stone or stones located distal to a stricture, or in patients with dramatically dilated ducts (>2 cm) with multiple stones. Choledochoenterostomy may be accomplished laparoscopically, but requires significant advanced laparoscopic suturing skills. These techniques are described elsewhere in this manual.

## Selected References

Arregui ME, Navarrete JL, Davis CJ, Hammond JC, Barteau J. the evolving role of ERCP and laparoscopic common bile duct exploration in the era of laparoscopic cholecystectomy. Int Surg. 1994;79:188–94.

Berci G, Cuschieri A. Bile ducts and bile duct stones. Philadelphia: WB Saunders; 1996.

Carroll BJ, Phillips EH, Daykhovsky L, Grundfest WS, Gershman A, Fallas M, et al. Laparoscopic choledochoscopy: an effective approach to the common duct. J Laparoendosc Surg. 1992;2:15–21.

DePaula A, Hashiba K, Bafutto M, Zago R, Machado M. Laparoscopic antegrade sphincterotomy. Surg Laparosc Endosc. 1993;3(3):157–60.

DePaula AL, Hashiba K, Bafutto M. Laparoscopic management of choledocholithiasis. Surg Endosc. 1994;8:1399–403.

Fielding GA, O'Rourke NA. Laparoscopic common bile duct exploration. Aust N Z J Surg. 1993;63:113–5.

Fletcher DR. Common bile duct calculi at laparoscopic cholecystectomy: a technique for management. Aust N Z J Surg. 1993;63:710–4.

Lezoche E, Paganini AM, Carlei F, Feliciotte F, Lomanto D, Guerrieri M. Laparoscopic treatment of gallbladder and common bile duct stones: a prospective study. World J Surg. 1996;20:535–42.

Millat B, Atger J, Deleuze A, Briandet H, Fingerhut A, Guillon F, et al. Laparoscopic treatment for choledocholithiasis: a prospective evaluation in 247 consecutive unselected patients. Hepatogastroenterology. 1997;44:28–34.

Perissat J, Huibregtse K, Keane FV, Russell CG, Neoptolemos JP. Management of bile duct stones in the era of laparoscopic cholecystectomy. BJS. 1994;81(6):799–810.

Petelin J. Laparoscopic approach to common duct pathology. Surg Laparosc Endosc. 1991;1(1):33–41.

Petelin JB. Laparoscopic ductal stone clearance: transcystic approach. In: Berci G, Cuschieri A, editors. Bile ducts and bile duct stones. Philadelphia: WB Saunders; 1996. p. 97–108.

Petelin JB. Laparoscopic common bile duct exploration: lessons learned from > 12 years experience. Surg Endosc. 2003;17(11):1705–15.

Phillips EH, Rosenthal RJ, Carroll BJ, et al. Laparoscopic trans-cystic duct common bile duct exploration. Surg Endosc. 1994;8:1389–94.

Rhodes M, Sussman L, Cohen L, Lewis MP. Randomised trial of laparoscopic exploration of common bile duct versus postoperative endoscopic retrograde cholangiography for common bile duct stones. Lancet. 1998;351:159–61.

Shapiro SJ, Gordon LA, Daykhovsky L, et al. Laparoscopic exploration of the common bile duct: experience in 16 selected patients. J Laparoendosc Surg. 1991;1(6):333–41.

Stoker ME, Leveillee RJ, McCann JC, Maini BS. Laparoscopic common bile duct exploration. J Laparoendosc Surg. 1991;1(5):287–93.

Traverso LW, Roush TS, Koo K. Common bile duct stones—outcomes and costs. Surg Endosc. 1995;9:1242–4.

Traverso LW. A cost-effective approach to the treatment of common bile duct stones with surgical versus endoscopic techniques. In: Berci G, Cuschieri A, editors. Bile ducts and bile duct stones. Philadelphia: WB Saunders; 1996. p. 154–60.

# 25. Laparoscopic Common Bile Duct Exploration via Choledochotomy*

*Richard A. Alexander, Jr., M.D.*
*Karla Russek, M.D.*
*Morris E. Franklin, Jr., M.D., F.A.C.S.*

## A. Indications and Preoperative Patient Assessment

Laparoscopic common bile duct (CBD) exploration has been proven to be a safe and effective manner of clearing the CBD of retained stones. *Indications* for laparoscopic CBD exploration currently are the following:

1. Large single (>6–8 mm) or multiple stones.
2. Stones proximal to the junction of the cystic duct and CBD.
3. Severe inflammation within the triangle of Calot (not including the CBD) may render cystic duct manipulation difficult.
4. Failure of transcystic approach, provided that CBD is greater than 8 mm.
5. Failure of endoscopic stone extraction for large or occluding stones.
6. Any or all of the above; if laparoscopic skills sufficient to achieve good operation.

There are conditions for which **LCBDE may be unsuitable**, and other means of clearing the CBD (i.e., endoscopic techniques) may be more suitable. These include: a **small diameter (<6 mm)** CBD. Choledochotomy is accompanied by an increased risk of stricture formation in this setting. These stones are best treated via endoscopic sphincterotomy and/or transcystic duct stone extraction. An issue of debate is

---

*This chapter was contributed by Alfred Cuschieri F.R.S.E., M.D., ChM F.R.C.S. FMedSci and Chris Kimber M.B.B.S. F.R.A.C.S. in the previous edition.

N.J. Soper and C.E.H. Scott-Conner (eds.), *The SAGES Manual: Volume 1 Basic Laparoscopy and Endoscopy*, DOI 10.1007/978-1-4614-2344-7_25, © Springer Science+Business Media, LLC 2012

the CBD that is 8 mm. In the past this situation was regarded as high risk for stricture formation; however, at our institution cholangiographic evidence of stones > 3 mm in a duct of 8 mm is still an indication for CBDE due to the possibility of a retained stone. It is commonly agreed upon that smaller stones will generally pass.

**Small stones (<3 mm)**—98% pass without problem, and choledochotomy is meddlesome.

**A grossly dilated duct (CBD > 2.5 cm)** generally indicates some form of distal CBD obstruction. This is generally secondary to stone obstruction, but it could also indicate malignancy in a small group of patients. Establishing adequate drainage is a mainstay to preventing recurrent stone formation. These patients should be evaluated with MRCP (magnetic resonance cholangiopancreatography) to delineate the biliary anatomy. Endoscopic choledochoduodenal stents may be used to decompress the area prior to a definitive drainage procedure.

**Patient preparation** includes presurgical antibiotic prophylaxis to cover most common biliary pathogens. First-generation cephalosporins are acceptable in those who are not penicillin allergic.

# B. Patient Positioning and Room Setup

Position the patient supine as for laparoscopic cholecystectomy, in reverse Trendelenburg, and slightly rotated to the left. Ensure that all of the instruments specifically needed for the procedure are readily available. These instruments include the following:

1. A selection of Fogarty catheters and baskets for extraction.
2. C-arm fluoroscopy with image intensifier for subsequent cholangiograms.
3. Cholangiography catheter.
4. Laparoscopic scissors.
5. 8 Fr T-tube for biliary decompression.
6. Separate monitors for laparoscopic and choledochoscopic viewing of the procedure.
7. Sutures for choledochotomy repair (we use 4–0 vicryl suture cut to 15 cm).
8. Extension tubing and bile drainage bag for T-tube.
9. 18-Gauge angiocath needle.
10. Choledochoscope (diameter of scope: 2.5 mm, 7.5 mm/3.3 mm, 10 Fr/5.0 mm, 15 Fr) with an instrument channel large enough to incorporate irrigation as well as instruments as large as 1.2 mm.

## C. Trocar Position and Choice of Laparoscope

We use four trocars for standard laparoscopic cholecystectomy: placing a 5-mm trocar in the RUQ in the anterior axillary line, a 10-mm trocar at or near the umbilicus, a second 5-mm trocar in the mid epigastrium, and a third 5-mm trocar in the RLQ anterior axillary line. The 10-mm port is the camera port where a 5-mm or 10-mm 0° scope is generally used. The mid epigastric port is used for introduction of the choledochoscope. We use an introducer with the choledochoscope and other flexible devices. This adds stability and protection from damage to the outer coating, which could occur if the instruments are passed directly through the trocar.

## D. Performing the Choledochotomy

The majority of CBDE's are performed with a concomitant cholecystectomy, and so dissection of Calot's triangle has preceded the CBDE. Leaving these structures intact enhances the ability to retract and visualize the CBD.

1.  Thus far the operation has involved: dissection in the triangle of Calot with visualization of the cystic artery (Fig. 25.1). The cystic duct has already been partially transected to allow for the IOC (Figs. 25.2 and 25.3).

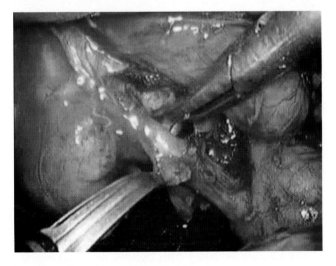

Fig. 25.1. Blunt dissection of cystic duct.

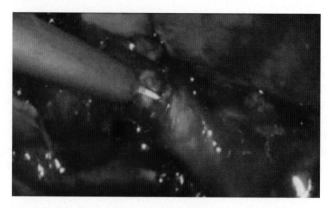

Fig. 25.2. Cholangiogram catheter introduction.

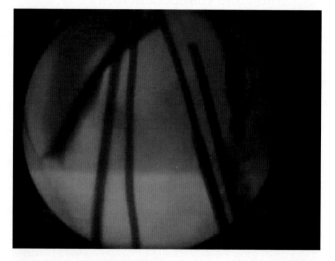

Fig. 25.3. Intraoperative cholangiogram showing a stone in the common bile duct.

2.  Identify the supraduodenal CBD as a bluish green tubular structure adjacent to the cystic duct.
3.  Bluntly dissect the peritoneum overlying the CBD with atraumatic graspers. If there is difficulty clearing the peritoneum, carefully use laparoscopic scissors to help divide the peritoneum. Care should be taken to avoid over dissection because of risk of vascular injury. This exposes the anterior wall of the

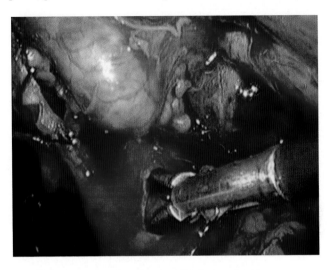

Fig. 25.4.  Choledochotomy for common bile duct exploration.

CBD. Clear the anterior surface of the CBD for approximately 1–2 cm.

4.   Make a longitudinal incision into the anterior wall of the CBD. A gush of bile should immediately occur. A longitudinal incision is preferred so as to not disrupt the blood supply to the CBD (Fig. 25.4). The incision length should be consistent and remain less than 1.5 cm because the CBD can distend and stretch, and thus the incision will tend to lengthen during subsequent manipulations. Keeping the incision within this range reduces the amount of suturing which will be required upon completion of the procedure. It is thought that this also limits the possibility of stricturing of the duct postoperatively.

## E.  Stone Extraction

Extraction of stones through the choledochotomy is accomplished with a variety of steps (Fig. 25.5):

1.   Place the suction irrigator into the choledochotomy and irrigate the duct. This accomplishes two things:
a.   Loose debris can be washed out of the duct with controlled irrigation.
b.   Bile and blood are cleared, maximizing visualization.

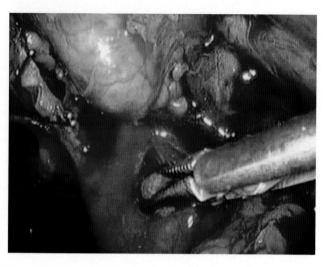

Fig. 25.5.  Stone extraction after common bile duct irrigation.

2. A Fogarty balloon catheter is inserted through the choledochotomy and guided distally. Resistance is generally met and the key is to guide the catheter past this area of resistance (which most of the time is the ampulla although a large stone could provide resistance). Inflate the balloon and gradually withdraw it through the choledochotomy. Suction and remove any loose debris encountered. Several passes may be necessary.

3. If the above attempts at clearing the duct are unsuccessful then directly visualizing the duct via choledochoscopy for stone clearance is indicated (Fig. 25.6). Connect irrigation to the scope and test it. Place the scope into the introducer and pass introducer and scope into the abdomen through the midepigastric port:

   a. Position the choledochoscope and guide it into the choledochotomy.

   b. Once the scope is in position, begin irrigation to allow visualization of the CBD.

   c. Slowly guide the scope distally with minimal flexion of the tip. Visualization is provided by manually rotating the scope through its descent while keeping the lumen in view (torque).

   d. Once the stone is in view, pass the extractor basket through the instrument port. Keep in mind that **the assistant** is in

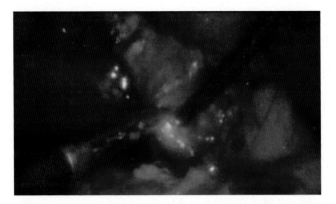

Fig. 25.6.  Choledoscope introduction.

charge of manipulating the basket while **the scope opera-tor** maintains visualization of the stone.

e.  Guide the extractor basket past the stone with the basket closed.

f.  Once the basket is past the stone, open it and slowly withdraw it proximally. Slight manipulation of the opened basket may be required to allow the stone to fall into the basket.

g.  Once the stone is inside the wires, close the basket just enough to fit snugly around the stone without crushing it. While closing the apparatus the natural tendency is for the catheter to migrate proximally, so slight inward pressure of the catheter is required to maintain visualization throughout the manipulation. Do not crush the stone, as this creates debris that can be dislodged upon withdrawing the stone causing proximal occlusion of intrahepatic ducts.

h.  Once in place, remove the scope with stone in tow through the choledochotomy.

i.  Release the stone and place in the abdomen for easy retrieval once the procedure is finished. We generally place the stone on the omentum where the omental fat helps prevent the stone from becoming lost in the abdomen.

4.  Once all stones have been removed, irrigate the CBD again.

5.  Perform completion choledochoscopy. We generally guide the scope distally until the ampulla (or duodenal mucosa) is visualized. Then manipulate the scope so that the proximal ducts can be visualized. Remove any residual fragments or sludge.

# F.  Closure of the Choledochotomy and Placement of a T-Tube

The choledochotomy can be closed in a variety of ways. **Primary closure** of the choledochotomy without biliary decompression is feasible. There is evidence that this technique: (1) reduces hospital stay, (2) reduces operative time, and (3) reduces overall hospital expense. However, it is the author's belief that instrumentation of the CBD, and the maneuvers utilized for stone extraction, result in edema of the papilla and elevated pressures in the biliary tree. These factors create an environment which places the closure at risk for biliary leak.

**Placement of a T-tube** arguably allows for resolution of edema and spasm while preventing biliary stasis (Fig. 25.7). It also provides a conduit for subsequent cholangiography and stone extraction for any retained stones.

Biliary decompression can also be accomplished via the **transcystic route**. The authors advocate placement of a T-tube because it allows for confirmed reliable anatomical structures. Cystic duct size and insertion anomalies can make fixation of the transcystic tube difficult. It is for these reasons that only the T-tube method is described.

1.  Once the duct has been cleared, prepare an 8 Fr T-tube for placement.
2.  Trim the crossbar of the T to approximately twice the size of the choledochotomy (2 cm) with one side of the crossbar slightly longer than the other and fillet it longitudinally.
3.  Grasp the junction of the T with a 2-mm grasper and introduce it through the epigastric port.

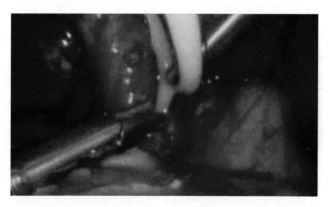

Fig. 25.7.   T-tube introduction at common bile duct.

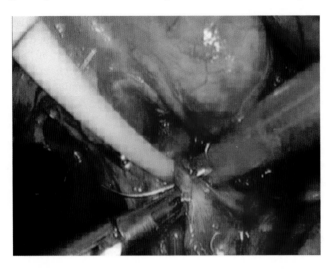

Fig. 25.8.   Sutures at the common bile duct after T-tube placement.

4.   Insert the tube into the duct with the long limb in the distal portion of the duct.
5.   Use a running suture of 4-0-vicryl to close the choledochotomy (Fig. 25.8). Take care in placing the first suture not to incorporate the tube. This first stitch is the most crucial in terms of anchoring the tube and preventing migration or leaking.
6.   Close the duct from above downward.
7.   Exteriorize the T-tube at the end of the surgical procedure through the RUQ 5 mm trocar site.

A completion cholangiogram is optional especially after choledochoscopic clearance of the duct. The authors always place a sub hepatic drain via the RLQ trocar, and position the tip of this drain adjacent to the choledochotomy. We generally avoid the use of internal stents due to the surgeon's inability to obtain subsequent cholangiograms and the need for a second procedure for removal of the stent.

# G.  Laparoscopic Holmium Laser

In the event that the initial exploration is unsuccessful there are adjuncts, which can be used to clear the duct prior to converting to open exploration. Holmium laser is an effective and safe way to clear impacted stones or large solitary stones of the CBD. The laser is emitted via a holmium:yttrium-aluminum-garnet laser fiber, which is approximately 270 μm. The fiber is guided through the instrument port of the scope. Since the light emitted by laser is invisible, eye protection is essential during use. Avoid contact with skin. The laser is equipped with a red "spotter" light that shows where the laser energy is being directed when fired. When triggered the laser emits light energy with a long pulse duration allowing the stone to be fragmented by photothermal ablation. This long duration minimizes collateral damage to the duct wall.

Once used, the resulting stone fragments can be cleared with saline irrigation.

# H.  Postoperative Management

1.  Continue perioperative antibiotics for approximately 24 h
2.  **Management of T-tube**:
    a.  Place the drainage bag on the floor for approximately 12 h and check the closed suction drain for any evidence of a bile leak. If the drainage is not bilious, reposition the bag at the level of the bed for another 12 h. After this time period, place the bag at the head of the bed. If bile is not seen in the closed suction drain, clamp the T-tube. It is the authors belief that the positional changes allow testing of the integrity of the repaired choledochotomy via various pressure gradients.
    b.  Remove the closed suction (subhepatic) drain before discharging the patient.
    c.  Schedule a cholangiogram at approximately 10–15 days after surgery. If there are no retained stones or leak, remove the T-tube.
    d.  Retained stones can be removed via endoscopy or through the T-tube tract.

## Selected References

Campagnacci R, et al. Is laparoscopic fiberoptic choledochoscopy for common bile duct stones a fine option or a mandatory step? Surg Endosc. 2010;24:547–53.

Dorman JP, Franklin Jr ME. Laparoscopic common bile duct exploration by choledochotomy. Semin Laparosc Surg. 1997;4:34–41.

El-Geidle AAR. Is the use of T-tube necessary after laparoscopic choledochotomy? J Gastrointest Surg. 2010;144:844–8.

Hanif F, Ahmed Z, Abdel Sanie M, Nassar AHM. Laparoscopic trancystic bile duct exploration: the treatment of first choice for common bile duct stones. Surg Endosc. 2010;24:1552–6.

Phillips EH. Laparoscopic common bile duct exploration: long-term outcome. Arch Surg. 1999;134:839–43.

Rogers SJ, et al. Prospective randomized trial of LC+LCBDE vs ERCP/S+LC for common bile duct stone disease. Arch Surg. 2010;145(1):28–33.

Varban O, Assimos D, Passman C, Westcott C. Laparoscopic common bile exploration and holmium laser lithotripsy: a novel approach to the management of common bile duct stones. Surg Endosc. 2010;24:1759–64.

Part IV

# Basic Laparoscopic Gastric Surgery

# 26. Laparoscopic Gastrostomy

*Sajida Ahad, M.D.*
*John D. Mellinger, M.D.*

## A. Indications

Indications for gastrostomy include access to the stomach for feeding or prolonged gastric decompression. Laparoscopic gastrostomy is indicated when a percutaneous endoscopic gastrostomy (PEG) cannot be performed or is contraindicated (see Chap. 42). Specific situations in which this is likely to occur include the following:

1. An obstructing oropharyngeal lesion
2. A lesion in the esophagus, when the stomach is not to be used for reconstruction
3. Concern that the colon, omentum, or liver is overlying the stomach, precluding adequate access via a percutaneous blind approach
4. Morbid obesity where transillumination may not be possible due to excessive adipose tissue

Other methods of achieving enteral nutrition (such as Dobhoff tube placement) should be considered, and pyloric obstruction and gastroesophageal reflux should be ruled out. If recurrent aspiration is a problem, a jejunal feeding tube may be more appropriate (but aspiration, including from oropharyngeal sources, may still occur). Laparoscopic visualization of the peritoneal cavity avoids iatrogenic fistula formation as may happen in PEG. It also allows the surgeon to identify optimal location for gastrostomy placement. An advantage of laparoscopic Gastrostomy over PEG placement is the ability to pexy the stomach to anterior abdominal wall reducing complications such as peritoneal gastric contents leakage, intraperitoneal catheter migration and necrosis of stomach wall. Laparoscopic visualization via a single port can also be used to help safely place a Percutaneous Endoscopic Gastrostomy (PEG) tube.

N.J. Soper and C.E.H. Scott-Conner (eds.), *The SAGES Manual: Volume 1
Basic Laparoscopy and Endoscopy*, DOI 10.1007/978-1-4614-2344-7_26,
© Springer Science+Business Media, LLC 2012

## B.  Patient Position and Room Setup

1. Position the patient supine on the operating room table with the arms tucked.
2. As with most upper abdominal procedures, some surgeons prefer a modified lithotomy position and operate from between the legs of the patient.
3. The surgeon generally stands on the left side of the patient, and the first assistant and scrub nurse on the right side.
4. The monitors are placed at the head of the bed and as close to the operating room table as the anesthesiologist permits.
5. The general setup is very similar to laparoscopic cholecystectomy in most respects, but less equipment is required.

## C.  Cannula Position and Choice of Laparoscope

Generally, only two cannulas are needed for a laparoscopic gastrostomy (Fig. 26.1).

1. Place the cannula for the 30° laparoscope below the umbilicus in short patients and at the umbilicus in tall patients. Estimate the working distance to the probable site of gastrostomy placement. Do not place the laparoscope too close, as a short working distance makes it difficult to proceed.
2. Place a second 5-mm cannula in the right subcostal region at the midclavicular line.

## D.  Performing the Gastrostomy

Two methods of laparoscopic gastrostomy have been described. The first method constructs a simple gastrostomy without a mucosa-lined tube. This is appropriate for most indications. The tract will generally seal without surgical closure when the tube is removed.

An alternative method utilizes the endoscopic stapler to construct a mucosa-lined tube in a fashion analogous to the open Janeway gastrostomy. This provides a permanent stoma that is easily recannulated. Both methods will be described here.

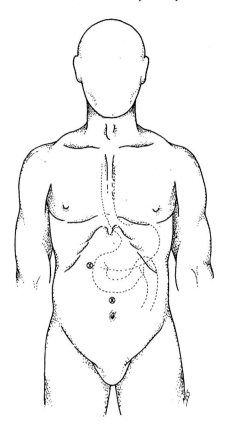

Fig. 26.1. Cannula placement for laparoscopic gastrostomy. Consider adequate working distance from anticipated site of gastrostomy placement.

## 1. Simple Gastrostomy

a.  Place a nasogastric tube into the stomach and insufflate air to distend the stomach. This helps prevent inadvertent T-fastener placement through the posterior gastric wall. Alternatively, a gastroscope can be used to simultaneously visualize and insufflate at the same time.

b.  Place the patient in reverse Trendelenburg position.

c.  Identify the anterior wall of the body of the stomach. Avoid the classic error of mistaking colon for stomach by confirming the absence of teniae.

d.   Select a location in the left subcostal area for gastrostomy
     construction.

e.   Pass an atraumatic grasper from the second cannula and grasp
     the mid portion of the selected region. Lift the gastric wall and
     simultaneously indent the selected region of the abdominal wall
     with one finger to determine the location of the gastrostomy
     site. Tip: The gastrostomy site should be selected towards the
     greater curvature of the stomach to ensure good laparoscopic
     visualization.

f.   Confirm that the area of the stomach selected for the gastros-
     tomy comfortably reaches the corresponding area selected in
     the left upper abdominal wall. Reassess and choose different
     sites if necessary.

g.   Reduce the pneumoperitoneal pressure to 7–10 mmHg to avoid
     tension on the stomach.

h.   Pass the T-fasteners though the skin and abdominal wall, and
     then through the anterior wall of the stomach (Fig. 26.2).

     i.   There is a slight give in resistance as the needle passes
          thought the gastric wall.

     ii.  Elevate the anterior gastric wall with a grasper to prevent
          passing the T-fastener through both walls of the stomach.

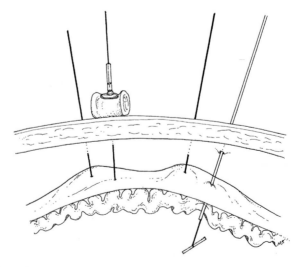

Fig. 26.2.  T-fasteners through the abdominal wall and anterior gastric wall.

   iii.  Insert the most proximal T-fasteners and pull up slightly to expose the distal sites of the T-fasteners. By pulling on the T-fasteners, the correct placement can usually be determined.

   iv.  Estimate depth of T-fasteners insertion by visualizing the external markings on the needle.

   v.  Place a total of four T-fasteners outlining a 2- to 3-cm square on the abdominal and gastric walls. Work towards the scope by placing the farthest T-fastener from the scope first to improve visualization.

i.  Make a 5- to 8-mm stab incision in the skin to adequately accommodate the diameter of the gastrostomy tube.

j.  Pass an 18-gauge needle through the center of the square of the T-fasteners in the abdominal wall and stomach with the stomach in apposition to the anterior abdominal wall.

k.  Pass a 0.35-mm guide wire through the lumen of the needle and thread at least 25 cm into the stomach.

l.  Enlarge the tract with dilators until the desired size stoma is created (18–24 Fr). Insert the dilators along the direction of insertion of guide wire to avoid kinking the latter.

m.  Check the gastrostomy tube balloon before insertion. Insert the stylet into the gastrostomy tube and slide the entire assembly over the guide wire into the stomach. Loosen the T-fasteners slightly to ensure the entire balloon is inside the stomach.

n.  Release the pneumoperitoneum and pull up the T-fasteners. Tie these to secure the gastric wall to the abdominal wall.

o.  Pull up the gastrostomy tube to approximate the gastric and abdominal walls. Secure the gastrostomy tube to the skin with sutures or with a Silastic plate.

p.  The sutures of the T-fasteners can be removed in 2 weeks.

## 2. Construction of Gastrostomy with Mucosa-Lined Tube (Janeway Gastrostomy)

a.  Place a 10-mm trocar above the umbilicus for camera insertion. Next place a 5-mm trocar in the right mid abdomen.

b.  Identify the preferred site on the stomach and gently pull towards anterior abdominal wall (site of gastrostomy) with atraumatic forceps or Endo Babcock.

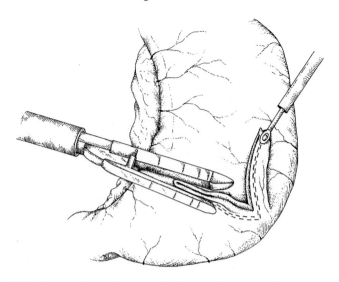

Fig. 26.3. Construction of mucosa-lined tube (Janeway-style gastrostomy). A fold of stomach is elevated and the endoscopic stapler applied. Approximately 1 cm of stomach must be included in the staple line to assure an adequate lumen. The tube is grasped and elevated and will be pulled out through the left upper quadrant cannula site.

   c.   Insert a 12-mm trocar where the gastrostomy site was marked on the left abdomen. Through this insert a linear cutting stapler and fire the stapler along the gastric fold so as to create a 6 cm long by 1 cm wide gastric tube (Fig. 26.3).

   d.   Grasp the end of the tube with atraumatic graspers and gently pull through the left trocars site releasing pneumoperitoneum at the same time.

       i.   Open the distal end and mature the gastric stoma with absorbable sutures

   e.   Insert a small Foley catheter through the stoma and inflate the balloon. Test the gastrostomy by instilling saline or methylene blue.

   f.   Reestablish a limited (6–8 mmHg) pneumoperitoneum sufficient to visualize the gastric wall with the laparoscope and confirm that the stomach lies comfortably against the anterior abdominal wall and that there is no leakage.

# E. Complications

## 1. Leakage of the Gastrostomy

a. **Cause and prevention**. Gastric contents and/or gastrostomy feeds can leak into the peritoneal cavity if the gastrostomy tube and T-fasteners are not approximated to the abdominal wall. Prevent this by directly observing the T-fasteners being pulled up and ensuring that the gastric wall is adherent to the abdominal wall. The balloon of the gastrostomy tube should be inflated and pulled with gentle traction to approximate the anterior gastric wall to the abdominal wall. This is confirmed by visualization though the laparoscope. If a stapled tube is constructed, an incomplete staple line may result in leakage.

b. **Recognition and management**. If visualization of the stomach to the abdominal wall is unsatisfactory at the time of operation, inject methylene blue through the gastrostomy tube while visualizing the gastric wall. If any dye is seen in the abdominal cavity, assume inadequate approximation between the stomach and abdominal wall. Fix this either by loosening the gastrostomy tube and inserting more T-fasteners around the gastrostomy site, or by using a gastrostomy tube with a larger balloon and applying sufficient retraction to provide a better seal between the stomach and abdominal wall.

## 2. Gastric Perforation

a. **Cause and prevention**. Gastric perforation may occur during laparoscopic gastrostomy if there is too much tension on the T-fasteners, or if the selected sites cannot be approximated without tension. Prevent this by careful site selection and by reducing the pressure of the pneumoperitoneum to 7–10 mmHg. Excessive use of electrocautery may produce a delayed perforation, and the patient may present with intra-abdominal sepsis 2–5 days after operation. If gastric tears occur due to tissue handling, these can be repaired intraoperatively by suturing laparoscopically.

b. **Recognition and management**. Confirm a suspected perforation by injecting water-soluble contrast through the gastrostomy tube under fluoroscopic observation. If no leak is seen and the patient is stable or improving, nasogastric decompression may be sufficient. Free leakage of contrast, clinical evidence of peritonitis, or clinical deterioration mandates exploratory laparotomy. Oversew the perforation or convert to a formal gastrostomy.

## 3. Stoma Necrosis (Janeway Gastrostomy)

**Cause and Prevention**. If a gastric tube is constructed so that it is too narrow at the base, the blood supply to the tip of the tube maybe compromised resulting in stoma necrosis and retraction. If the gastric tube looks compromised intraoperatively, the tube should be stapled off and alternative site and/or technique selected for gastrostomy placement.

**Recognition and management**. If discovered postoperatively, a necrosed stoma carries the risk of peritonitis. Such patients should be reexplored and necrosed gastric tube resected. Select an alternate site on the stomach and/or another technique for gastrostomy placement.

## Selected References

Arnaud J-P, Casa C, Manunta A. Laparoscopic continent gastrostomy. Am J Surg. 1995;169:629–30.

Brink M, Hagan K, Rosemurgy AS. Laparoscopic insertion of the Moss feeding tube. J Laparoendosc Surg. 1993;3:531–4.

Duh Q-Y, Way LW. Laparoscopic gastrostomy using T-fasteners as retractors and anchors. Surg Endosc. 1993;7:60–3.

Duh QY, Senokozlieff-Englehart AL, Choe YS, Siperstein AE, Rowland K, Way LW. Laparoscopic gastrostomy and jejunostomy: safety and cost with local vs. general anesthesia. Arch Surg. 1999;134:151–6.

Edelman DS, Unger SW. Laparoscopic gastrostomy. Surg Gynecol Obstet. 1991;173:401.

Peitgen K, von Ostau C, Walz MK. Laparoscopic gastrostomy: result of 121 patients over 7 years. Surg Laparosc Endosc Percutan Tech. 2001;11:76–82.

Ritz JP, Germer CT, Buhr HJ. Laparoscopic gastrostomy according to Janeway. Surg Endosc. 1998;12:894–7.

Yu SC, Petty JK, Bensard DD, Patrick DA, Bruny JL, Hendrickson RJ. Laproscopic-assisted percutaneous gastrostomy in children and adolescents. JSLS. 2005; 5:302–4.

# 27. Laparoscopic Plication of Perforated Ulcer

*I. Bulent Cetindag, M.D.*
*John D. Mellinger, M.D.*

## A. Indications

Laparoscopic plication of perforated ulcer is indicated in patients with a suspected or confirmed perforated duodenal ulcer when laparoscopic access to the perforation is possible. It is an alternative to the standard open Graham patch plication and is appropriate whenever this procedure would be considered.

## B. Patient Position and Room Setup

Laparoscopic exposure for treatment of a perforated duodenal ulcer is analogous to that used for laparoscopic cholecystectomy. Some surgeons prefer to stand between the legs of the patient for all upper abdominal laparoscopic procedures.

## C. Cannula Position and Choice of Laparoscope

The cannula position and laparoscope are shown in Fig. 27.1. The use of an angled (30° or 45°) laparoscope is preferred to facilitate visualization.

N.J. Soper and C.E.H. Scott-Conner (eds.), *The SAGES Manual: Volume 1 Basic Laparoscopy and Endoscopy*, DOI 10.1007/978-1-4614-2344-7_27,
© Springer Science+Business Media, LLC 2012

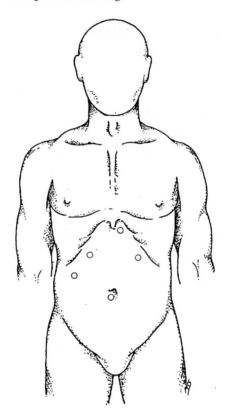

Fig. 27.1.  Cannula placement for laparoscopic placation of perforated ulcer.

## D.  Performing the Laparoscopic Plication

1.  Perform a careful, thorough exploration and lavage the abdominal cavity. If the liver has sealed the perforation, leave this seal undisturbed until the remainder of the abdomen has been explored and lavaged. This minimizes contamination.
2.  Pass an irrigating cannula into the right cannula and a Babcock or other atraumatic grasping instrument in the left cannula and irrigate any fibrin away to expose the site of perforation.
3.  If the liver is adherent to the site of perforation, a fan, balloon, or noodle retractor passed through an additional trocar may be necessary.

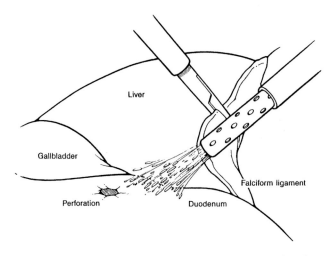

Fig. 27.2. Exposure of a typical perforated duodenal ulcer using the suction irrigator to wash away fibrin.

4.  Assess the size, location, and probable cause of perforation. Large perforations, particularly those for which all borders cannot be clearly identified (e.g., large duodenal perforations that extend onto the back wall of the duodenum) are difficult to plicate. Always consider the possibility of gastric malignancy or gastric lymphoma if the perforation is on the stomach. Exercise good judgment and convert to an open surgical procedure if the situation is not conducive to simple Graham patch closure (Fig. 27.2). As a general rule, perforated gastric ulcers should be excised and not simply plicated because of the risk of malignancy.

5.  Close the perforation with three or four sutures placed 8–10 mm from the edge of the perforation.

6.  Tie these sutures as they are placed.

7.  Place omentum over the plication, if possible. The authors prefer to close the perforation first and then overlay omentum, rather than placing omentum in the perforation, depending on the size of the defect, tissue integrity, and caliber of the adjacent duodenal lumen (Fig. 27.3). The sutures are retied over the omentum to secure it to the plication site.

8.  If the omentum is surgically absent or insufficient, the ligamentum teres and adjacent falciform ligament may be mobilized

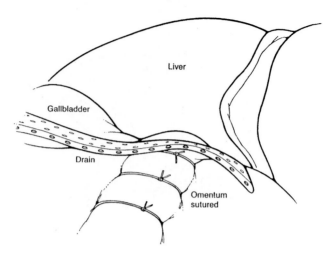

Fig. 27.3.  Completed plication buttressed with omentum. A drain may be placed if desired.

and used for the tissue patch. Irrigate the area with saline to dilute and remove as much of the gastric contents as possible.

9.  Air insufflation via a nasogastric tube with gentle manual compression of the duodenum distal to the plication site may be used to test the integrity of the closure.

## E.  Complications

1.  In general, the complications of laparoscopic plication are similar to those previously described for laparoscopic gastrostomy (Chap. 26) and recognition, prevention, and management are similar.

2.  Additional problems with this procedure are incorrect diagnosis (which can be avoided if the laparoscopist is scrupulously careful to visualize the site of perforation), recurrent ulcer (which is likely to occur in 30% of cases if treatment of the underlying ulcer diathesis is not followed), and inadvertent plication of a malignancy or lymphoma. These complications can be avoided by exercising good surgical judgment and converting to formal

laparotomy if the diagnosis is unclear or plication does not appear feasible.

3.  Gastric outlet obstruction may result if the plicating sutures are placed too deep or if the ulcer has produced significant pyloric stenosis.

4.  A recent meta-analysis has documented a 12% conversion rate for laparoscopic placation, with perforation diameter being the main reason for conversion to an open approach. The laparoscopic approach conferred less pain, morbidity, and hospital length of stay in comparison to open plication, but recurrent leakage and longer operating times were more likely in the laparoscopically managed patients. Overall mortality was lower with laparoscopic management, with the likelihood that this was related at least in part to patient selection bias.

# Selected References

Bertleff MJOE, Lange JF. Laparoscopic correction of perforated peptic ulcer: first choice? Surg Endosc. 2010;24:1231–9.

Lorand I, Molinier N, Sales JP, Douchez F, Gayral F. Results of laparoscopic treatment of perforated ulcers. Chirurgie. 1999;124:149–53.

Mouret P, François Y, Vignal J, Barth X, Lombard-Platet R. Laparoscopic treatment of perforated peptic ulcer. Br J Surg. 1990;77:1006.

Munro WS, Bajwa F, Menzies D. Laparoscopic repair of perforated duodenal ulcers with a falciform ligament patch. Ann R Coll Surg Engl. 1997;79:156–7.

Part V

# Basic Laparoscopic Procedures
# of the Small Intestine, Appendix, Colon

# 28. Small Bowel Resection, Enterolysis, and Enteroenterostomy

*Bruce David Schirmer, M.D., F.A.C.S.*

## A. Indications

**Laparoscopic small bowel resection** has been used for essentially all situations for which a small bowel resection might otherwise be done via celiotomy, where circumstances allow the favorable technical performance of the procedure using a laparoscopic approach. Specific indications include the following:

1. Inflammatory bowel disease (Crohn's disease)
2. Diverticula
3. Ischemia or gangrenous segment of bowel
4. Obstructing lesions
5. Stricture (postradiation, postischemic, etc.)
6. Neoplasms

Nonresectional laparoscopic small bowel procedures and their indications include **laparoscopic enterolysis** for acute small bowel obstruction, **"Second look" diagnostic laparoscopy** for possible ischemic bowel, and **laparoscopic palliative enteroenterostomy** for bypassing obstructing nonresectable tumors.

## B. Patient Positioning and Room Setup

1. Position the patient supine. Tuck the arms, if possible, to create more space for surgeon and camera operator.
2. The surgeon should stand facing the lesion:
   a. On the patient's right for lesions in the patient's left abdominal cavity or those involving the proximal bowel.

b.   On the patient's left for lesions in the patient's right abdominal cavity, or those involving the terminal ileum.
3.   The camera operator stands on the same side as the surgeon.
4.   The assistant stands on the opposite side as the surgeon.
5.   Two or more monitors should be set up if possible if the lesion location is in doubt or there is likelihood the lesion may be manipulated from side to side within the peritoneal cavity. Monitors should be situated to face the surgeons as they stand facing the lesion area.
6.   Follow the basic principles of laparoscopic surgery setup: the surgeon should stand in line with the view of the laparoscope, and have within comfortable reach a port for each hand. The primary monitor should be directly opposite the surgeon and facing the line of view of the telescope. Secondary monitors are for the assistant's view or for the view of a second operative field if needed.
7.   An ultrasound machine with laparoscopic probe should be available for use if a condition such as intestinal ischemia or neoplasm (requiring hepatic assessment) is encountered.

## C.  Trocar Position and Instrumentation

1.   In a previously unoperated abdomen, where the lesion location is unclear, place the initial trocar in the umbilical region and insert the laparoscope. The reader is referred to the previous chapters on access to the abdomen for tips on gaining access in the previously operated or difficult abdomen. We often add a second trocar in the quadrant opposite the small intestinal lesion, once located, for maximum view of the abdomen while performing the operation.
2.   **For distal intestinal lesions:**
a.   Place the monitor by the patient's right hip.
b.   Place additional trocars in the right upper quadrant for the assistant, and lower midline or left lower quadrant for the surgeon. Larger 12-mm ports are needed to accommodate the stapler. An example of port placement is given in Fig. 28.1.
3.   **For proximal intestinal lesions:**
a.   Place the monitor near the left shoulder.
b.   The surgeon stands near the right hip.

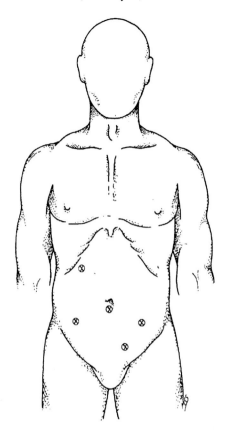

Fig. 28.1. Suggested trocar placement for resection of small bowel lesions. Right and left lower-quadrant trocars are per the surgeon's preference.

    c.  Place trocars to the right and left of the telescope for the surgeon, and in the left abdomen for the assistant (Fig. 28.1).

4.  An angled (we prefer 45°) laparoscope gives the best view of the small bowel mesentery and is much preferred over a 0° scope. New flexible laparoscopes are also now available for improved angle of viewing.

5.  Other essential equipment includes atraumatic graspers for safe handling of the bowel. Laparoscopic intestinal staplers, both linear dividing [gastrointestinal anastomosis (GIA)-type] and linear closing (TA type) greatly facilitate anastomosis. Mesenteric division may be accomplished using a combination

of vascular endoscopic staplers for larger vascular pedicles and the ultrasonic scalpel for smaller vessels. Clips should be available if needed for isolated well defined vessels, but should be avoided to control bleeding in an area that may require the stapler, since stapling over clips is impossible. On rare occasion, we still use Roeder loops to control a bleeding pedicle of tissue where the vessel is poorly defined. Laparoscopic scissors are also useful in performing enterolysis when that is required.

# D. Technique of Small Bowel Resection

When feasible, small bowel resection should be preceded by a thorough exploration and visualization of the entire small bowel, to rule out other lesions or multifocal lesions. If preoperative studies localize a lesion well, and there are extensive adhesions which preclude "running" the entire small bowel, then this rule may not apply.

1. **Laparoscopic-assisted small bowel resection**
   a. Let gravity assist in visualizing the bowel.
      i. Use initial Trendelenburg position if needed. Locate and grasp the transverse colon and maintain upward traction.
      ii. While maintaining upward traction, change the position to slight reverse Trendelenburg, again if needed. The small intestine will slip down, away from the transverse colon, allowing identification of the ligament of Treitz. Often, this identification is possible without table position change.
   b. Run the small intestine between a pair of atraumatic bowel clamps or endoscopic Babcock clamps. Identify the segment to be resected. Lyse adhesions to surrounding loops of bowel if needed for mobilization.
   c. Mark and suspend the section of bowel. This may be done using the following technique, or the surgeon may choose to simply move directly to bowel division with the stapler if the lesion is well defined and exposure of the bowel is good. One method of optimal exposure of the bowel is to place traction sutures through the mesentery just below the mesenteric side of the bowel at the proximal and distal points of intended resection.

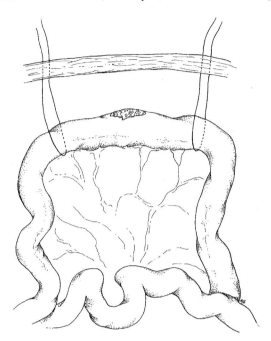

Fig. 28.2. The small bowel segment chosen for resection has been suspended by traction sutures passed through the anterior abdominal wall. This facilitates subsequent dissection of mesenteric vessels and provides traction without additional graspers or trocars.

i. These sutures are most easily placed by using large straight needles passed through the abdominal wall, through the mesentery, and back through the same area of abdominal wall, thereby suspending the bowel near the anterior abdominal wall.

ii. This suspends the segment of small bowel like a curtain (Fig. 28.2).

iii. Silastic vessel loops may be used if preferred, but must be passed through trocars.

iv. Choose the site for suspension near one of the large size trocars, which will be enlarged for extracorporeal anastomosis.

d. Score the peritoneum overlying the mesentery, on the side facing the surgeon, with scissors or ultrasonic scalpel along the line of intended resection. This outlines the V-shaped part of small bowel and mesentery that will be resected.

Make the V just deep enough for the intended purpose (e.g., wide mesenteric excision is appropriate when operating for cancer, but unnecessary when a resection is performed for a benign stricture).

e.  Next, divide the mesentery along one vertical limb using a combination of the ultrasonic scalpel and a linear stapler with a vascular load (white or gray cartridge). The stapler should be used for larger vessels and major vascular pedicles (vessels 4 mm or over in size).

f.  Divide the bowel using the linear stapler with the intestinal size (usually 3.5 mm or blue load) cartridge. The end of the bowel is now free for removal through the abdominal wall.

g.  Grasp the divided bowel end just proximal to the stapled division with an atraumatic grasper, for easy subsequent identification. Do the same with the distal end.

h.  Enlarge the adjacent trocar site (usually to around 4 cm) to allow removal of both ends of bowel. Eliminate the pneumoperitoneum and pull the end of the segment to be resected (and associated mesentery) out through the incision. Use wound protection if neoplasm is suspected (Fig. 28.3).

i.  Divide the remaining portion of scored mesentery extracorporeally using a standard technique. Divide the bowel extracorporeally using an intestinal stapler.

j.  Remove the other end of the bowel through the incision and perform an extracorporeal anastomosis with a stapler (functional end-to-end, Fig. 28.4), or by hand suturing technique.

k.  Close the mesenteric defect extracorporeally (if possible) or intracorporeally after reestablishment of pneumoperitoneum.

l.  Return the reanastomosed bowel to the peritoneal cavity. Close the small incision in layers, and then reestablish the pneumoperitoneum, confirm hemostasis, and inspect the bowel anastomosis. Perform any additional mesenteric suturing needed at this time.

2.  **Laparoscopic small bowel resection**. The totally laparoscopic technique uses an intracorporeal anastomosis. Begin as outlined in Steps 1a through 1d above.

a.  Divide the remaining mesentery to completely devascularize the segment to be resected.

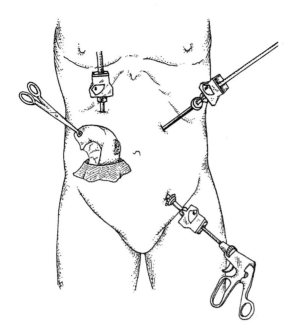

Fig. 28.3. The small bowel segment to be resected is brought out through a small incision for extracorporeal resection and reanastomosis. A wound protector is advisable.

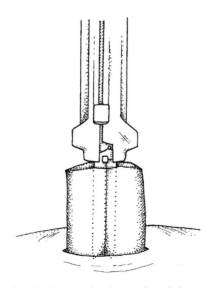

Fig. 28.4. Performing the functional end-to-end stapled anastomosis of the ends of the small intestine for reconstruction. The jaws of the stapler are advanced into the enterotomies. Traction sutures help control the bowel position during this process.

b.   Use a laparoscopic stapler loaded with the 3.5-mm staples to divide the bowel at the proximal and distal points of resection.

c.   Enlarge a trocar site, using wound protection as needed, and remove the specimen. Close the trocar site and reestablish pneumoperitoneum.

d.   Align the divided bowel ends with stay sutures placed through the antimesenteric surface of the bowel just proximal and distal to the intended anastomosis.

e.   Cut off a corner from the staple line of each segment, then pass one limb of the 45 mm or longer endoscopic gastrointestinal stapler loaded with a blue cartridge into each enterotomy, approximating the segments. Close the stapler and verify correct alignment.

f.   Fire the stapler and remove it.

g.   Use the traction sutures to inspect the anastomotic staple line for bleeding. Control any bleeding sites with intracorporeally placed figure-of-8 sutures of absorbable suture material along the staple line.

h.   Close the enterotomies with an endoscopic TA type linear stapler.

   i.   Place three traction sutures (one at each end and one in the middle) to approximate the enterotomy and elevate the edges.

   ii.   Place the endoscopic TA stapler just beneath the cut edges. Be careful to ensure that both edges are completely enclosed within the stapler, but avoid including excessive amounts of the bowel (which can narrow the enteroenterostomy).

   iii.   Fire the stapler and remove excess tissue from the staple line using scissors.

   iv.   Alternatively, the defect from the stapler may be closed using one or two layers of interrupted sutures. These sutures are best placed and tied in an intracorporeal fashion, since extracorporeal tying may place excessive tension on the suture as the knot pusher is being advanced.

   v.   A running suture line may be used as an alternative, but the surgeon must take great care to maintain the appropriate degree of tension on the suture line as subsequent sutures are placed. This also requires an intracorporeal technique.

    i.    Close the mesenteric defect with interrupted sutures carefully placed in a superficial subperitoneal location (so as not to injure the blood supply).

# E. Technique of Enterolysis

Enterolysis is performed for acute small bowel obstruction or as an initial step in performing any intra-abdominal laparoscopic procedure where previous adhesions preclude adequate visualization or access to abdominal organs. Each procedure is different, but here are some general rules, followed by details of the technique for enterolysis in the presence of small bowel obstruction.

1.    Use laparoscopic scissors to sharply lyse adhesions between the intestine, omentum, other viscera, and abdominal wall. The use of energy devices to divide adhesions involving the intestine should be discouraged, as unrecognized, or delayed, injury to the bowel may result.

2.    Use atraumatic graspers to carefully grasp the viscera or omentum, providing traction and assisting in division. Do not rely simply on traction to tear adhesions, as damage to viscera or bleeding may result.

3.    The main precaution to take against visceral damage is adequate visualization of all surfaces to be cut before actual division with the scissors.

4.    It may be necessary to reposition the laparoscope to begin work in an area of less dense adhesions, and then move into other areas as exposure is obtained.

5.    **Enterolysis for acute small bowel obstruction.**

    a.    The usual limiting factor is bowel distention. A laparoscopic approach is feasible only if distension is not excessive.

    b.    Use the Hasson technique to place the first trocar if significant distention is present. Optical viewing trocars or Veress needle and pneumoperitoneum creation in the left subcostal area are alternative options for gaining access.

    c.    Trace the bowel from the area of proximal distention to the transition point, identifying the site of obstruction and the distal decompressed bowel.

d.   Sometimes it is easier to work retrograde from the decompressed area. In any case, a clear transition point should be identified and freed, if possible.

e.   Finally, perform full examination of the entire small intestine if at all possible.

## F. Technique of Enteroenterostomy

The performance of an enteroenterostomy essentially mimics the anastomotic portion of small bowel resection. In most cases, the anastomosis will need to be performed intracorporeally, since mobilization of both bowel segments proximal and distal to the obstructing point will usually be technically difficult. In addition, the proximal bowel is often dilated and not amenable to exteriorization through a limited size incision. The anastomosis may be performed using a stapled or a sutured technique.

1.   **Stapled enteroenterostomy**

a.   Define the segments of bowel proximal and distal to the obstruction point and mobilize these sufficiently to approximate without tension.

b.   Place traction sutures to maintain alignment. Do not tie these, as bowel mobility facilitates insertion of the endoscopic linear stapler.

c.   Make an enterotomy in each segment of bowel. Suction enteric contents and contain spillage as much as possible.

d.   Insert one limb of the endoscopic linear stapler into each enterotomy. Close the stapler and verify good alignment. Fire the stapler to create the anastomosis. Inspect the inside of the staple line for hemostasis and close the enterotomies as previously outlined.

e.   Reinforce the corners of the GIA staple line, if necessary, with seromuscular interrupted sutures placed and tied intracorporeally.

f.   A **double-stapled technique**, firing the linear stapler in both directions from the same enterotomy site, gives an even wider anastomosis less subject to stenosis. The enterotomy defect is closed in a similar fashion as with a single stapled technique.

2. **Hand-sewn enteroenterostomy**
    a. Approximate the bowel as described above for stapled anastomosis.
    b. Perform a one- or two-layer anastomosis as per surgeon's preference. A standard two-layer closure is feasible. All sutures should be placed and tied intracorporeally.

# G. Complications

1. **Anastomotic leak**
    a. **Cause and prevention**: Anastomotic leak most frequently results from technical error, excess tension on the anastomosis, or poor blood supply to the anastomosis. A number of technical errors can occur:
        i. Incomplete closure of the enterostomies with the linear stapler. This is particularly likely if the two ends of the staple lines are opposed in the center rather than at the end points (resulting in poor tissue approximation at the double staple site). Prevent this by always placing these two staple lines at the two ends of the stapled enterotomy closure.
        ii. Similar technical problems can occur if the enterostomy is hand-sewn and the sutures are not placed carefully.
        iii. Take care that the anastomosed ends have adequate blood supply and are not under tension. Evidence of ischemia mandates further resection back to clearly well-vascularized intestine. Excessive tension requires mobilization of additional length of bowel.
        iv. Edematous bowel is best approximated by a hand-sewn, rather than a stapled, anastomosis. This may require an extracorporeal technique.
    b. **Recognition and management**: Maintain a high index of suspicion. A small leak may seal and present with minimal symptoms. The more classic presentation includes postoperative fever, abdominal tenderness, and leukocytosis. Treatment is based on the clinical condition of the patient. Small leaks occasionally seal, or manifest as low volume enterocutaneous fistulae through an abdominal wound.

Favorable conditions (absence of distal obstruction, intravenous antibiotics, limiting oral intakes) may allow the situation to resolve without surgery.

Clinical deterioration, sepsis, persistence of the fistula, high-volume or proximal location of the fistula, or the presence of conditions likely to prevent fistula closure (such as distal obstruction, foreign body, or neoplasm) are all indications for reoperation as treatment for anastomotic leak.

In general, suture closure of the leak will not work as the tissues are too edematous and friable to hold suture, and there is an intense local inflammatory reaction. Recurrence of the fistula is the norm when this is the treatment. Give strong consideration to proximal diversion of the enteric stream (through creation of an ileostomy or jejunostomy), or repair plus drainage of the fistula to control an anticipated postoperative leak. The former is more definitive and hence greatly preferred unless precluded by condition of the intestinal tissue itself (e.g., intestinal loops virtually "frozen" by severe intra-abdominal adhesions). On rare occasions, a tube placed into the fistula as a jejunostomy type tube may be used as a last resort to control the fistula if repair or closure or diversion is not possible. Proximal diversion may require placement of a feeding tube distal to the fistula for administration of an elemental formula, or even total parenteral nutrition. Occasionally, bypass of the leaking anastomosis may be feasible; adequate diversion of the enteric stream should be assured by this technique to prevent likely further leakage. Do not attempt to restore intestinal continuity for at least 3 months. It is prudent to wait longer if severe inflammation and adhesions were encountered at the second operation. These management principles are no different from those followed when an open small bowel resection results in leak.

2. **Anastomotic stricture**
   a. **Cause and prevention**: Anastomotic stricture is usually caused by one of three factors—technical error, ischemia, or tension on the anastomosis—probably in that order of frequency.
      i. The technical errors that most frequently result in anastomotic stricture include creation of an inadequate size opening, including the opposite side of the

bowel wall in a suture (thereby effectively closing the opening at that point), turning in too much bowel wall, incorporating excess bowel wall in a staple enterotomy closure (hence narrowing the outflow), and creation of a hematoma at the anastomotic site (which may produce transient stenosis).

ii.   Prevent these errors through diligence and careful visualization of tissues as sutures are placed.

iii.  In some situations it is possible to pass a dilator through the anastomosis to prevent inadvertent inclusion of the back wall in a suture when the front walls are being approximated to complete the anastomosis.

iv.   Remember, during intracorporeal anastomosis it is not possible to palpate the anastomosis to confirm patency. Exercise vigilance and inspect the anastomosis carefully.

v.    Ischemia results from resecting excess mesentery relative to the length of bowel wall resected, or from sutures placed in the mesentery to reapproximate it or control hemorrhage.

vi.   In situations where low-flow states or thromboembolic events resulted in bowel ischemia requiring resection, the potential for anastomotic ischemia postoperatively remains high due to persistence of the conditions causing thromboembolic events or low-flow status. Prevention of this low-flow state is often impossible, as it usually results from intrinsic cardiovascular disease and its complications.

vii.  Tension on the anastomosis will often result in leakage or complete disruption. When it does not, it may result in excessive scarring and narrowing of the anastomotic lumen.

b.  **Recognition and management**: Recognize intraoperative technical errors by vigilance and by testing the anastomosis for patency afterward (milk succus or intestinal gas across the anastomosis and observe the result). If an error is recognized, redo the anastomosis.

i.    When anastomotic strictures are recognized during the postoperative period, the severity of obstructive symptoms dictates whether reoperation and revision of the anastomosis is indicated.

ii.  Usually in this situation, a picture of mechanical postoperative bowel obstruction arises. Confirm the site with contrast studies such as barium small bowel follow-through, but take care to avoid vomiting and aspiration. Confirmation of postoperative obstruction at the anastomotic site demands reoperation and anastomotic revision.

Intestinal ischemia, if recognized at the time of the original procedure, must be addressed by further resection of ischemic intestine and performance of an anastomosis only in well-vascularized bowel if the ischemia resulted from a technical error. Ischemia from low-flow mandates careful correction of the underlying hemodynamic abnormality with optimization of cardiopulmonary status to prevent recurrence. A second look procedure should be performed 24 h later. Depending on the severity of the condition and the potential for rethrombosis, primary anastomosis may be contraindicated and the patient better served by anastomosis at the time of second look. Alternatively, if a primary anastomosis was performed, the integrity can be assessed at the second look.

Anastomotic tension is often appreciated at the time of anastomotic construction. If present, the anastomosis should be abandoned until adequate mobilization has been performed to allow construction without tension. If tension is unrecognized and anastomotic stricture results, reoperation is indicated if obstructive symptoms of significant severity arise, since they almost always will persist or worsen.

3.  **Small bowel obstruction**
   a.  **Cause and prevention**: The majority of small bowel obstructions occur as a result of postoperative adhesions. There is no certain way to avoid this problem, but limiting the amount of dissection and hemorrhage intraoperatively will usually limit the extent of postoperative adhesions. On occasion, a technical error will result in obstruction, such as failure to close a mesenteric defect with resultant internal herniation of bowel and obstruction.

b. **Recognition and management**: Bowel obstruction presents with the typical picture of nausea, vomiting, distention, and cramping abdominal pain. Radiographic confirmation is helpful. Partial small bowel obstruction, particularly in the early postoperative period, is usually successfully managed with bowel rest, decompression, and intravenous fluid support until spontaneous resolution. In cases of significant mechanical small bowel obstruction, surgical intervention is indicated. Reoperation should be done emergently if there is any concern that tissue compromise (strangulation obstruction) exists.

4. **Prolonged postoperative ileus**
   a. **Cause and prevention**: Postoperative ileus is a normal response after abdominal surgery. While its severity is often lessened using a laparoscopic approach, it nevertheless does occur, even if subtle enough to have few clinical manifestations. The etiology of postoperative ileus is unknown, as are factors that govern its usual spontaneous reversal. Postoperative ileus is particularly likely in settings of ongoing intra-abdominal sepsis and inflammation, and should raise the suspicion of a postoperative infection, particularly an anastomotic leak.
   b. **Recognition and management**: The signs and symptoms of postoperative ileus typically include lack of signs of intestinal peristalsis, abdominal bloating and distention, nausea, and vomiting. The condition must be differentiated from mechanical obstruction. Treatment for ileus is nonoperative and consists of intravenous fluids and bowel rest until peristalsis begins. Prokinetic agents may, on occasion, be of some help in treatment.

5. **Hemorrhage**
   a. **Cause and prevention**: Intra-abdominal hemorrhage almost always arises as a result of technical error from inadequately securing vascular structures as they are divided. Less frequently, it may arise as a result of delayed trocar-site bleeding. On occasion, it results from postoperative anticoagulation. Prevention of this problem relies on careful assessment of vascular structures for hemostasis intraoperatively, and use of appropriate ligature or hemostatic measures for vascular structures. Cautery is an inadequate means of dividing significant-sized vessels.

Instead, vascular staples, clips, or ligatures are required. The ultrasonically activated scissors may be used to safely divide vessels up to 3 mm in diameter; larger ones require the above measures. Trocar sites should be checked for hemostasis as the pneumoperitoneum is being decompressed and the trocars are being removed. Postoperative anticoagulation is rarely indicated for the first few days. If it is, care should be taken to administer heparin or Coumadin in conservative doses with careful monitoring of clotting parameters.

b. **Recognition and management**: A drop in hematocrit, abdominal distention, and hemodynamic instability with hypotension and tachycardia are the symptoms, either singularly or in combination, that suggest postoperative hemorrhage. An abdominal wall hematoma may also be detected for trocar-site bleeding. Management is based on the severity of the problem: hemorrhage of a significant enough quantity to cause hemodynamic instability requires reoperation, while a simple drop in hematocrit of five points may be best treated conservatively with fluids and, if necessary, transfusions. The time course is also important: the earlier the problem arises after surgery, the more likely significant-sized vessels are involved and the more urgent the need for reoperation.

Bleeding arising as a result of excessive anticoagulation should be treated by correcting the clotting factors, transfusion, and then determination if hemorrhage is ongoing. If it is not, nonoperative treatment is indicated.

6. **Inadvertent enterotomy (during enterolysis)**

a. **Cause and prevention**: Most enterotomies result from technical errors and are more likely in the previously operated abdomen or when extensive tumor is present (e.g., carcinomatosis). Prevention involves careful sharp dissection in the proper plane. When extremely difficult dissection is encountered, consider converting to open laparotomy.

b. **Recognition and management**: Usually a full-thickness enterotomy is recognized at the time of surgery. Sutured repair is immediately indicated. When tissue quality precludes adequate repair and closure, a diverting ostomy or tube drainage via the site to create a controlled fistula may be the only options. When partial-thickness violation of the bowel wall has occurred but an enterotomy has not been done, attempt to ascertain the likelihood of the injured area converting to a full-thickness injury in the postoperative period. Many partial-thickness injures require suture reinforcement. Small deserosalized segments usually do not require such repair, and overzealous reinforcement of such areas may do more harm than good. This is no different than the open situation, but the laparoscopic surgeon may have greater difficulty judging the degree of injury. Delayed recognition of an enterotomy (in the postoperative period) is treated in the same manner as an anastomotic leak.

# Selected References

Canedo J, Pinto RA, Regadas S, et al. Laparoscopic surgery for inflammatory bowel disease: does weight matter? Surg Endosc. 2010;24:1274–9.

Cirocchi R, Abraha I, Farinella E, et al. Laparoscopic versus open surgery in small bowel obstruction. Cochrane Database Syst Rev. 2010;1:CD007511; UI:20166096.

Desari BV, McKay D, Gardiner K. Laparoscopic versus open surgery for small bowel Crohn's disease. Cochrane Database Syst Rev. 2011;1:CD006956; UI:21249684.

Khoury W, Stocchi L, Geisler D. Outcomes after laparoscopic intestinal resection in obese versus non-obese patients. Br J Surg. 2011;98:293–8.

Koppman JS, Li C, Gasandas A. Small bowel obstruction after laparoscopic Roux-en-Y gastric bypass: a review of 9527 patients. J Am Coll Surg. 2008;206:571–84.

Lange V, Meyer G, Schardey HM, et al. Different techniques of laparoscopic end-to-end small-bowel anastomoses. Surg Endosc. 1995;9:82–7.

Nguyen SQ, Teitelbaum E, Sabnis AA, et al. Laparopscopic resection for Crohn's disease: an experience with 335 cases. Surg Endosc. 2009;23:2380–4.

Simmons JD, Rogers EA, Porter JM, Ahmed N. The role of laparoscopy in small bowel obstruction after previous laparotomy for trauma: an initial report. Am Surg. 2011;77:185–7.

Simon T, Orangio G, Ambroze W, et al. Laparoscopic-assisted bowel resection in pediatric/adolescent inflammatory bowel disease: laparoscopic bowel resection in children. Dis Colon Rectum. 2003;46:1325–31.

Soper NJ, Brunt LM, Fleshman Jr J, et al. Laparoscopic small bowel resection and anastomosis. Surg Laparosc Endosc. 1993;3:6–12.

# 29. Laparoscopic Placement of Jejunostomy Tube

*Bruce David Schirmer, M.D., F.A.C.S.*

## A. Indications

Placement of a jejunostomy tube is indicated in situations where the proximal gastrointestinal system is unable to be used safely as a route for delivery of enteral nutrition, but intestinal function is otherwise unimpaired. Tube placement may be the sole indication for the operation, or may accompany another procedure. Where tube placement is the sole procedure, the indications include the following:

1. Documented gastroparesis with nutritional compromise.
2. Proximal gastrointestinal obstruction precluding percutaneous gastrostomy placement and/or warranting jejunostomy rather than gastrostomy (such as inoperable duodenal obstruction).
3. Inadequate nutritional intake after certain bariatric operations such as sleeve gastrectomy.
4. Specific requirements for a jejunostomy rather than a gastrostomy, such as for the delivery of L-dopa to treat Parkinson's disease (where the medication is less effective if exposed to an acid environment).

Jejunostomy tube placement may also be incorporated as part of a larger operation. Common indications for its placement include the following:

1. Major upper gastrointestinal reconstruction where postoperative anastomotic problems, if present, will preclude enteral feeding. Examples include esophagogastrostomy, total gastrectomy, and pancreaticoduodenectomy.
2. Operations to treat pancreatic or duodenal trauma, and severe pancreatitis.

N.J. Soper and C.E.H. Scott-Conner (eds.), *The SAGES Manual: Volume 1 Basic Laparoscopy and Endoscopy*, DOI 10.1007/978-1-4614-2344-7_29,
© Springer Science+Business Media, LLC 2012

# B. Patient Positioning and Room Setup

1.  Position the patient supine with the right arm tucked. Place a monitor near the patient's left shoulder.
2.  The surgeon stands by the patient's right hip, with the camera operator on the same side. The assistant may stand on the opposite side.

# C. Trocar Position and Instrumentation

1.  Place the initial trocar in the infraumbilical region. Where jejunostomy accompanies another procedure, this may already have occurred.
2.  Place a second trocar in the left lower quadrant. This must be of sufficient size to allow intracorporeal suturing (10–12 mm, or smaller depending upon instrumentation and needle size).
3.  Place the final trocar in the right upper quadrant, not far from the midline, in a comfortable position for use by the surgeon's left hand (Fig. 29.1).
4.  While standard laparoscopy instruments should be available, only a 45° telescope, a needle holder, two atraumatic bowel graspers, a knife with an #11 or #15 blade, and a suture passing device similar to those used to pass sutures to close trocar sites are the essential instruments needed for this technique.
5.  A commercially available gastrostomy or jejunostomy kit is helpful. These consist of a silastic catheter with an inflatable balloon, separate channels for decompression and feeding, and an outer bolster to secure it to the skin. Serial dilators and a percutaneous needle and guide wire for tube insertion via a Seldinger technique are to be found in such kits and are also required using the technique described here.

# D. Technique of Jejunostomy Tube Placement

1.  Initially the patient is positioned supine. Elevation of the omentum with upward retraction of the transverse colon helps visualize the ligament of Treitz. It is essential that clear identification of the proximal jejunum occur. If the omentum is not free,

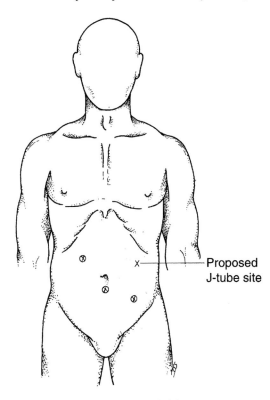

Proposed
J-tube site

Fig. 29.1.  Trocar placement for laparoscopic jejunostomy.

adhesiolysis may be necessary to free it. Division of the omentum usually requires an energy source instrument such as an
ultrasonic scalpel.

2.  Once the ligament of Treitz is seen, place the patient in slight
reverse Trendelenburg to allow easier tracing of the bowel and
the remainder of the distal intestine to fall away. Trace the proximal jejunum to a convenient point, usually 1–2 ft beyond the
ligament, where the bowel can be elevated to touch the left
upper quadrant abdominal wall.

3.  Place four anchoring sutures in a diamond configuration on
the antimesenteric surface of the jejunum at this location. The
author uses 2–0 permanent suture on a curved needle to perform
a seromuscular bite through the jejunal wall at each of the four
locations of the diamond. The suture attached to the needle is
left long, about 24 in. or longer (Fig. 29.2).

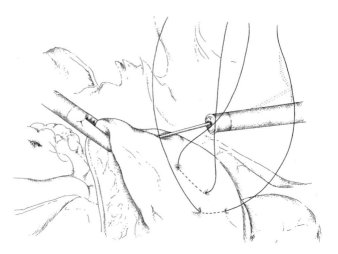

Fig. 29.2. The anchoring sutures are being placed. The suture is pulled through the abdominal wall using a suture passer. Four sutures are placed in a diamond-shaped configuration, providing both retraction and anchoring.

4.  Determine the location for the tube site in the left upper quadrant (see Chap. 26 for more information about tube siting).
5.  As each suture is placed on the jejunum, cut off the needle and use a suture passer to pull the two ends of the suture separately through the abdominal wall at each of the designated sites on the abdominal wall corresponding to the diamond configuration on the intestinal surface.
6.  Additional sutures, if necessary, may be placed to anchor any portion of the bowel wall to the underside of the abdominal wall and safeguard against leakage. Usually, however, the four diamond configuration sutures are adequate. We will also usually place another permanent suture about 1 in. proximal to the most proximal of the diamond configuration sutures, in the middle of the antimesenteric surface of the jejunum, to prevent jejunal kinking proximal to the tube site
7.  Insert the jejunostomy tube via a Seldinger technique.
    a.  Pass the percutaneous hollow needle through the abdominal wall in the center of the diamond configuration of anchoring sutures.

b.  Take care to position the bowel and advance the needle
    only far enough to penetrate into the lumen. Do not allow
    the needle to pierce the back wall. The anchoring sutures
    are helpful in providing counter-traction as the needle is
    passed through the bowel wall.

c.  Pass the guidewire through the needle, into the lumen of the
    jejunum. Laparoscopic visualization of intestinal movement
    from wire manipulation is used to confirm the wire's position
    within the lumen of the bowel. Turn the bowel and inspect it
    to confirm that penetration or injury to the back wall has not
    occurred. If needed, a 5-mm telescope passed through either
    of the other ports may facilitate this maneuver.

d.  With the guide wire in place, enlarge the skin site with a
    knife and pass serial dilators percutaneously to dilate the
    track for the tube (Fig. 29.3). Take care to avoid passage of
    the stiff dilators too far into the jejunum as perforation of
    the posterior bowel wall may result.

e.  Once the largest of the dilators has been passed and with-
    drawn, pass the tube into the jejunum under laparoscopic
    vision, using the stent available in the kit (Fig. 29.4).
    Remove the stent.

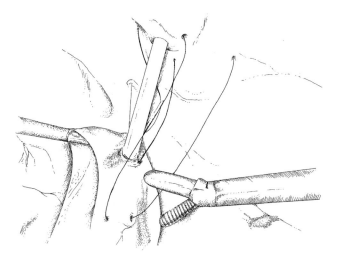

Fig. 29.3. Passing one of the dilators through the abdominal wall and into the
lumen of the jejunum. Care is taken to pass the dilator just into the lumen of the
bowel (under laparoscopic visualization) and not so far as to risk posterior intestinal wall perforation.

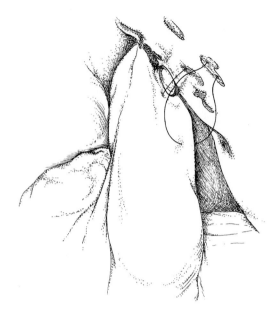

Fig. 29.4. Passing the silastic feeding tube into the lumen of the jejunum.

8. Inflate the balloon with 3 ml of saline. Overdistention of the balloon may cause intestinal obstruction. Position the catheter so that the balloon is snug against the abdominal wall within the lumen of the jejunum.

9. Tie the anchoring sutures so the knots are in the subcutaneous space. Laparoscopic vision is essential to determine the degree of tightness in pulling up on the sutures. If additional sutures are needed, these may be placed and tied at this point rather than earlier. If they are placed, it is advisable to deflate the balloon, to prevent perforation of the balloon, and then reinflate the balloon.

10. Adjust the outer bolster to the skin level and secure it with nylon skin sutures. Close the incisions for the sutures with glue or steri-strips (Fig. 29.5).

11. Test the catheter for ease of gravitational flow of saline into the jejunum, and observe the resulting flow into the bowel with the laparoscope. Methylene blue may be used if there is concern about leakage or bowel injury.

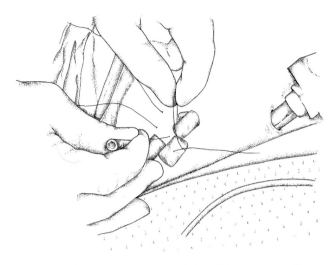

Fig. 29.5.  The abdominal wall upon completion of the procedure. The externals and anchoring sutures are secured to the skin.

# E.  Complications

1. **Intestinal perforation**
   a. **Cause and prevention**: Intestinal perforation may result if the guide wire or dilator is passed too far, injuring the back wall. Careful attention to technique as described should prevent this complication.
   b. **Recognition and management**: Intraoperative recognition is the goal; this requires careful intraoperative inspection of the posterior intestinal wall. Any injuries that are recognized need immediate suture repair and confirmation that the repair is watertight. Absence of leakage of methylene blue from the repaired site provides good reassurance that the repair is sound.
2. **Intestinal obstruction**
   a. **Cause and prevention**: The most common cause of postoperative intestinal obstruction is overinflation of the intraluminal balloon. Do not use more than 3 (or at most 4) ml of saline to prevent this problem.
   b. **Recognition and management**: Maintain a high index of suspicion for this problem. Balloon deflation is both diagnostic and therapeutic.

3. **Leakage from jejunostomy**
   a. **Cause and prevention**: The most likely causes are inadequate fixation of the bowel to the abdominal wall or an unrecognized perforation. Prevention is through careful technique.
   b. **Recognition and management**: A high index of suspicion for this problem should occur when signs and symptoms of peritonitis result postoperatively. A water-soluble contrast study through the tube is indicated to help determine if a leak is present. If the study is negative and strong suspicion still exists that the tube is the source of the peritonitis, reexploration is indicated.

      If a tube site leak is identified, it must be repaired operatively with sutures or even reconstruction if needed. On occasion, the leak may result from balloon deflation, and balloon reinflation to the appropriate size should be performed and the contrast study repeated to determine if the leak has been corrected.

4. **Dislodgment of catheter**
   a. **Cause and prevention**: Most often this results when a disoriented patient pulls on the tube. When the patient's condition predisposes to such action, protect all but the very end of the tube under an occlusive dressing or abdominal binder. Make connections to external feeding or drainage tubes **loose** so that a pull on the tube results in disruption of the external connection rather than tube dislodgment. Careful intraoperative securing of the tube and postoperative protective dressing with a binder should prevent this problem. However, it is always wise to carefully instruct the individual caring for the patient about this danger.
   b. **Recognition and management**: Recognition is usually obvious clinically. Management depends on the time course after surgery and after tube dislodgment. In all cases, an attempt to replace the tube into the intestinal lumen should be made immediately. If this is felt to be successful, radiographic confirmation of correct tube positioning and absence of tube site leak is mandatory in the first 10 days after surgery or if a question as to tube position remains at any time thereafter. If the tube cannot be replaced, and the patient is less than 10 days from tube placement, emergent reoperation for tube replacement and to prevent potential

intraperitoneal contamination is indicated. If the tube has been in place for more than 10 days, elective reoperation to replace it may be performed.

## Selected References

Allen JW, Ali A, Wo J, et al. Totally laparoscopic feeding jejunostomy. Surg Endosc. 2002;16:1802–5.

Duh QY, Senokozlieff-Englehart AL, Siperstein AE, et al. Prospective evaluation of the safety and efficacy of laparoscopic jejunostomy. West J Med. 1995;162:117–22.

Han-Guerts IJM, Lim M, Stignen T, Bonjer HJ. Laparoscopic feeding jejunostomy: a systematic review. Surg Endosc. 2005;19:951–7.

Hotokezaka M, Adams RB, Miller AD, et al. Laparoscopic percutaneous jejunostomy for long term enteral access. Surg Endosc. 1996;10:1008–11.

Nagle AP, Murayama K. Laparoscopic gastrostomy and jejunostomy. J Long Term Eff Med Implants. 2004;14:1–11.

Rosser Jr JC, Rodas EB, Blancaflor J, et al. A simplified technique for laparoscopic jejunostomy and gastrostomy tube placement. Am J Surg. 1999;177:61–5.

# 30. Laparoscopic Appendectomy[*]

*Jessica K. Smith, M.D.*

## A. Indications

1. Laparoscopic appendectomy is indicated for patients in whom the diagnosis of acute appendicitis is clinically suspected or confirmed on radiographic studies including computed tomography (CT) or ultrasound. Appendiceal diameter, wall changes, and fat stranding are the three CT findings most suggestive of appendicitis. Laparoscopic appendectomy is acceptable even in cases of complicated and perforated appendicitis. Overall complication rates are comparable to open series with lower wound infection rates and decreased hospital length of stay.

2. Laparoscopic appendectomy should be performed even in the case of a normal-appearing appendix if the procedure is being performed for right lower quadrant pain. This issue is controversial though, in that others would advise that the normal-appearing appendix should only be removed if no other cause for the patient's right lower quadrant pain is found at diagnostic laparoscopy.

   The differential diagnosis of right lower quadrant pain is extensive and includes regional adenitis, gastroenteritis, Crohn's, ulcerative colitis, terminal ileitis, urinary tract infection, torsion of an appendix epiploica, diverticulitis of the sigmoid colon lying in the right lower quadrant, perforated duodenal ulcer, cholecystitis, and Meckel's diverticulitis. The laparoscopic method is especially useful in these cases as the ideal location of incision, if open surgery is needed, may change based on pathology found at initial diagnostic laparoscopy.

---

[*]This chapter was contributed by Keith N. Apelgren M.D. in the previous edition.

N.J. Soper and C.E.H. Scott-Conner (eds.), *The SAGES Manual: Volume 1 Basic Laparoscopy and Endoscopy*, DOI 10.1007/978-1-4614-2344-7_30, © Springer Science+Business Media, LLC 2012

It should be kept in mind that there is a 25–33% incidence of pathology in an appendix that appears normal at laparoscopy. Removal of a normal-appearing appendix in the absence of other pathology is not equivalent to an incidental appendectomy.

3. Most do not recommend incidental laparoscopic appendectomy when another procedure is being performed for a different indication.

4. Laparoscopic appendectomy is the preferred operation for morbidly obese patients, women of child-bearing age in whom the diagnosis is uncertain and in the pediatric population.

5. Although controversial, laparoscopic appendectomy is indicated for interval appendectomy in cases where appendiceal abscess or phlegmon has previously been managed nonoperatively or with percutaneous drainage. Some authors suggest that interval appendectomy is unnecessary after successful conservative management of periappendiceal abscess or phlegmon because the recurrence rate is low (13.7%) and the complication risk high (18%) in some studies. Further data are needed before a consensus is reached.

6. Contraindications to laparoscopic appendectomy include lack of surgeon experience, inability to tolerate general anesthesia, refractory coagulopathy, or diffuse peritonitis with hemodynamic compromise. Relative contraindications include extensive previous surgery, portal hypertension, severe cardiopulmonary disease, and advanced pregnancy.

# B. Patient Position and Room Setup

1. Position the patient supine with the left arm tucked for the standard left-sided approach.

2. If it is anticipated that alternative port placement may be utilized, both arms should be tucked so that the surgeon, the camera operator, and/or the assistant may stand in a cephalad position near the shoulder of the patient if needed.

3. The patient should be fully secured to the operating table as steep positioning may be helpful or required.

4. Some surgeons prefer to use the lithotomy position in women to allow access to the perineum in the event the pelvic organs may be involved and need to be accessed.

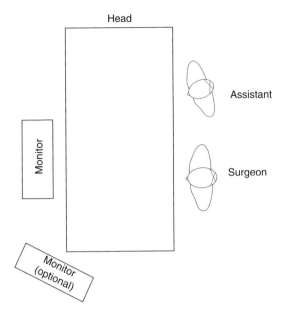

Fig. 30.1. Patient position and room set-up.

5. In the standard position, the surgeon and the camera operator both stand on the patient's left side (Fig. 30.1).
6. Place the monitor at the patient's hip on the right side or directly below the feet. Usually a single monitor is sufficient.
7. Place a Foley catheter to decompress the bladder in the event that a supra-pubic port will be used.
8. Antibiotics with anaerobic and gram negative coverage are given prior to skin incision as they have been shown to decrease post-operative wound infection and intra-abdominal abscess regardless of the pathologic state of the appendix.

## C. Trocar Position and Choice of Laparoscope

1. Place an initial port at the umbilicus via either a Veress or Hassan technique. This port may be either a 5 or 10/12-mm trocar depending on the instrumentation you are intending to use. Placing two 10/12-mm trocars to accommodate the endoscopic linear stapler from two different angles may be helpful.

2. Establish pneumoperitoneum and insert a 30° or 45° angled laparoscope.

3. Place two additional ports based on surgeon preference with appropriate triangulation to the right lower quadrant. The typical configuration is a periumbilical, a suprapubic, and a lateral left lower quadrant trocar. Place the left lower quadrant trocar lateral to the rectus abdominus muscle to avoid injury to the inferior epigastric vessels (Fig. 30.2). Alternative configurations commonly used are shown in Figs. 30.3–30.5. Figure 30.3 shows a variation using bilateral suprapubic ports which may be of cosmetic appeal. Figure 30.4 shows a variation using a right upper quadrant port in place of the left lateral port. Figure 30.5 is a combination of the standard technique with the addition of a fourth, right upper quadrant port, which can be helpful if an additional hand is needed for retraction.

4. If a suprapubic port is placed it can be helpful to place this last because of laxity of the underlying peritoneum, especially in younger patients. Counter-pressure with an instrument from the

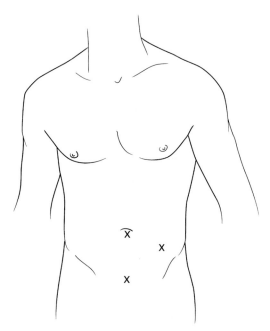

Fig. 30.2. Standard trocar position for laparoscopic appendectomy.

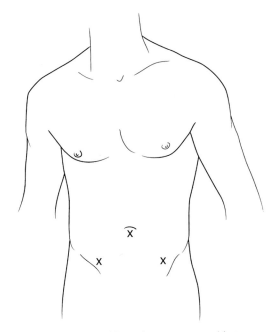

Fig. 30.3. Alternative trocar position using two suprapubic trocars.

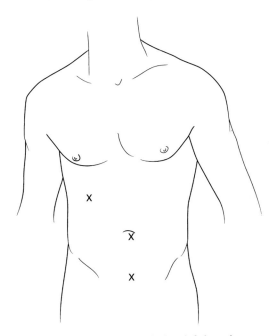

Fig. 30.4. Alternative trocar position replacing left lateral trocar with a right upper quadrant port.

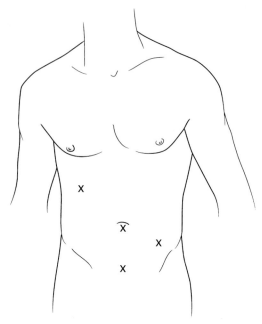

Fig. 30.5. Alternative trocar position adding a fourth right upper quadrant port to the standard orientation.

left lower quadrant port can be helpful. Take care to avoid the dome of the urinary bladder.

5.  Additional fourth or fifth ports, if needed, can be placed in the upper midline or right upper quadrant.

6.  Perform laparoscopic exploration and evacuate any purulent or murky-appearing fluid. Routine fluid cultures are unnecessary and unhelpful.

7.  Rotate the patient into a slight left lateral decubitus and Trendelenburg position to allow the ascending colon and small intestine to fall away from the area of dissection.

## D. Performing the Appendectomy

1.  Identifying and mobilizing the appendix can be the most challenging part of the operation. Begin by identifying the cecum and following the tenia coli to their confluence to identify the base of appendix.

2.  The cecum may be mobilized if needed by incising its lateral attachments and the white line of Toldt. This is especially helpful for a retrocecal appendix or if a periappendiceal phlegmon is present.

3.  Retract the cecum medially to allow the appendix to roll toward the operating surgeon.

4.  Grasp the appendix with an atraumatic grasper or Babcock clamp placed through the suprapubic trocar (Fig. 30.6). Alternatively, an extremely inflamed appendix may be lassoed with a pretied suture ligature used as a handle for manipulation. Elevate the appendix anteriorly and identify the mesoappendix. Create a window at the base of the appendix in preparation for division of the mesoappendix (Fig. 30.7).

5.  The appendix is then transected at its base using a tissue load on the endoscopic GIA stapler. In the correct position this removes a short cuff of cecum (Fig. 30.8). Alternatively, two pretied suture ligatures can be used to doubly ligate the base of the appendix, which is then divided between the ligatures. If the appendiceal necrosis extends to the base of the appendix, it is best to perform a partial cecal resection.

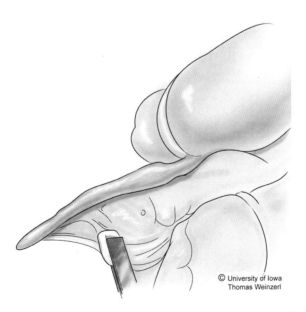

© University of Iowa
Thomas Weinzerl

Fig. 30.6.  Identification and mobilization of the appendix. © 2011 University of Iowa Board of Regents.

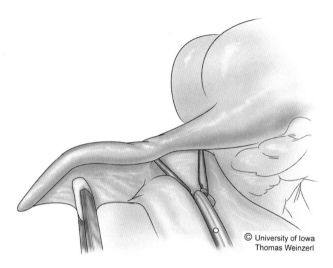

Fig. 30.7. The base of the appendix is identified and a window is created.
© 2011 University of Iowa Board of Regents.

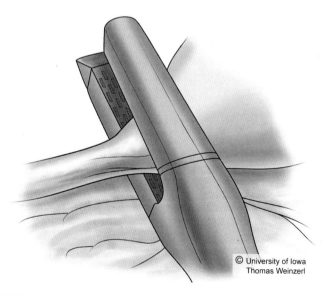

Fig. 30.8. Division of the appendix with a linear GIA endoscopic stapler.
© 2011 University of Iowa Board of Regents.

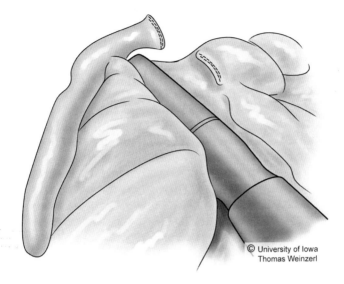

© University of Iowa
Thomas Weinzerl

Fig. 30.9.  Division of the mesoappendix with a linear GIA endoscopic stapler.
© 2011 University of Iowa Board of Regents.

6.  Divide the mesoappendix using a vascular load on the endo-
    scopic GIA stapler (Fig. 30.9). Clips or harmonic scalpel can
    also be used to serially divide the mesoappendix down to the
    base. Occasionally in early appendicitis or when the base is
    uninvolved a single 3.5-mm staple load can be used to divide
    both the appendix and mesoappendix but hemostasis must be
    ensured.

7.  Insert a specimen retrieval bag via the 10/12 mm trocar, place
    the appendix inside the bag and close securely (Fig. 30.10).
    Remove the appendix with the bag intact.

8.  Only if there is a defined, well-formed abscess cavity and there
    is concern for re-accumulation should a closed-suction drain be
    left within this space.

9.  Examine all staple lines carefully for hemostasis and continuity.
    Irrigate and suction as necessary to remove any gross
    contamination.

10. Remove all ports under direct visualization, closing fascia of
    larger ports if cutting trocars were used or port sites dilated for
    specimen retrieval.

11. Close skin with absorbable monofilament suture or staples as
    desired.

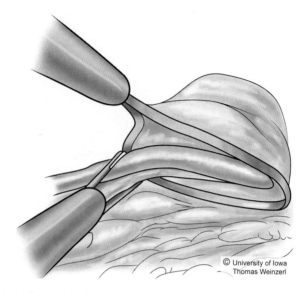

Fig. 30.10. Removal of the appendix in a specimen retrieval bag. © 2011 University of Iowa Board of Regents.

# E. Intra-operative Complications

## 1. Bleeding

Bleeding can occur during dissection of the mesoappendix from small branches of the appendiceal artery or from avulsion of the artery itself if dissection is too aggressive. Several maneuvers should allow for laparoscopic control, including suction with endoloop or endoclip or careful cautery control of the vessel. Additional ports can always be placed in one of the alternative positions suggested to aid in exposure or control. If visualization is severely impaired and control cannot be obtained laparoscopically, it is unlikely due to the appendiceal artery only and the operation should be quickly converted to an open procedure.

Bleeding can also stem from omental vessels or the inflamed retroperitoneum. Careful dissection with early control of the mesoappendix with minimal dissection should prevent this complication.

## 2. *Leakage of Appendiceal Pus or Fecalith*

Iatrogenic perforation of the appendix may occur with grasping or even with simple manipulation of a tensely distended and inflamed appendix. Spillage of pus, stool, or fecaliths can occur. It is important to limit spillage to the immediate area and remove any fecaliths as soon as they are seen by placing them in a specimen retrieval bag. Irrigation should be avoided until leakage is controlled and fecaliths removed. After appendectomy is completed the field should be irrigated and suctioned free until there is no evidence of gross contamination. All staple lines or the looped appendiceal stump should be carefully inspected to ensure there is no ongoing leakage. There is no indication for drainage for intra-operative perforation or leakage. Length of hospital observation and/or antibiotic coverage in these cases should not change provided the clinical course does not dictate otherwise.

## 3. *Incomplete Appendectomy*

This problem is seen with both open and laparoscopic appendectomy and may lead to recurrent appendicitis. It is caused by ligation and division of the appendix distant from the cecum. Careful dissection and identification of landmarks including the junction of the base of the appendix with the cecum must be ensured before ligating and dividing the appendix. Any patient who has undergone laparoscopic or open appendectomy may later present with signs and symptoms of appendicitis and should be thoroughly evaluated for recurrence secondary to this complication.

# F. Post-operative Complications

Post-operative complications of laparoscopic appendectomy include intra-abdominal abscess, appendiceal stump leak, surgical site infection, small bowel obstruction, and fistula. Post-operative mortality is less than 1% and is increased in patients with perforated appendicitis.

# G. Unusual Findings at Appendectomy and How to Manage Them

## 1. Appendiceal Phlegmon or Abscess

If appendiceal phlegmon and/or abscesses are unexpectedly encountered at diagnostic laparoscopy, the best course of action is to remove all grossly purulent material and perform laparoscopic washout and drainage of any well-formed abscess cavities found. IV antibiotics are continued until symptoms resolve. Interval appendectomy is still the subject of current debate and can be done at the surgeon's discretion approximately 6 weeks later or once all acute processes have resolved.

## 2. Crohn's/Terminal Ileitis

Crohn's disease which is limited only to the appendix or inflammation of the terminal ileum with extension to the appendix may occasionally be found. In general, it is advised that if the base of the appendix appears to be involved, it should not be resected and inflammation should instead be managed with standard medical therapy for IBD. If there is no cecal involvement, appendectomy can be performed and consideration should be given to ileocecectomy or simple laparoscopic washout.

## 3. Appendiceal Masses

Primary tumors of the appendix include mucoceles, mucinous cytadenoma, mucinous adenocarcinoma, and carcinoid tumors. Although it is uncommon to diagnose a primary tumor of the appendix at initial laparoscopy, any unusual masses seen require specific precautions depending on their size and location. It must be emphasized if at any time the surgeon is unsure about ability to perform complete oncologic resection laparoscopically or if tactile feedback is needed open conversion should occur. General recommendations for appendiceal masses encountered at laparoscopy are as follows: Lesions less than 1 cm located at the tip of the appendix can be treated with laparoscopic appendectomy. Lesions greater than 1 cm or those that involve the base of the appendix should prompt consideration of open conversion and possible intra-operative frozen section.

# H.  Interval and Incidental Appendectomy

A patient with a right lower quadrant mass, pain and fever should be believed to have a periappendiceal abscess until proven otherwise. If the patient is stable and a fluid collection is confirmed on imaging, it is recommended the patient undergo percutaneous drainage and possibly interval appendectomy after negative colonoscopy has ruled out colitis or malignancy. Patients with a large phlegmon or abscess should not be explored due to significant morbidity and decreased likelihood of being able to successfully perform laparoscopic or open appendectomy. They should instead be treated with IV antibiotics, bowel rest, percutaneous drainage, and serial imaging. The utility of interval appendectomy is still to be determined and is at the discretion of the individual surgeon.

There are currently no indications for prophylactic removal of the appendix in conjunction with another procedure, the so-called "incidental appendectomy." Some suggest appendectomy should be performed even in the event of another pathology being found if the incisions used are typical of appendectomy to avoid future confusion.

# I.  Laparoscopic Appendectomy in Pregnancy

Laparoscopic appendectomy may be safely performed in pregnant women in any trimester. CT scan or MRI may be needed to confirm a diagnosis that is in question. The patient should be positioned in the left lateral recumbent position to maximize venous return. Insufflation pressure should be kept at 10–15 mmHg. Any insertion technique can be used but should be based on the experience of the laparoscopist and consideration should be given to the gravidity of the uterus. Open Hasson technique is usually preferred but has not been shown superior to other techniques.

# J.  Single-Incision Laparoscopic Appendectomy/NOTES

The technical details of single-incision appendectomy and NOTES appendectomy are discussed elsewhere in this book. Currently, data suggest similar outcomes for single incision and conventional laparoscopic appendectomy. Both techniques should be reserved for the more advanced laparoscopic surgeon.

# Selected References

Affleck DG, Handrahan DL, Egger MJ, Price RR. The laparoscopic management of appendicitis and cholelithiasis during pregnancy. Am J Surg. 1999;178(6):523–9.

Ball CG, Kortbeek JB, Kirkpatrick AW, Mitchell P. Laparoscopic appendectomy for complicated appendicitis: an evaluation of postoperative factors. Surg Endosc. 2004;18(6):969–73. Epub 21 Apr 2004. Review.

Cueto J, D'Allemagne B, Vázquez-Frias JA, et al. Morbidity of laparoscopic surgery for complicated appendicitis: an international study. Surg Endosc. 2006;20(5):717–20. Epub 16 Mar 2006.

Enochsson L, Hellberg A, Rudberg C, et al. Laparoscopic vs. open appendectomy in overweight patients. Surg Endosc. 2001;15(4):387–92. Epub 6 Feb 2001.

Guidelines Committee of the Society of American Gastrointestinal and Endoscopic Surgeons, Yumi H. Guidelines for diagnosis, treatment, and use of laparoscopy for surgical problems during pregnancy: This statement was reviewed and approved by the Board of Governors of the Society of American Gastrointestinal and Endoscopic Surgeons (SAGES), September 2007. It was prepared by the SAGES Guidelines Committee. Surg Endosc. 2008;22(4):849–61. Epub 21 Feb 2008.

Korndorffer Jr JR, Fellinger E, Reed W. SAGES guideline for laparoscopic appendectomy. Surg Endosc. 2010;24(4):757–61. Epub 29 Sep 2009.

Long KH, Bannon MP, Zietlow SP, et al., Laparoscopic Appendectomy Interest Group. A prospective randomized comparison of laparoscopic appendectomy with open appendectomy: clinical and economic analyses. Surgery. 2001;129(4):390–400.

Nguyen DB, Silen W, Hodin RA. Interval appendectomy in the laparoscopic era. J Gastrointest Surg. 1999;3(2):189–93.

Pedersen AG, Petersen OB, Wara P, Rønning H, Qvist N, Laurberg S. Randomized clinical trial of laparoscopic versus open appendicectomy. Br J Surg. 2001;88(2):200–5.

Sweeney KJ, Keane FB. Moving from open to laparoscopic appendicectomy. Br J Surg. 2003;90(3):257–8.

# 31. Laparoscopic Colostomy<sup>*</sup>

*John Byrn, M.D.*

## A. Indications

1. Laparoscopic colostomy is an effective tool whenever fecal diversion is required. Applying the laparoscopic technique to colostomy formation allows the surgeon to perform a thorough exploration of the abdomen, biopsy any suspicious areas, and adequately mobilize and assure correct orientation of the intestinal loop of interest; creating a tension free stoma without the patient morbidity and recuperation time of a formal laparotomy. Laparoscopic colostomy formation is indicated in the following circumstances:

   a. Oncologic
      Gynecologic pelvic cancer (palliation for unresectable disease).
      Cancers of the colon, rectum, or anus rendering the patient incontinent or obstructed (prior to neoadjuvant therapy or for palliation).

   b. Incontinence/Perianal Sepsis/Constipation
      Fecal Incontinence-refractory to medical or definitive surgical management
      Rectovaginal fistula
      Complex fistula-in-ano
      Severe anorectal Crohn's Disease
      Obstructed Defecation Syndrome (pelvic outlet obstruction)

---

*This chapter was contributed by Anne T. Mancino, MD in the previous edition.

N.J. Soper and C.E.H. Scott-Conner (eds.), *The SAGES Manual: Volume 1 Basic Laparoscopy and Endoscopy*, DOI 10.1007/978-1-4614-2344-7_31, © Springer Science+Business Media, LLC 2012

    c.    Trauma
         Extraperitoneal rectal injuries
         Severe perineal trauma
         Perineal necrotizing infections requiring diversion for wound care

2. In cases of a proximal colon obstruction or an immobile sigmoid colon from carcinomatosis or prior surgery, a **laparoscopic loop ileostomy** or transverse colostomy can be formed in a similar manner, with similar advantages.

## B. Patient Position and Room Setup

1. The site of the planned colostomy should be marked preoperatively by a stoma therapist, or utilizing a site that will not lie in major creases of the abdominal wall when sitting upright.
2. Position the patient supine or in the modified lithotomy position (low stirrups) with both arms tucked and the patient secured to the bed (preventing sliding of the patient if steep Trendelenburg is required).
3. After trocar placement, tilt the operating table to the Trendelenburg position and rotate the table to left side up, to move the small intestine out of the pelvis and expose the desired segment of colon.
4. The surgeon and assistant stand on the patient's right.
5. Monitors are positioned toward the foot of the bed or toward upper right if transverse colostomy is planned.
6. If an ileostomy or transverse colostomy is planned the surgeon/assistant stand on the patient's left.

## C. Trocar Placement and Choice of a Laparoscope

1. The first trocar is placed at or just superior to the umbilicus (Fig. 31.1). A 0-degree or 30-degree laparoscope is used to explore the abdomen and verify that the planned ostomy site is free of adhesions.

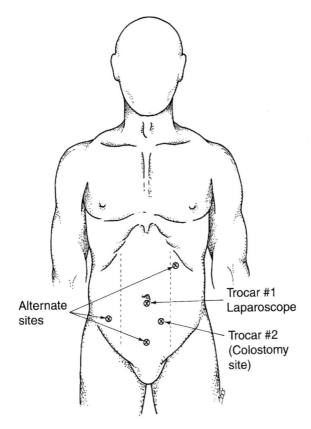

Fig. 31.1. Trocar placement for colostomy. The laparoscope should be placed through trocar #1 and the site for trocar #2 inspected for suitability prior to port insertion. The other trocar sites should be used as needed to facilitate exposure and mobilization. If a loop ileostomy is planned, the port sites will be reversed (mirror image).

2.  The second trocar is a 10- to 12-mm port placed at the planned ostomy site. This site should be identified and marked by an enterostomal therapist or surgeon prior to the procedure.

3.  Further trocars can be positioned in the opposite iliac fossa lateral to the rectus muscle, in the midline suprapubic area, or in the ipsilateral upper quadrant to allow for better mobilization of the bowel. If intracorporeal stapling is planned for the

construction of an end stoma, one of these ports should be 12 mm to accommodate an endoscopic stapler. Otherwise 5-mm ports are in order.

## D.  Technique of Colostomy

1.  Insert the laparoscope through the umbilical port and perform a thorough inspection of the abdominal contents and perform any needed biopsies (see Chap. 18).
2.  Assess the suitability of the predetermined stoma site and ascertain that a proximal loop of sigmoid colon or transverse colon will reach without tension.
3.  If the site is acceptable, excise a disk of skin and divide the subcutaneous tissue down to the anterior fascia and insert a 10- to 12-mm port through the center of the incision.
4.  Pass an atraumatic clamp such as a Babcock into the port, grasp the colon, and pull it toward the abdominal wall to assess mobility.
5.  If there are adhesions or mesenteric attachments to the paracolic gutters, a third trocar is inserted to allow countertraction. The lateral attachments or greater omentum can be dissected through the left lower quadrant port using coagulating scissors.
6.  Once mobilized, the colon is again grasped with the Babcock clamp (Fig. 31.2a).
7.  Back the trocar out over the clamp, withdraw the laparoscope into its trocar, and remove other instruments (except for the Babcock) from the abdomen.
8.  Enlarge the fascial defect to allow the colon to be exteriorized. At this point, pneumoperitoneum will be lost.
9.  Construct an end colostomy by dividing the colon with a linear stapler, either extracorporeally, which is the simplest method, or under laparoscopic vision using a linear stapling device.
10.  Place the distal colon back into the peritoneal cavity and fashion an end stoma in the usual manner (Fig. 31.2b).
11.  If an end stoma is not desired, the loop of colon may be matured as a loop colostomy.

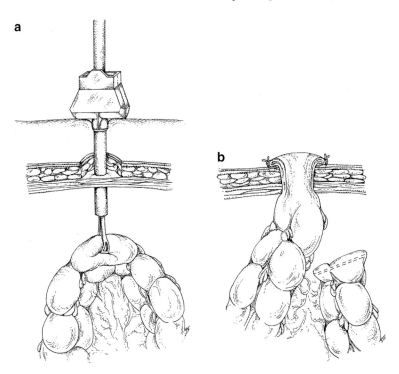

Fig. 31.2. Laparoscopic colostomy. (**a**) The preselected colostomy site has been prepared by excising a disk of skin and subcutaneous tissue down to fascia. Fascia is left intact to prevent loss of pneumoperitoneum. A trocar is placed through the center of the ostomy site and a loop of sigmoid colon is grasped. The fascial defect is enlarged and the colon exteriorized. (**b**) The loop has been divided extracorporeally with a linear stapler and the distal segment dropped back into the abdomen. An end stoma has been fashioned in the usual manner. Alternatively, a loop colostomy could be constructed.

12. Do not fully mature the stoma at this point.
13. Reestablish pneumoperitoneum and inspect the intestine to verify:
    a. Absence of any tension or twist
    b. Adequacy of hemostasis
    c. Correct identification of proximal and distal segments
14. Remove the trocars, close the fascial defects, and mature the ostomy.

# E. Complications

The full spectrum of stoma complications can afflict a laparoscopically created ostomy. This includes, but is not limited to: stoma ischemia and necrosis, mucocutaneous separation, stenosis and retraction, and parastomal hernia or prolapse. The discussion of these complications is beyond the scope of this chapter and the etiology and management is not unique to the laparoscopically performed stoma. Of particular concern in laparoscopically prepared stomas is the complication of stoma malrotation or twist.

## 1. Malrotation of Intestinal Loop

a. **Cause and prevention**: On occasion the intestinal loop becomes twisted as it is pulled through the abdominal wall. This malrotation can usually be identified intraoperatively therefore re-insufflating the abdomen and evaluating the position of the loop by direct visualization is paramount. The proximal and distal limbs can be marked prior to exteriorization using sutures, staples, or methylene blue injected through a long spinal needle. If a sigmoid colostomy is being created a flexible sigmoidoscopy per anus will definitively identify the distal loop of bowel.

b. **Recognition and management**: In the unfortunate circumstance that the malrotation is not identified in the operating room postoperatively the patient will exhibit signs of bowel obstruction with minimal output. If the obstruction appears to be proximal to the stoma on digital exam, then evaluation with endoscopy or water-soluble contrast through the stoma is indicated. If a malrotation of the intestine is identified, it should be repaired operatively.

## Selected References

Bogen GL, Mancino AT, Scott-Conner CEH. Laparoscopy for staging and palliation of gastrointestinal malignancy. Surg Clin North Am. 1996;76:557–69.

Hellinger MD, Al Haddad A. Minimally invasive stomas. Clin Colon Rectal Surg. 2008; 21:53–61.

Ludwig KA, Milsom JW, Garcia-Ruiz A, Fazio VW. Laparoscopic techniques for fecal diversion. Dis Colon Rectum. 1996;59:285–8.

Lyerly HK, Mault JR. Laparoscopic ileostomy and colostomy. Ann Surg. 1994; 219:317–22.

Milsom JW, Lavery IC, Church JM, Stolfi VM, Fazio VW. Use of laparoscopic techniques in colorectal surgery. Dis Colon Rectum. 1994;37:215–8.

Oliveira L. Laparoscopic stoma creation and closure. Semin Laparosc Surg. 2003; 10:191–6.

Oliviera L, Reissman P, Nogueras J, Wexner SD. Laparoscopic creation of stomas. Surg Endosc. 1997;11:19–23.

Part VI

# Hernia Repair

# 32. Laparoscopic Inguinal Hernia Repair: Transabdominal Preperitoneal and Totally Extraperitoneal Approaches[*]

*Nathaniel Stoikes, M.D.*
*L. Michael Brunt, M.D.*

## A. History

Surgical approaches to the preperitoneal space were initially described in the late 1700s for the treatment of iliac artery aneurysms. The preperitoneal space for vascular surgery was further clarified by Bogros (1823) with the subsequent evolution of open preperitoneal techniques for hernia described by Cheatle, Henry, McEvedy, and Nyhus (1921–1959). The first person to describe the placement of mesh from a posterior preperitoneal approach was Estrin (1963). This was further modified and popularized by Rives (1967), Stoppa (1972), and Wantz (1989).

The advent of laparoscopy for general surgery starting with laparoscopic cholecystectomy in the late 1980s translated to hernia repair in the early 1990s resulting in two different laparoscopic surgical approaches to the preperitoneal space: transabdominal preperitoneal (TAPP) and totally extraperitoneal (TEP). TAPP was first described by Ger in 1990, and TEP was subsequently described in 1991 by Dulucq.

---

[*]This chapter was contributed by Muhammed A. Memon MD and Robert J Fitzgibbons Jr MD in the previous edition.

N.J. Soper and C.E.H. Scott-Conner (eds.), *The SAGES Manual: Volume 1 Basic Laparoscopy and Endoscopy*, DOI 10.1007/978-1-4614-2344-7_32, © Springer Science+Business Media, LLC 2012

414 N. Stoikes and L.M. Brunt

## B. Preperitoneal Anatomy

The key to successful laparoscopic inguinal hernia repair relies on superior knowledge of the preperitoneal space (Fig. 32.1). The view of the preperitoneal space via the laparoscope allows for examination of all types of inguinal hernias which include: direct defect (medial to inferior epigastric vessels), indirect defect (lateral to epigastric vessels), and the femoral defect (bordered by femoral vein laterally, the iliopubic tract anteriorly and medially, and Cooper's ligament). Lateral to the cord structures, inferior to the inguinal ligament, and overlying the psoas muscle lie the femoral branch of the genitofemoral nerve and the lateral femoral cutaneous nerve. This area is known as the "Triangle of Pain,"

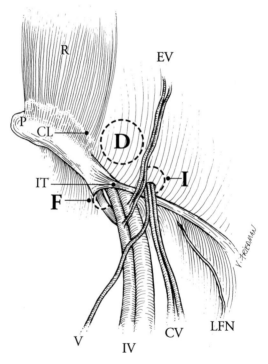

Fig. 32.1. Preperitoneal anatomy for right inguinal hernia displaying vital structures and their relationships to indirect, direct, and femoral hernia spaces. *I* indirect space, *D* direct space, *F* femoral space, *EV* epigastric vessels, *R* rectus muscle, *P* pubic bone, *IT* iliopubic tract, *CL* Cooper's ligament, *V* vas deferens, *CV* cord vessels, *IV* iliac vessels, *LFN* lateral femoral cutaneous nerve.

which should be avoided in mesh fixation to avoid nerve injury and risk of chronic pain. The "Triangle of Doom" refers to the region in which the iliac vessels are located; its borders include the vas deferens, the cord vessels, and the peritoneal reflection. Other important landmarks include the midline pubis and iliopubic tract.

# C. Indications

For many patients, either a laparoscopic or open approach to inguinal hernia repair is appropriate to consider. In experienced hands, outcomes are similar in terms of hernia recurrence. The laparoscopic approach may offer some advantage in terms of postoperative pain and earlier return to unrestricted activity. Meta-analyses (Chung et al. and Schmedt et al.) have contributed to understanding the differences between an open repair and laparoscopic repair. Study parameters for these topics can be quite varied. With respect to recurrence, laparoscopy was found to have similar recurrence rates in experienced hands. Postoperative pain and return to activities trended in favor of laparoscopy. Other issues such as chronic pain, other morbidity such as hematoma and seroma, and operative time are subject to debate.

Both approaches to inguinal hernia repair are typically outpatient procedures and the decision to choose a particular approach is best based on physician preference, patient preference, and the clinical situation. However, there are certain clinical scenarios in which one or the other may be preferred. For example, chronically incarcerated hernias, large scrotal hernias, patients who have had prior lower midline or open preperitoneal operations (e.g., radical prostatectomy) and those who have medical comorbidities that place them at increased risk for general anesthesia are usually managed with an open anterior approach under local anesthesia with sedation. In addition, most women with inguinal hernias are approached in an open fashion. The advantages of the laparoscopic approach are more apparent in the following situations:

1.  Bilateral inguinal hernias.
2.  Recurrent inguinal hernia after a prior open anterior approach.
3.  Patients who are undergoing another laparoscopic procedure who also have an inguinal hernia. For this to be considered:
    a.  The primary procedure must not incur any risk of contamination of the preperitoneal space or risk of mesh contamination.

b.  Placement of additional trocars may be required. Hernia repair should not be performed using trocars in suboptimal positions. Access and appropriate angles for dissection are critical for laparoscopic surgery.

# D.  Patient Position and Room Setup: TAPP or TEP

1.  The patient is supine with both arms tucked so that the surgeon has room to move cephalad in order to work down toward the pelvis.
2.  Surgeon stands on the side opposite of the hernia.
3.  Placement of a urinary catheter is optional and is according to surgeon preference.
4.  Placing the patient in the Trendelenberg position helps the peritoneum and viscera to fall away from the operative field.
5.  The monitor should be positioned at the foot of the bed.

# E.  Transabdominal Preperitoneal Approach

Distinctive features to the transabdominal laparoscopic approach include the ability to inspect the intra-abdominal cavity and the contralateral groin. The hernia sac itself is easier to recognize as its origin is identified. Finally, the landmarks are in a setting more familiar to the general surgeon.

1.  Laparoscopic inguinal hernia repair may result in significant pneumoscrotum due to dissection into the preperitoneal space in the inguinal region. This consequence may be avoided by lightly wrapping the scrotum and penis with a gauze roll prior to prepping and draping the patient. Patients are typically given intravenous antibiotics within 1 h prior to skin incision and receive compression devices for deep venous thrombosis prophylaxis.
2.  Initial port placement is a 10-mm port at the umbilicus. This facilitates visualization and provides a site for mesh insertion into the abdomen.
3.  Two subsequent 5-mm ports are placed at the level of the umbilicus and lateral to the semilunar line on either side of the 10-mm port (Fig. 32.2).

## TAPP Port Placement

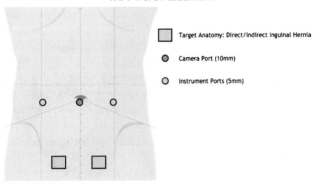

Fig. 32.2.  Transabdominal preperitoneal (TAPP) port (Courtesy of Dr. Michael Awad).

4.  Use a 30 or 45° angled laparoscope for the procedure and evaluate both inguinal regions for hernia defects with the patient in Trendelenberg position.

5.  Using laparoscopic scissors or a hook electrosurgery device, incise the peritoneum laterally by the anterior superior iliac spine at a distance of approximately 3 cm over the internal ring all the way to the median umbilical ligament.

6.  Sweep the peritoneum down to view the preperitoneal space.

7.  Medially, identify the symphysis pubis and Cooper's ligament. Pay special attention to the iliac vessels, as these structures lie within the operative field.

8.  At the level of the internal ring, identify the epigastric vessels and leave them on the abdominal wall.

9.  It is important to create a lateral space for mesh placement. Potential nerve injury can occur dissecting this space as the femoral branch of the genitofemoral nerve and the lateral femoral cutaneous nerve course here.

10.  Then, dissect the peritoneum off the cord structures posteriorly such that the divergent courses of the vas deferens and cord vessels may be seen proximal to the internal ring.

    i.  Indirect hernias must be separated from the cord structures. It is also important to evaluate for cord lipomas as they can be mistaken as associated fatty tissue on the cord vessels. Large indirect sacs that track down into the scrotum should be transected at the level of the internal ring to prevent displacement of the testicle out of the scrotum or testicular devascularization.

ii. Direct hernia sacs are medial to the epigastric vessels and should be reduced manually.

iii. Femoral hernias can be manually reduced as well.

11. Select a large (10 cm by 15 cm) piece of mesh (usually polypropylene or polyester based) and place it into the abdomen via the 10-mm port.

12. Position the mesh so that the entire myopectineal orifice is covered with good superior, medial, and lateral overlap. The mesh necessarily overlaps the cord structures in order to cover the indirect space completely. It is important that the peritoneum and sac be reduced proximal to where the inferior border of the mesh will lie so that it cannot slip back under the mesh and lead to a recurrence.

13. Anchor the mesh with spiral tacks at three major places (Fig. 32.3):

i. Laterally and superiorly about 2 cm medial to the anterior superior iliac spine and above the inguinal ligament (so that the cutaneous nerve branches to the thigh are avoided).

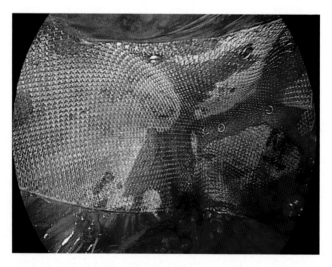

Fig. 32.3. Mesh fixation with spiral metal tacks for left inguinal hernia repair placement.

ii. Midline and medial to the inferior epigastric vessels on the abdominal wall.

iii. Just above the pubic tubercle and into Cooper's ligament along the superior border of the pubic ramus. The location of the femoral vessels should be clear at all times in order to avoid injury to these structures. It is important not to place tacks directly into the pubic bone at any point because of the risk of periostitis and increased postoperative pain.

14. The peritoneal flap is closed back over the mesh either using a staple fixation device or an absorbable suture. It is important that there be no gaps in the peritoneal closure through which bowel could herniate. It may be beneficial to decrease the pneumoperitoneum prior to closure to decrease tension and prevent tenting of the peritoneal flap over the mesh.

15. For bilateral hernias, perform a similar dissection and mesh placement on the contralateral side.

16. Local anesthetic can be injected into the operative site.

17. The 10-mm fascial defect is typically closed in an open manner under direct vision or using a fascial closure device.

# F. Totally Extraperitoneal Approach

The extraperitoneal approach is a more direct route to the preperitoneal space and eliminates the need to open and close the peritoneum. For this reason, it is usually faster to perform and the balloon does much of the dissection of the space. The main disadvantages are that the working space is smaller, understanding the anatomy requires experience, and small peritoneal tears that can compromise the working space occur frequently. Because of these factors, the learning curve for the TEP approach may be longer than for the TAPP approach.

1. Incision and access: make a 1.5–2 cm incision below the umbilicus, and incise the anterior rectus sheath just off the midline toward the side of inguinal hernia. Retract the rectus muscle laterally and identify the posterior sheath.

2. Development of the preperitoneal space: the preperitoneal space is most often developed with a specialized dissection balloon but some surgeons use blunt dissection to perform this step. Place the dissection balloon along the posterior rectus sheath and guide it into the preperitoneal space below the arcuate line

**TEP Port Placement**

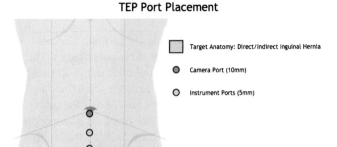

Fig. 32.4. Total extraperitoneal (TEP) port placement (Courtesy of Dr. Michael Awad).

anterior to the peritoneum and down to and 1–2 cm under the pubis. Expand the balloon under direct vision with either a 0 or 30° laparoscope.

3. Deflate the balloon and replace it by a balloon-tipped trocar. Insufflate the space with $CO_2$ to a pressure of 12–15 mmHg[++].

4. Place two 5-mm ports in the lower midline under direct laparoscopic vision. Alternatively, first bluntly dissect the lateral space after the first 5 mm port is inserted and then place one of the ancillary ports laterally (Fig. 32.4). Use two blunt, atraumatic graspers for the dissection. Unlike most other procedures, the dissection is largely done using blunt techniques with atraumatic laparoscopic graspers without the need for a surgical energy source. A key initial component to the dissection is creation of a large lateral space up to almost the level of the umbilicus.

5. The remainder of the dissection, mesh placement, and fixation is similar to the described TAPP procedure. It is important to continually confirm anatomic landmarks in this space in order to maintain orientation and avoid injury to other structures. For direct sacs, the balloon completes much of the hernia dissection. Indirect sacs must be carefully teased away from the cord structures and vas deferens and reduced for several centimeters proximal to the internal ring (Fig. 32.5).

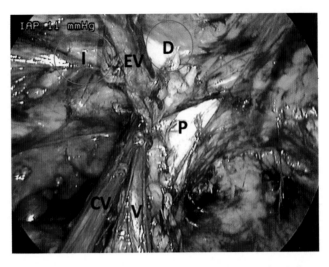

Fig. 32.5. Dissected preperitoneal space for left inguinal hernia. *D* direct space, *I* indirect space, *P* pubic bone, *EV* epigastric vessels, *V* vas deferens, *CV* cord vessels.

6. For dissection of the contralateral side, the same ports are used and the space is bluntly dissected under direct vision, keeping the inferior epigastric vessels anterior on the posterior rectus.

7. Anchor the mesh in a similar fashion as for the TAPP approach. Inspect the field for hemostasis and evacuate the space of $CO_2$ while keeping the inferior borders of the mesh flat. This maneuver reduces the chance that the leading peritoneal edge will slip back under the mesh during desufflation.

8. Close the anterior rectus sheath at the umbilicus with an absorbable suture and close the skin. Local anesthetic can be infiltrated at the port sites either during placement or at the conclusion of the procedure.

## G. Complications

Major complications after laparoscopic inguinal hernia repair are uncommon and are best avoided by a detailed knowledge of preperitoneal anatomy and a precise and careful anatomic dissection. Most other complications are similar to those for open inguinal hernia repair but with some differences. In experienced hands, complications are infrequent.

## 1. Bleeding/Vascular Injuries

a.  **Cause and Prevention**: Overall, major vascular injuries have been reported in 0.4–0.6% of patients. The most common vessel to be injured during laparoscopic inguinal hernia repair is the inferior epigastrics, although cord vessels and iliac vessels are also potentially vulnerable. Another potential source of bleeding is from small arteries and veins that run transversely along the superior pubic ramus and the obturator vessels which lie deep to the femoral canal. Injuries to these vessels often occur because of inappropriate identification of the anatomy or confusing anatomy, which may be secondary to hernia size, prior surgery, or surgeon inexperience. Understanding the key features of the preperitoneal space, creation of an adequate working space, and a gentle, precise dissection technique are important variables in avoiding vascular injury. Dissection and/or mesh fixation in the region of the iliac vessels (see "Triangle of Doom" above) can also lead to major bleeding events.

b.  **Recognition and Management**: One should be suspicious of any bleeding during laparoscopic inguinal hernia repair. It is important to keep in mind that insufflation of the preperitoneal space may actually mask bleeding; therefore, one must carefully examine the operative field for any active bleeding prior to closure. Bleeding from small vessels will stop and rarely requires reoperation. However, injuries to the epigastric and iliac vessels can be life threatening events that require prompt intervention. The inferior epigastric vessels can be ligated either with clips or by percutaneous suture placement in the event of an injury, but iliac vessel injuries require immediate open repair. Unlike open inguinal hernia repair where bleeding typically results in visible swelling and hematoma, patients who bleed after LIHR may harbor a substantial amount of blood in the preperitoneal space with minimal exam findings. Symptoms may include pain out of proportion to the procedure, difficulty with urination, weakness, and dizziness. Aggressive reevaluation in the office or emergency room that includes cross-sectional imaging is warranted to make the diagnosis.

## 2. Urologic Complications

a. **Cause and Prevention**: Postoperative urinary retention is one of the most common complications after LIHR and occurs in approximately 2–7% of patients. Factors that my impact the rate of urinary retention include a history of prostate or urinary symptoms, general anesthetic, and administration of excessive intravenous fluids both intraoperatively and early postoperatively. Urinary tract infection should be rare unless the bladder has been instrumented with a catheter. Injury to the urinary bladder or distal ureter is the most serious urologic complications reported during LIHR. History of prior violation of the preperitoneal space (e.g., prostatectomy) potentially increases the risk of urologic injury making the preperitoneal approach relatively contraindicated. There can be chronic urologic complications as well, which are related to the placement and migration of mesh in the preperitoneal space. Reports of erosion or fixation of mesh into the bladder leading to chronic infection, pain, and hematuria have also occurred. Postoperative symptoms of urinary frequency, urgency, pain with urination, or hematuria after LIHR should be evaluated aggressively for the cause.

b. **Recognition and Management**: Urinary retention is treated by catheterization; if more than 500 ml is returned, the catheter may need to be left in place for 2–3 days until bladder detrusor function recovers. Extraperitoneal bladder injuries should be repaired if identified at the index procedure with catheterization postoperatively. Delayed diagnosis presents a problem because of potential mesh contamination. The spectrum of treatment can range from catheterization only to mesh explantation with primary hernia repair with autologous tissue. Symptoms of recurrent UTI, pain with urination, urinary frequency, and hematuria should undergo evaluation for the cause. Cystoscopy and imaging with computed tomography (CT) scan should be performed if mesh erosion into the bladder is a possibility. Management of this complication requires mesh explantation and bladder repair.

## 3. Nerve Injury

a. **Cause and Prevention**: Chronic pain has replaced recurrence as the most common complication after either open or laparoscopic hernia repair. Chronic pain is usually defined as inguinal pain or discomfort lasting greater than 3 months postoperatively. With laparoscopic repair, the incidence of chronic pain is low and has been reported as 1–2% in some series. Causes of postoperative pain manifest from three potential sources: mesh, mesh fixation, and the dissection of the preperitoneal space itself. Mesh selection for inguinal hernia has trended toward the use of lightweight mesh which contracts less and creates a less dense scar plate which may result in less postoperative symptoms. Methods of mesh fixation include the use of spiral metal tacks, absorbable tacks, fibrin sealants, or no fixation at all (see Sect. H). Misplaced tacks in the triangle of pain (borders include the inguinal ligament, cord structures and the lateral peritoneal dissection) predisposes one to injury of the femoral nerve branches and the lateral femoral cutaneous nerve. Nerve injury may also occur during dissection of the hernia and peritoneum as well. During creation of the lateral space, one must take care to leave the fine layer of fat that covers the abdominal wall musculature to ensure that the blunt dissection is not carried too deep, thereby exposing the nerves to potential injury. Whether the approach is laparoscopic or open, the groin nerves should not be skeletonized, which exposes them to fibrosis from the adjacent mesh.

b. **Recognition and Management**: The initial management for chronic pain is conservative measures which include a course of rest and nonsteroidal anti-inflammatory medications (NSAIDS). Injections with combinations of local anesthetic and steroids can be both diagnostic and therapeutic. For those patients refractory to these measures, surgical intervention can be up to 80% effective in resolving or decreasing symptoms. Aims of surgical management are to remove possible offending tacks or the mesh itself if necessary.

## 4. Testicular and Fertility Complications

a. **Cause and Prevention**: Some degree of testicular discomfort related to dissection of the cord structures is not unusual after LIHR. This typically is self-limited and resolves within a few weeks of the repair. Injuries to the cord structures including the vas deferens can occur during the dissection of the hernia sac but are uncommon. These injuries can be avoided by using minimal electrosurgery during the dissection and doing fine blunt dissection of the hernia sac off the cord. There are reports of mesh placement in the preperitoneal space causing obstructive azoospermia, but this has been mainly associated with keyholing the mesh around and the cord structures. Ischemic orchitis is a rare complication of LIHR and is usually associated with large hernias. This complication can occur when a large sac is dissected along the full extent of the cord leading to vascular disruption and ischemia.

b.  **Recognition and Management**: Patients may have some temporary scrotal swelling from the pneumoperitoneum which usually resolves quickly but beyond that scrotal swelling is uncommon. Pneumoscrotum can be avoided by wrapping the testicles with gauze preoperatively (see operative descriptions). Some patients may experience testicular discomfort that is usually self-limited. Pain control and scrotal support is the preferred management. Ischemic orchitis is best avoided by not dissecting the entire sac down into the scrotum and transecting it more proximally instead. If injury to the vas deferens occurs, it can be repaired primarily.

## 5.  *Recurrence*

a.  **Cause and Prevention**: Recurrence after laparoscopic hernioplasty has become less frequent compared to the era of primary suture repair. Recurrences may be secondary to technical failures at the index procedure. Established causes of recurrence include: lateral recurrence, medial recurrence, missed cord lipoma, and mesh selection. Lateral recurrence can be secondary to failure to create a large enough lateral space, inadequate fixation laterally, or an inadequately sized mesh. Medial recurrences may happen for similar reasons. Inadequate dissection of the cord structures including inadequate identification of an indirect sac or a missed lipoma is another cause of recurrence. Finally, use of a smaller mesh that does not completely cover the myopectineal orifice with enough overlap can also lead to recurrence as the mesh contracts.

b.  **Recognition and Management**: Clinical exam is usually sufficient to make the diagnosis of a recurrent inguinal hernia. It is important to do a thorough exam because the characteristic reducible bulge may not occur in the usual location of the external ring. In some cases, the patient may have vague complaints and an unconvincing exam. Such a scenario may necessitate ultrasound or a CT scan to assist in the diagnosis. A preferred surgical strategy for recurrent hernia is to use the anterior approach to avoid reentering the operative field of the preperitoneal space.

## 6. *Miscellaneous*

a.  Seroma: The incidence of seroma has been found to be higher in LIHR compared to open inguinal hernia repair. The postoperative incidence can be as high as 16% and is often associated with a large direct sac. Patients should be reassured about this finding as most of these fluid collections resolve with time. Symptomatic or large fluid collections can be aspirated in the office under sterile conditions.

b.  Future prostatectomy: There has been concern that dissection of the preperitoneal space and placement of mesh for inguinal hernia may create a contraindication for future extraperitoneal radical prostatectomy. While it has been documented that prior LIHR with mesh increases the technical difficulty of prostatectomy, there has been controversy over whether there are increased adverse outcomes.

## H. Technical Controversies

There are technical subtleties to all surgical procedures that are widely a product of opinion and preference and laparoscopic inguinal hernia repair is no exception in this regard. Two major points of contention include methods of (or need for) mesh fixation (TAPP or TEP) and the closure of peritoneal tears during TEP repairs.

1.  **Mesh Fixation**: There are three main options for mesh fixation: spiral tacks, fibrin glue, and no fixation. Spiral tack fixation is the classic method used for LIHR and is the gold standard for

comparison. Some groups have advocated the use of a fibrin sealant to avoid potential issues of pain and other complications that may be associated with tack fixation. The rationale for this method is that the sealant provides temporary fixation and because the mesh is also held in place to some extent by the pressure of the peritoneum and contents on the inguinal floor until tissue ingrowth occurs. One theoretical advantage of fibrin glue is reduced risk of chronic postoperative pain since there is no tissue penetration. No mesh fixation at all has also been described, although this approach is less accepted.

2. **Peritoneal Tears**: Peritoneal tears at the time of TEP hernia repair occur not infrequently. There has been much debate regarding the management of these tears. Large tears can result in insufflation of the intraperitoneal cavity, thereby leading to decreased working space and loss of insufflation in the preperitoneal space. The general management of this problem is to lower $CO_2$ pressure and if the space or visualization is compromised, to place a Veress needle into the peritoneal cavity to decompress the pneumoperitoneum. The defect should be closed when feasible with a pretied loop suture in order to maintain the working space. Large tears may require suturing to close or even conversion to a TAPP approach. Potential risks of not repairing a tear are herniation of bowel through the defect, which can result in obstruction or exposure of uncoated mesh to intestine leading to fistulization. Though these theoretical risks exist, proponents of leaving peritoneal tears believe that after desufflation the redundant peritoneum folds upon itself and seals quickly, leaving the mentioned risks unlikely to occur. Currently, management of peritoneal tears is based on surgeon preference.

## Selected References

Chung R, Rowland D. Meta-analysis of randomized controlled trials of laparoscopic vs conventional inguinal hernia repairs. Surg Endosc. 1999;13:689–94.

Felix E, Harbertson N, Vartanian S. Laparoscopic hernioplasty. Surg Endosc. 1999; 13:328–31.

Felix E, Scott S, Crafton P, et al. Causes of recurrence after laparoscopic hernioplasty. Surg Endosc. 1998;12:226–31.

Ferzli G, Edwards E, Al-Khoury G, et al. Postherniorraphy groin pain and how to avoid it. Surg Clin N Am. 2008;88:203–16.

Hamouda A, Kennedy J, Grant N, et al. Mesh erosion into the urinary bladder following laparoscopic inguinal hernia repair; is this the tip of the iceberg? Hernia. 2010; 14:317–9.

Hindmarsh A, Cheong E, Lewis N, et al. Attendance at a pain clinic with severe pain after open and laparoscopic inguinal hernia repairs. Brit J Surg. 2003;90:1152–4.

Katkhouda N. A new technique for laparoscopic hernia repair using fibrin sealant. Surg Technol Int. 2004;12:120–6.

Kato Y, Yamataka A, Miyano G, et al. Tissue adhesives for repairing inguinal hernia: a preliminary study. J Lap Adv Surg Tech. 2005;15:424–8.

Keller J, Stefanidis D, Dolce C, et al. Combined open and laparoscopic approach to chronic pain after inguinal hernia repair. Am Surg. 2008;74:695–701.

Kocot A, Gerharz E, Riedmiller H. Urological complications of the laparoscopic inguinal hernia repair: a case series. Hernia. 2010; Hernia. 2011;15:583–6.

Kumar S, Wilson R, Nixon J, et al. Chronic pain after laparoscopic and open mesh repair of groin hernia. Brit J Surg. 2002;89:1476–9.

Lo Menzo E, Spector S, Iglesias A, et al. Management of recurrent inguinal hernias after total extraperitoneal herniorrhaphies. J Lap Adv Surg Tech. 2009;19:475–8.

Messaris E, Nicastri G, Dudrick S. Total extraperitoneal laparoscopic inguinal hernia repair without mesh fixation: prospective study with 1 year follow up results. Arch Surg. 2010;145:334–8.

Moore J, Hasenboehler E. Orchiectomy as a result of ischemic orchitis after laparoscopic inguinal hernia repair: case report of a rare complication. Patient Saf Surg. 2007;1:3.

Morena-Egea A, Paredes P, Perello J, et al. Vascular injury by tacks during totally extraperitneal endoscopic inguinal hernioplasty. Surg Laparosc Endosc Percutan Tech. 2010;20:129–31.

Muzio G, Bernard K, Polliand C, et al. Impact of peritoneal tears on the outcome and late results (4 years) of endoscopic totally extraperitoneal inguinal hernioplasty. Hernia. 2006;10:426–9.

Nagler H, Belletete B, Gerber E, et al. Laparoscopic retrieval of retroperitoneal vas deferens for postinguinal herniorraphy obstructive azoospermia. Fertil Steril. 1842; 2005(83):e1–3.

Pavlidis T. Current opinion on laparoscopic repair of inguinal hernia. Surg Endosc. 2010;24:974–6.

Peeters E, Spiessens C, Oyen R, et al. Laparoscopic inguinal hernia repair in men with lightweight meshes may significantly impair sperm motility. Ann Surg. 2010; 252:240–6.

Read R. Crucial steps in the evolution of the preperitoneal approaches to the groin: a historical review. Hernia. 2010; Hernia. 2011;15:1–5.

Schmedt C, Sauerland S, Bittner R. Comparison of endoscopic procedures vs Lichtenstein and other open mesh techniques for inguinal hernia repair. Surg Endosc. 2005; 19:188–99.

Schopf S, von Ahnen T, von Ahnen M, et al. Chronic pain after laparoscopic transabdominal preperitoneal hernia repair: a randomized comparison of light and extralight titanized polypropelene mesh. World J Surg. 2011;35(2):202–10.

Shpitz B, Lansberg L, Bugayev N, et al. Should peritoneal tears be routinely closed during laparoscopic total extraperitoneal repair of inguinal hernias? Surg Endosc. 2004; 18:1771–3.

Stolzenburg J, Ho K, Rabenalt R, et al. Impact of previous surgery on endoscopic extraperitoneal radical prostatectomy. Urology. 2005;65:325–31.

Takata M, Duh Q. Laparoscopic inguinal hernia repair. Surg Clin N Am. 2008;88:157–78.

Voeller G. Laparoscopic approach to inguinal hernia repair. Prob Gen Surg. 2002;19:42–50.

Winslow E, Quasebarth M, Brunt LM. Perioperative outcomes and complications of open vs. laparoscopic extraperitoneal inguinal hernia repair in a mature surgical practice. Surg Endosc. 2004;18:221–7.

# 33. Laparoscopic Repair of Ventral Hernia[*]

*Michael J. Rosen, M.D.*

## A. Indications and Contraindications

1. **The general indication** for a laparoscopic repair of a ventral hernia is the presence of a hernia in patients who would otherwise meet the criteria for a traditional open surgical repair. Identifying the most appropriate patient for the laparoscopic repair can be more challenging. The laparoscopic approach clearly provides the primary advantage of reduced wound morbidity and potential mesh infection than an open approach. However, after any bridging mesh repair (including laparoscopic ventral herniorrhaphy) the abdominal wall is often not functionalized and large sheets of adynamic prosthetics span the abdominal wall. This can result in an unsightly bulge, and lack of core strength in young thin active patients. Recognizing these limitations, I feel that laparoscopic ventral hernia repair is best reserved for obese, or elderly patients with small to medium (<15 cm wide) defects in which the bulge is often imperceptible, and reducing the chance of wound morbidity outweighs the potential advantage of medializing the rectus muscles. Young, active, manual labor patients are often offered a more formal reconstruction of the abdominal wall. Abdominal wall hernias in the midline or in the upper and lower quadrants are equally accessible by the laparoscopic approach. Special conditions include the following.

   a. **Incarcerated hernias**: Care must be taken to not injure the bowel while manually reducing the hernia contents. Using

---

[*] This chapter was contributed by Gerald M. Larson, MD in the previous edition.

bimanual palpation on the abdominal wall or extending the defect internally can aid safe reduction. Finally, if this cannot be achieved, a small open incision can be made over the defect, and the contents reduced and the skin closed and the mesh can be deployed laparoscopically.

b.  In the **multiply operated abdomen**: Safe adhesiolysis is the most important step to a successful laparoscopic ventral hernia repair. The extent of intra-abdominal adhesions is unpredictable, and multiply reoperative abdomens can successfully be completed laparoscopically. However, careful attention to prior operative reports, location of mesh, type of prior mesh, and surgeon comfort with difficult adhesiolysis should all be factored into choosing the most appropriate operation.

c.  **Suprapubic Hernias**: These can safely be approached laparoscopically. Placing a 3-way Foley catheter and instilling 300 cc of saline into the bladder aids in confirming the location of the bladder and safe mobilization. The mesh can be secured to the pelvis using sutures and tacks.

d.  **Subxiphoid Hernias**: These hernias are common after median sternotomy and can also be repaired laparoscopically. Key technical points include complete mobilization of the falciform ligament, and allowing the mesh to drape over the diaphragm. It is important to avoid placing any fixation above the xyphoid process for fear of injuring the pericardium.

2.  **Contraindications** to laparoscopic repair of ventral hernia include the densely scarred abdomen (in which it is impossible to safely introduce a trocar or establish a pneumoperitoneum), and the acute abdomen with strangulated or infarcted bowel. Large hernias with defects over 20 cm in width are also relative contraindications to the laparoscopic approach.

## B.  Patient Preparation and Room Setup

1.  Place the patient supine on the operating table. Tucking the patient's arms bilaterally allows the surgeon's to stand on either side along with the assistant. When performing pelvic dissections this is particularly helpful.

2.  For most midline hernias, the surgeon stands on the patient's left side. If the splenic flexure has been mobilized the surgeon can stand on the right. Two monitors are placed bilaterally at the head of the patient. If a suprapubic hernia is present, one monitor should be placed at the foot of the bed.

3.  The assistant stands opposite the surgeon, and a second monitor is placed in a suitable position.

4.  We no longer use preoperative bowel preparation, as it often induces an ileus, or distended bowels, and does not sterilize the intestines sufficiently to make synthetic mesh safe in cases of an enterotomy.

# C.  Trocar Position and Choice of Laparoscope (Fig. 33.1)

1.  The author prefers open access with a Hasson cannula because of the likelihood of adhesions and bowel fixed to the abdominal wall. Place the initial port in the lateral abdominal wall, typically just off the tip of the 11th rib. Placing ports as far laterally as possible aids in dissection and avoids overlapping with large pieces of prosthetic mesh. It is not advisable to place the first port in the midline, as these are often reoperative cases and one risks bowel injury at the site of prior midline incisions. Some surgeons use a direct vision trocar in the left upper quadrant as the initial port. This is another option to the open or Veress needle technique, and while many authors have reported excellent outcomes with these ports, major retroperitoneal vascular injuries can occur.Establish pneumoperitoneum. A 30° 5-mm laparoscope is helpful to visualize adhesions on the anterior abdominal wall.

2.  Place two 5-mm ports in the lateral abdominal wall on the same side as the Hasson. This allows the surgeon to operate two handed in line with the camera. After complete adhesiolysis, place an additional 5 mm port on the opposite side to allow fixation of the mesh on one side (Fig. 33.1).

3.  The surgeon can perform adhesiolysis using one hand to provide counter traction and the other hand using scissors to lyse adhesions. Utilizing a 5 mm scope allows the surgeon to change ports freely during the dissection. We strictly avoid the use of

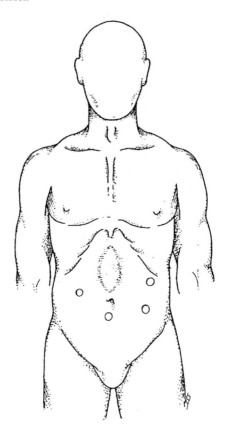

Fig. 33.1. Demonstration of port placement for repair of a ventral hernia in the upper abdomen. Place the first trocar in the lower midline, 2 or 3 in. inferior to the ventral hernia. Ventral hernias in the lower abdomen require placement of the camera port in the upper abdomen.

electrocautery, ultrasonic dissection, or LigaSure during adhesiolysis. Instead, 5-mm clips are utilized if necessary to avoid inadvertent thermal injury to the bowel. The minimal bleeding that can result is rarely disruptive as it often runs down out of the field.

4.  It is important to perform a complete adhesiolysis of the entire anterior abdominal wall to avoid missing any occult hernias. It is technically challenging to perform additional adhesiolysis once the prosthetic mesh is in the abdomen (Fig. 33.2).

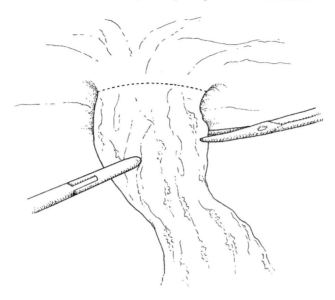

Fig. 33.2.  Laparoscopic view of a ventral hernia with incarcerated omentum. The hernia contents must be dissected free from the abdominal wall to expose the hernia defect.

## D. The Technique of Laparoscopic Hernia Repair

Laparoscopic hernia repair is an intra-abdominal, intraperitoneal repair that uses a mesh prosthesis to secure and cover the hernia defect. The hernia defect itself is typically not closed and therefore it is more of a patch of the defect. Given this limitation, it is important to adequately size the mesh for sufficient overlap and provide durable fixation. There is little general agreement as to the ideal size of the overlap necessary. It is the authors' opinion that overlap should depend on defect and patient characteristics. Large defects in obese patients require additional overlap (at least 5 cm) and more transfascial fixation. However, smaller defects, or swiss cheese defects probably require 4–5 cm of overlap and only four transfascial sutures. The mesh is anchored and held in position with transfascial mattress sutures (0-PTFE); usually four mattress sutures, but for larger hernias twelve or more mattress sutures placed at 5- to 6-cm intervals, is appropriate. The sutures are tied through a small stab incision in the skin and tied subcutaneously. In between the mattress sutures the mesh is tacked to the abdominal wall fascia at 1-cm intervals with special hernia spiral tacks. Recently several absorbable fixation devices have been introduced to reduce pain and adhesion formation. Little data exists detailing any benefit to these fixation devices.

An important principle of laparoscopic ventral hernia repair is appropriate mesh sizing and fixation. The mesh should be placed under moderate tension to avoid excessive buckling when releasing the pneumoperitoneum. Many techniques have been described to place the prosthetic, but the author likes to consider two steps in this process: measuring to size the mesh, and appropriately centering the mesh during deployment.

1.  **Sizing the Mesh**: Measuring the size of the defect and determining the appropriate sized mesh can be done using multiple techniques. Because the skin can be at a variable distance away from the fascia (particularly in obese patients), one can obtain falsely elevated measurements if performed on the skin. In small hernias, this is of little consequence; however, in larger defects, excess mesh can become very difficult to appropriately place without buckling (Fig. 33.3).

    a.  Measure the length of the defect using 22 gauge spinal needles, and a 15-cm ruler with the inches cut off to fit down a 5-mm port. Place the spinal needles through the abdominal wall at the longest point of the hernia in a cephalad to caudad orientation. The tips of the needles are then measured from within the abdomen using the ruler. Before removing the needles, draw a line on the outside of the patient to mark their location. This will be used later during centering measurements.

    b.  Measure the defect at its widest point in a medial to lateral direction using the needles and a ruler. Again, draw an external line on the skin to mark the widest point of the hernia. The two internal measurements are used to size the mesh. I typically add 10 cm to each of the numbers to provide a 5-cm overlap in all directions. It is important to point out that using this technique, some areas of the hernia will be overlapped with more than 5 cm of coverage, while no area will be less than 5 cm. It is tempting to tailor the mesh to fit the defect exactly, however, this makes it very difficult to adequately center the mesh, because if it doesn't come up exactly on the line one side might not be adequately overlapped.

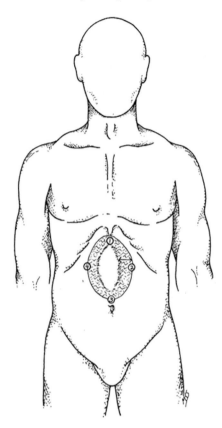

Fig. 33.3.  Cut the mesh prosthesis to the desired size and mark its intended location on the anterior abdominal wall. The shaded area indicates the approximate outline of the ventral hernia, and the mesh is indicated by crosshatches. The mesh should extend beyond the hernia defect by 3 cm or more on all sides. This 3-cm cuff will be used to anchor the mesh to the solid tissue surrounding the defect for the repair.

c.  Cut the mesh to size. We then fold the mesh in half one way and draw a line, and then fold in half the other orientation and draw another line. These lines mark the center point of the mesh. Place a 0-PTFE suture on each of these lines near the edge of the mesh as a mattress. Roll the mesh upon itself, protecting the anti-adhesive barrier if necessary, and pass it into the abdomen.

2. **Center the Mesh**: It is crucial to find the center point of the hernia to appropriately orient the mesh. Accomplish this by measuring the external lines drawn at the location of the spinal needles. Measure each of these points and draw a line across the entire abdomen at the half way point a line is drawn across the entire abdomen. By doing so, you have found the actual center point of the hernia defect via external measurements. Recall that you have also found the center point of the mesh during the prior steps by marking another cruciate line on the mesh. A suture has also been placed in the mesh on each of these lines. These marks on the anterior abdominal wall will correlate where the transfascial sutures are to be retrieved that are placed on the lines of the. The key to this system is that the mesh is centered by using lines on the skin to prevent any difficulty using laparoscopic visualization and alignment.

3. Bring the first suture at the point where one is most limited by overlap, typically based on proximity to the xyphoid or pubis bone. Using the center lines drawn externally, pass a spinal needle into the abdomen to mark the superior extent of the hernia defect. A standard small bowel grasper opened up is 4 cm. Use this device to measure 4 cm of overlap and pass a second spinal needle through the abdominal wall, on the center line to retrieve the transfascial suture tails at that site (Fig. 33.4). Repeat the procedure on the opposite side of the abdomen—use another needle to mark this center point at the edge of the hernia defect, measure 4 cm with the opened grasper, and pass a second spinal needle. To overcome any errors in measurements of the mesh, pull these two sutures tightly, while grasping the third pretied knot on the mesh and to stretch it taut. The spinal needle is placed on the center line localizing this knot, and the suture ties retrieved. These three sutures are tied, with the knots buried under subcutaneous tissue. The fourth suture is then grasped and stretched tightly across the abdominal wall, localizing the area to retrieve and secure this suture in a similar manner.

4. Secure the edges of the mesh to the abdominal wall using a spiral tacker every one centimeter. If necessary, place additional transfascial sutures of 1–0 Prolene every 4–5 cm.

5. Close the cutdown trocar site with a Vicryl suture and the small skin incisions in the usual fashion.

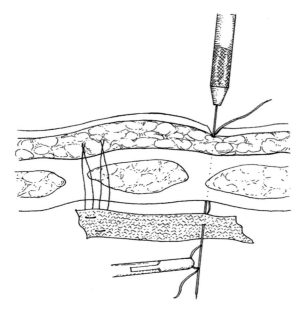

Fig. 33.4.  Method of mesh fixation with a suture passer. Use the suture passer to introduce the suture through the musculofascial layer, the mesh, and then back out through all layers as a mattress suture. Use 4–8 mattress sutures to anchor the mesh, depending on the size of the hernia and the surgeon's preference. Knot the sutures subcutaneously. Use hernia tackers or staples to fix the mesh to the abdominal wall between the mattress sutures.

# E.  Complications

Complications include trocar site wound infection, seroma, enterotomy, urinary retention, and postoperative ileus. Dissection of adhesions and manipulation of bowel may result in injury (see Chap. 10.2, Previous Abdominal Surgery). Unlike most laparoscopic procedures, laparoscopic ventral hernia repair typically results in significant postoperative discomfort. These procedures are rarely outpatient procedures in my practice, and for larger hernia, the average length of stay is typically 3–4 days.

All patients develop some form of a seroma and patients should understand this is not a recurrent hernia. I typically advise wearing an abdominal binder for 4–6 weeks to compress the hernia sac and limit seroma formation.

**Recurrence** is the complication unique to hernia repair. The risk can be minimized by adhering to sound surgical principles, clearly identifying all fascial defects, and placing the mesh properly with solid fixation to sound tissue. The mesh must be sufficiently large, and it must be sutured under some (but not excessive) tension.

The **wound infection** rate should be no greater than for other laparoscopic procedures of similar magnitude. Infections can generally be treated by opening the wound. This must be done in a timely fashion so that the anchoring sutures are not jeopardized.

**Mechanical bowel obstruction** may result from internal herniation of bowel between anchoring sutures or clips. This may require laparotomy for repair. A high index of suspicion for any patient presenting with bowel obstruction early after this procedure should prompt relaparoscopy.

Missed enterotomy is a devastating complication associated with all ventral hernia repairs. Its management is controversial; however, it is critical to recognize early and intervene before systemic sepsis. Any patient with unexplained tachycardia, fever, or elevated white blood cell count after postoperative day two should be given consideration for second look laparoscopy.

# Selected References

Heniford BT, Ramshaw BJ. Laparoscopic ventral hernia repair. Surg Endosc. 2000; 14(5):419–23.

Holzman MD, Puret CM, Reintgen K. Laparoscopic ventral and incisional hernioplasty. Surg Endosc. 1997;11(1):32–5.

Larson GM. Ventral hernia repair by the laparoscopic approach. Surg Clin North Am. 2000;80(4):1329–40.

LeBlanc KA. The critical technical aspects of laparoscopic repair of ventral and incisional hernias. Am Surg. 2001;67:809–12.

MacFadyen BV, Arregui ME, Corbitt JD. Complications of laparoscopic herniorrhaphy. Surg Endosc. 1993;7:155–8.

Park A, Gagner M, Pomp A. Laparoscopic repair of large incisional hernias. Surg Laparosc Endosc. 1996;6(2):123–8.

Temudom T, Siadati M, Sarr MG. Repair of complex giant or recurrent ventral hernias by using tension-free intraparietal prosthetic mesh (Stoppa technique): lessons learned from our initial experience (fifty patients). Surgery. 1996;120(4):738–44.

# Part VII
# Pediatric Laparoscopy and Endoscopy

# 34. Pediatric Minimally Invasive Surgery: General Considerations

*John J. Meehan, M.D.*

## A. Applications

Pediatric general surgeons perform a wide variety of procedures in the abdomen and chest. Several pediatric MIS procedures are similar to MIS procedures for adults. However, there are some procedures that are unique to pediatric general surgery. The following three chapters focus on the differences between pediatric and adult techniques for MIS and highlight several common MIS procedures in children.

1. Basic procedures which are commonly performed in children but covered more extensively elsewhere in this manual include appendectomy, cholecystectomy, splenectomy, and adrenalectomy.
2. The following additional laparoscopic procedures are commonly performed in children:
   a. Contralateral exploration for inguinal hernia repair
   b. Pyloromyotomy
   c. Fundoplication
   d. Undescended testicle
   e. Laparoscopic assisted anorectal pull-through (Hirschprung's and imperforate anus)
   f. Resection of Meckel's diverticulum
   g. Reduction of Intussusception
3. The following thoracoscopic procedures are commonly performed in children:
   h. Empyema drainage and decortication
   i. Blebectomy for spontaneous pneumothorax
   j. Thoracoscopically assisted repair of pectus excavatum (Nuss procedure)

N.J. Soper and C.E.H. Scott-Conner (eds.), *The SAGES Manual: Volume 1* 443
*Basic Laparoscopy and Endoscopy*, DOI 10.1007/978-1-4614-2344-7_34,
© Springer Science+Business Media, LLC 2012

> k.  Congenital diaphragmatic hernia (CDH) repair
> l.  Pulmonary lobectomy (for pulmonary sequestration or congenital cystic adenomatoid malformation-CCAM)
> m.  Repair of esophageal atresia and tracheoesophageal fistula

## B.  Contraindications

Contraindications for laparoscopy in children have been dwindling over the years. While absolute contraindications may still exist, such as hemodynamic instability or resection of certain tumors (where risk of rupture is unacceptably high), many issues that were previously thought to be contraindications have been dismissed. There are now very few procedures which have yet to be accomplished using MIS. However, individual surgeons should each evaluate their own skill level and be sure they do not compromise the principles of a given procedure in an attempt to stay with the MIS approach. New MIS technologies have been enabling surgeons to perform more and more complex procedures. Robotics has made tremendous impact on the advancement of complex MIS procedures. Meanwhile, single incision laparoscopic surgery is finding a new niche in pediatrics, but it has been fairly limited to date. Robotic single incision surgery has now even been accomplished in kids and may be the perfect melding of both of these platforms.

## C.  Patient Position and Preparation

Ergonomic principles are crucial in planning any minimally invasive surgery. In pediatric surgery, these principles are even more important owing to the smaller intracorporeal environment inside the pediatric patient.

The arrangement and planning of every laparoscopic case can be compared to the alignment of a baseball field (Fig. 34.1).

1.  The camera is placed at home plate.
2.  The target of interest is at second base.
3.  The working ports are typically located at first and third bases.
4.  Monitors should be placed in centerfield directly behind the target at second base
5.  Accessory ports and assistants come in from the lateral fields (foul ground) as necessary.

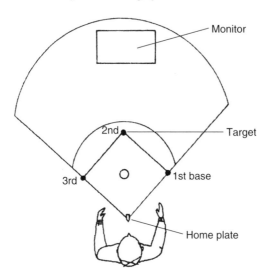

Fig. 34.1. Position the trocars and monitors using the baseball analogy. The camera is at home plate, instrument ports are at first and third bases, and the target lesion is at second base. Place the monitor directly in the surgeon's line of sight.

## D. Instrumentation and Port Size

The procedure planned will dictate port selection and size. For example, cholecystectomies and splenectomies may still require at least one larger port (10–12 mm) to extract the specimen. Although 5-mm instruments are probably the most popular for adult surgeons, the 3-mm instruments are now commonly used in pediatrics. Linear staplers, ultrasound probes, and specimen bags currently require ports which are 10–12 mm in size. Unfortunately, most current stapler designs are too large for neonates and small children, partially due to their diameter but mainly due to the lack of room for adequate articulating length. Argon beam coagulators, thermal sealing devices, bipolar technology, and a variety of other energy source options are now available in 5 mm form. Optics continues to improve with HD visualization now available even in small scope sizes. Most procedures in children are performed utilizing either a 3- or 5-mm scope using viewing angles of 0 and 30 degrees. Occasionally, a 70-degree scope may be useful which may be selected for the contralateral inguinal hernia exploration. Robotic surgery is now also used more frequently which has the distinct advantage of HD visualization in 3D with scopes as small as 8.5 mm and articulating instrumentation down to 5 mm.

# E.  Port Placement

1.  The smaller anterior-to-posterior distance in a child highlights the need for exercising extreme caution while placing trocars. Bladed and non-bladed trocars can both cause injury if not placed carefully. Access can be gained by inserting a Veress needle under controlled guidance or placing a Hasson blunt-tipped trocar.

    a.  To gain access using a Veress needle,

        i.  Anterior retraction on the abdominal wall is critical. Place a Kocher clamp securely on the fascia and retract upward. Alternate techniques include use of a piercing towel clamp or a monofilament suture to lift and retract the abdominal wall anteriorly.

        ii.  Insert the needle and listen for the "click" indicating the spring loaded retraction of the sharp needle blade.

        iii.  Test the placement by sweeping the needle back and forth torquing it upward against the anterior abdominal wall. It should move freely. If not, it may still be in the subcutaneous tissues.

        iv.  Further test the placement by injecting saline through the Veress needle port. A 5 or 10 cc syringe is perfect for this step. Upon disconnecting the syringe, residual saline in the clear plastic hub should fall into the abdomen by gravity.

        v.  Insufflate to desired pressure.

    b.  To gain access using a Hasson cannula, make a small fascial incision under direct visualization. Insert the blunt-tipped cannula into the abdomen under direct vision.

        vi.  Gain access to the fascia under direct visualization and incise the fascia a short distance. It is particularly important to make the trocar incisions as small as possible in children to limit $CO_2$ escape and loss of the pneumoperitoneum.

        vii.  Place two large 0 or 2–0 absorbable sutures into the fascia and hold upward traction.

        viii.  Insert the blunt tipped Hasson trocar in through the open incision and secure the large absorbable sutures to the Hasson.

        ix.  Insufflate to desired pressure.

2. While adults can usually tolerate a pneumoperitoneum of 15 cm $H_2O$, small children may have significant hemodynamic compromise with pressures of that magnitude. Size is the most important factor but can also hinge on the patient's underlying disease. Other patient related issues may also factor into the selected pressures. For example, CDH patients often have significant $CO_2$ retention and further $CO_2$ compromise may be too much to tolerate. Although many factors ultimately determine whether a pneumoperitoneum will be tolerated, the following suggestions are reasonable guidelines:

    a. Infants, newborns, and patients less than 10 kg: May only tolerate 7–8 cm of $H_2O$.

    b. Children between 10 and 20 kg: 12 or 13 cm $H_2O$.

    c. Children larger than 20 kg: 15 cm $H_2O$.

3. Closure of 5-mm trocar sites in adults is rarely necessary. That is not true for children. Incisional hernias may occur in small children with unclosed port sites as small as 5 mm. We recommend that all trocar sites 5 mm or larger should be formally closed at the fascial level if the fascia can be reached by locally exploring the wound. Port sites that are 2- and 3-mm sites usually do not require fascial closure.

# Selected Readings

Garrett D, Emami C, Anselmo DM, Torres MB, Nguyen N. Single-incision laparoscopic approach to management of splenic pathology in children: an early experience. J Laparoendosc Adv Surg Tech A. 2011;21(10):965–7.

Muensterer OJ, Puga Nougues C, Adibe OO, Amin SR, Georgeson KE, Harmon CM. Appendectomy using single-incision pediatric endosurgery for acute and perforated appendicitis. Surg Endosc. 2010;24(12):3201–4. Epub 2010 May 19.

Oltmann SC, Garcia NM, Ventura B, Mitchell I, Fischer AC. Single-incision laparoscopic surgery: feasibility for pediatric appendectomies. J Pediatr Surg. 2010;45(6): 1208–12.

Ponsky TA, Rothenberg SS. Minimally invasive surgery in infants less than 5 kg: experience of 649 cases. Surg Endosc. 2008;22(10):2214–9. Epub 2008 Jul 23.

Rothenberg SS, Shipman K, Yoder S. Experience with modified single-port laparoscopic procedures in children. J Laparoendosc Adv Surg Tech A. 2009;19(5):695–8.

# 35. Pediatric Minimally Invasive Surgery: Specific Surgical Procedures

*John J. Meehan, M.D.*

## Section I: Laparoscopy

## A. Appendectomy

1.  General considerations. Laparoscopic appendectomy is becoming more and more frequent for treating acute appendicitis in both pediatric and adult patients. In small thin children, a few surgeons still prefer the open technique because the procedure can be performed through a small 2–3 cm incision. Laparoscopic exploration, however, gives excellent visualization and may allow for improved suctioning of the right gutter, right lower quadrant, and deep pelvis in perforated patients. A Foley catheter is recommended prior to trocar placement.

2.  Positioning and trocar placement. The patient is supine with the table in Trendelenberg and tilted to the patient's left. Three trocars are generally required, and two popular techniques can be used (Figs. 35.1 and 35.2). Although both methods are equally effective, we prefer the trocar placement outlined in Figure 35.1. In this arrangement, the video tower is off to the right of the operating table and the surgeon and the assistant both stand on the patient's left, giving both caregivers the same visual perspective. The surgeon and the assistant may need to be on opposite sides of the table in the other method (Fig. 35.2).

3.  Details of operative procedure. Surgical technique is similar to that employed in adults (see Chap. 30) and is summarized here.
    a.  Suction out purulent fluid if present. Although the data has been debated, recent evidence suggests that suctioning alone is superior to irrigation and suction.

N.J. Soper and C.E.H. Scott-Conner (eds.), *The SAGES Manual: Volume 1 Basic Laparoscopy and Endoscopy*, DOI 10.1007/978-1-4614-2344-7_35, © Springer Science+Business Media, LLC 2012

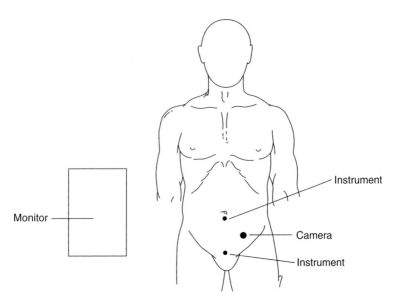

Fig. 35.1.  Port placement for laparoscopic appendectomy (preferred placement) with a single monitor to the right of the operating table, directly opposite the surgeon. Surgeon and assistant stand on patient's left.

b. Take any adhesions down bluntly or with cautery until the appendix is mobilized and free from the retroperitoneum.

c. Dissect through the mesoappendix to isolate the appendiceal artery with a curved dissector.

d. The mesenteric vessels may be secured with an ultrasonic dissector, stapler, LigaSure, bipolar, or standard cautery. When using the stapler, a finer vascular load is ideal.

e. After dividing the mesoappendix, amputate the appendix with a stapler or ligate it with a pretied suture ligature such as an Endoloop™. If pretied ligatures are used, we recommend using two loops on the patient side near the base of the appendix, followed by one on the specimen side.

f. Amputate the appendix and remove it through the umbilical port. Recent evidence suggests that the use of a specimen retrieval bag is associated with a lower rate of umbilical wound infection.

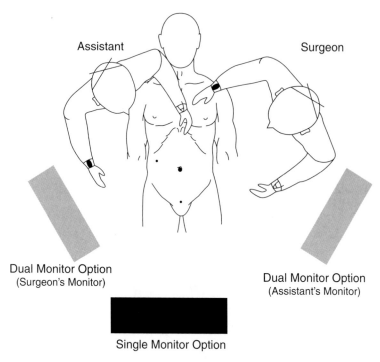

Fig. 35.2. Port placement for laparoscopic appendectomy (alternate placement) with two monitors. The surgeon stands to the left, and the assistant may need to stand to the patient's right.

## B. Cholecystectomy

1. General considerations. Laparoscopic cholecystectomy is very similar in pediatric patients to the corresponding adult procedure (see Chaps. 20–22). In addition to symptomatic cholelithiasis, other causes of cholecystitis in children include the following:
   a. Cystic fibrosis.
   b. Sickle cell anemia.
   c. Chronic use of total parenteral nutrition.
2. Patient positioning and trocar placement:
   a. The patient is placed supine in reverse Trendelenberg.
   b. For most patients, four trocars are used, placed in a manner similar to that used in adults (Fig. 35.3). However, slight

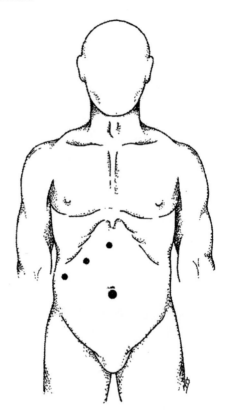

Fig. 35.3. Port placement for laparoscopic cholecystectomy.

modifications of the trocar placement may be required in smaller patients.

3.  Details of procedure (see Chap. 20).

   a.  Grasp the gallbladder through the retracting port and push it cephalad and over the liver to expose the porta hepatis.

   b.  Use a grasper through the midclavicular port to retract the infundibulum of the gall bladder laterally and the majority of the dissection is carried out from the midline port.

   c.  Begin the dissection laterally and proceed medially to safely identify structures.

   d.  Identify the cystic duct and dissect it to expose an adequate length. Lateral traction of the fundus of the gallbladder should be maintained during this dissection to help expose the proper dissecting angle.

    e. If a cholangiogram is desired, only partially divide the duct to facilitate cannulation (see also Chap. 22).

       i. Advance the cholangiogram catheter into the cystic duct. A Kumar camp is an example of a 5-mm laparoscopic instrument that can be useful as an adjunct for performing the cholangiogram.

      ii. Place a clip lightly over the proximal duct and catheter to prevent back-leakage from the open ductomy, taking care not to occlude the catheter. We recommend using contrast that has been diluted 1 to 1.

    f. After completing the cholangiogram, remove the temporary clip, retrieve the catheter, and secure the proximal and distal cystic duct with the clip applier. We recommend two clips on the patient side and one on the specimen side. Complete the division of this structure.

    g. The cystic artery is usually located in close proximity to the duct, slightly medial and superior. Dissect this structure in a similar manner holding lateral traction on the fundus of the gallbladder. Clip and divide it in a similar fashion. Electrocautery has also been used successfully and can be applied in smaller vessels.

    h. The gallbladder is taken down in a retrograde fashion using hook cautery.

    i. Remove the specimen through the umbilical port site. An endocatch bag is recommended. Occasionally, the incision will need to be extended or dilated slightly to retrieve the specimen if large stones are present.

# C. Laparoscopic Splenectomy

1. General considerations. Postsplenectomy sepsis is far more common in children than in adults. Whenever possible, vaccinations for *Pneumococcus*, *Meningococcus*, and *Hemophilus* should be completed preoperatively. They can be given postoperatively following emergent splenectomies but have not been as effective.

2. Patient positioning and trocar placement. Flexibility in port placement should be tailored on a case-by-case basis as some patients may have a significantly larger spleen than others. Adaptability is key while maintaining the ergonomic relationships of the working space.

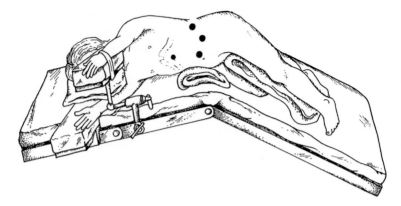

Fig. 35.4. Patient position and port placement for pediatric laparoscopic splenectomy. Note that the patient is in the lateral position, and the operating table has been flexed to increase the distance between costal margin and superior iliac crest.

    a. Place the patient in a right lateral decubitus position. Alternatively, the patient can be supine with a bump under the left hip to elevate the left side about 45°.

    b. Positioning the patient over the break in the table and flexing the table a small amount can help, particularly if the lateral decubitus position is desired.

    c. Port placement is shown in Fig. 35.4.

3.  Details of procedure (also see Volume II, Chap. 26).

    a. Begin by taking down the splenic attachments including the splenocolic, splenorenal, and splenophrenic ligaments. This can be accomplished with either a hook cautery, the LigaSure, a bipolar, or an ultrasonic dissector.

    b. Divide the short gastric vessels in a similar fashion, preferably reserving dissection of the splenic hilum for last.

    c. Elevate the spleen using a retractor or grasper from the accessory port and completely mobilize any remaining attachments to the spleen.

    d. Dissect and expose the hilar vessels. Ideally, the artery should be ligated before the vein. This avoids potential significant congestion of the spleen which is inevitable if the vein is taken before the artery.

        i. A wide variety of options exist for taking down the hilar vessels. These include use of an endoscopic stapler with a vascular load, endoclips, an ultrasonic dissector, stapler, or the LigaSure. We prefer the LigaSure as long as the vessels are smaller than the maximal allowable vessel for the LigaSure (7 mm or smaller).

e. Place the specimen in an endocatch bag. Removal of the spleen will require morcellation. This step can be facilitated if ringed forceps are used to help break the specimen down. Extending the extraction trocar site a short distance can reduce unnecessary frustration during this final tedious step.

# D. Laparoscopic Adrenalectomy

Pediatric Adrenalectomy should follow the same recommendations as found in adults in Chap. 27.

# E. Contralateral Exploration for Inguinal Hernia

Controversy continues to surround exploration for a possible contralateral inguinal hernia in children less than 6 months of age. Open exploration carries a risk of injury to the vas deferens or testicular vessels. Laparoscopic exploration offers an alternative to the open contralateral incision and may have less risk of testicular damage. The justification of contralateral exploration has also been recently challenged as infertility rates in patient who had bilateral surgery as children have now shown to be significantly higher than patients who had unilateral procedures. The perceived justification of bilateral incidence of 8–10% previously quoted has also now come under fire, as the true incidence may be substantially lower. Advocates of the laparoscopic exploration claim the use of the scope has all but eliminated this risk but the procedure still carries a risk of ipsilateral hernia sac disruption while trying to inspect the contralateral internal ring.

Description of procedure:

1. Isolate the ipsilateral hernia sac via open exploration.
2. The hernia sac is entered and a 3–5 mm trocar inserted into the abdomen through the open tunica vaginalis (hernia sac). Care should be taken to be sure not to tear the hernia sac.
3. Insufflate with 5–10 cm of pressure.

4. Preferentially, a 70° scope is ideal to visualize the contralateral internal ring. A 30° scope will suffice if a 70° is unavailable.

5. After the determination has been made, remove the trocar and allow the abdomen to desufflate and ligate the ipsilateral hernia sac in the usual fashion.

6. If a hernia is present, the contralateral side can be explored and a standard open repair performed immediately.

## F. Laparoscopic Pyloromyotomy

1. Patient positioning and trocar placement:
   a. Position the patient supine. We recommend that the baby, not the table, be rotated 90° so that they lay across the table transversely instead of inline longitudinally.
   b. Optionally, a small roll can be placed under the back transversely to slightly hyperextend the spine, allowing better access to the pylorus.
   c. The surgeon and assistant stand at the patient's feet.
   d. The table is rolled slightly toward the surgeon and the assistant.
   e. Place one 3-mm trocar at the umbilicus and two small stab incisions in the left upper and right upper quadrants as shown in Fig. 35.5. The stab incisions are made using an 11 blade directly through the abdominal wall (trocars will not be needed). Care should be taken not to make the stab incisions too large as insufflation will be lost.

2. Details of procedure:
   a. Place a grasper directly through the right upper quadrant stab incision and grasp the duodenum just distal to the pylorus.
   b. Pass a pyloromyotomy knife, commonly referred as a pyloro-tome, through the left upper quadrant incision. Make a longitudinal incision into the serosa of the pylorus. The pylorotome is designed so that it only makes an incision about 2 mm in depth (Fig. 35.6a).
      i. A commonly used alternative to the pylorotome is a cautery blade which is used as a blunt cutting instrument. NOTE: use of the thermal energy source is not recommended for this step, just the cautery blade itself.

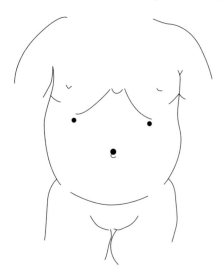

Fig. 35.5.  Port placement and stab incisions for laparoscopic pyloromyotomy.

 

 

c. Use blunt dissection to break the pyloric muscle down longitudinally.

d. Spread the pyloric muscle with a laparoscopic pyloromyotomy spreader (Fig. 35.6b, c). Adequate spreading will demonstrate an uninterrupted but visibly apparent mucosa in the bed of the pyloromyotomy incision.

e. Confirm completeness of the pyloromyotomy by using graspers to grab the upper half of the pyloromyotomy and the lower half and be sure each half moves independently.

f. Insufflate air into the stomach from the nasogastric tube while watching the pyloromyotomy bed for the presence of bubbles. Absence of bubbles in the bed of the pyloromyotomy may be reassuring that a perforation has not occurred but is not entirely reliable. Careful inspection should also be employed.

g. Patients can be placed on ad lib feeds immediately following surgery.

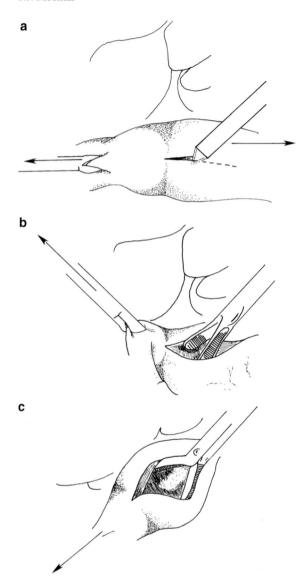

Fig. 35.6. (**a**) The myotomy is created with a laparoscopic myotome. (**b**) A pyloromyotomy spreader is used to divide the hypertrophied circular muscle fibers. (**c**) This division is continued through the hypertrophied segment, but not onto the duodenum.

# E. Laparoscopic Fundoplication

1. Overview:
   a. There are some significant differences in the indications for an antireflux procedure in children when compared to adults. While they are certainly not mutually exclusive, adults usually deal with acid burning problems, while children deal with a volume problem.
   b. Neurologically impaired children comprise the majority of kids requiring a fundoplication.
   c. A gastrostomy tube is often placed following a fundoplication, particularly in the neurologically impaired children with failure to thrive.
   d. Preexisting gastrostomy tube sites may have to be temporarily taken down in order to perform a fundoplication using laparoscopic instrumentation. This additional step is almost never required in a robotic fundoplication due to the articulating instrumentation and ease with navigating around a preexisting gastrostomy site.
2. The Nissen, Toupet, and Thal fundoplications are the most popular pediatric antireflux techniques.
   a. The Nissen fundoplication is probably the most popular and consists of a full 360° wrap.
   b. The Toupet is a partial posterior wrap.
   c. The Thal fundoplication is a partial anterior wrap.
   d. Each technique has its own set of complications and issues. Failure rates are roughly similar. Despite many heated debates among their respective advocates, no single technique has been definitively shown to be superior to another.
3. Patient positioning and trocar placement.
   a. Position the patient in a slight reverse Trendelenberg position to allow the bowel to fall into the pelvis.
   b. Bring the patient down to the foot of the bed as far as possible. Infants and small children can have their legs taped over small rolls while larger children may require a lithotomy position.
   c. The surgeon should stand at the foot of the bed; the assistant is usually toward the patient's right, but still at the foot of the bed.
   d. Place ports as shown in Fig. 35.7 with the camera at the umbilicus and the working ports along the left and right midclavicular lines.

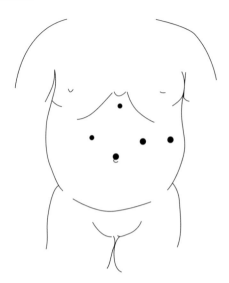

Fig. 35.7. Port placement for laparoscopic fundoplication.

    e. A fourth port is placed along the right anterior axillary line and used for liver retraction. Kite, fan, or snake retractors are all good choices for this function. A table-mounted securing clamp is recommended to hold the selected retractor throughout the case.

    f. A fifth port is sometimes required which is often used to pass suture or retract the stomach. The exact location of this site is variable but is often strategically placed at the site of potential gastrostomy tube if one is needed.

4.    Details of procedure (see also Volume II, Chap. 10).

    a. Select an appropriately sized bougie. Care must be employed in placing the bougie, especially in the thinned wall stomach of infants and small children.

    b. Takedown of the short gastric vessels can help mobilize the fundus but is optional in many cases depending on the laxity of the fundus. This can be accomplished with the hook cautery, ultrasonic scalpel, or the LigaSure.

    c. Once the stomach has been adequately mobilized, incise the peritoneum overlying the gastroesophageal junction and identify the esophagus and vagus nerve.

d. For a complete or partial posterior wrap, create a window behind the esophagus by blunt dissection usually by starting to the right of the esophagus and passing an instrument behind the esophagus. Have the anesthesiologist temporarily pull the bougie back out of the stomach to make the dissection easier during this step. This posterior window should be adequate in size to accept the fundus. Care should be taken to avoid overdissection which can result in a hiatal hernia or pneumothorax.

e. Temporarily pass the stomach through the window to confirm that an adequate amount of stomach will be available for the wrap. Let the wrap fall back.

f. Before creating the wrap, reapproximate the crura and repair any hiatal defect with a permanent suture.

g. Have the anesthetist pass the bougie back down into the stomach and confirm its location.

h. Repass the stomach back behind the esophagus and construct the wrap using interrupted permanent sutures. A minimum length of 2.5–3 cm is required for an adequate wrap. The sutures are placed at the 12:00 h position for the Nissen procedure and the 04:00 and 10:00 h positions for the Toupet.

i. To create a Thal fundoplication, suture the fundus anteriorly in either a running or interrupted technique with reconstruction of the angle of His.

j. Complete the procedure by securing the wrap to underside of the diaphragm with permanent sutures.

# F. Laparoscopic Surgery for Undescended Testes

1. The laparoscope can be used to assess the location of an undescended testicle in a child with an empty scrotum and nonpalpable testis.

2. A 30° scope is inserted through an umbilical port. Working ports are slightly inferior to the umbilicus and a few centimeters lateral to the midline in both directions, as shown in Fig. 35.8.

   a. The testicle is most commonly found at the internal ring or nearby.

   b. If the testicle is adequate in size, the vessels will also appear normal in caliber.

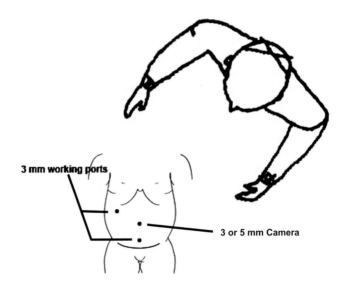

**Port placement for undescended right testicle**

Fig. 35.8. Port placement for laparoscopic exploration for the undescended testicle.

     c. Occasionally, a vas is seen entering the canal and only rudimentary strands of vessels are seen, yet nothing is palpable within the inguinal canal. This is usually indicative of a prenatally torsed or absent testicle, and inguinal exploration with orchiectomy of the remnant is indicated.

     d. If no vas or vessels are seen entering the internal ring, then exploration along the tract of descent is required. The gonad could reside anywhere from the internal ring all the way up the inferior pole of the ipsilateral kidney.

3. Once the gonad has been found and its viability determined, a decision must be made whether this gonad can be safely brought down to the scrotum during the current operation or whether a staged procedure will be required. If the testicle is at the internal ring, it is reasonable to attempt an orchiopexy during this time; proceed to make an inguinal incision with mobilization in the standard fashion.

4. If the testicle is too far from the inguinal canal, then a staged procedure is required.

a. Ligate and divide the vessels to the testicle close to the gonad. That concludes the operation for the first stage. The patient will undergo gonad mobilization laparoscopically 3–6 months later after the gonad has had an opportunity to develop an adequate secondary blood supply from the vas.

b. During the second procedure, develop a wide strip of peritoneum as a flap on three sides, preserving the vas, testicle, and the peritoneum around these structures.

c. This mobilized peritoneal flap with the vas and testicle attached is then brought up through the inguinal ring via a standard inguinal incision and eventually down to the scrotum for the orchidopexy.

# G. Laparoscopic Pull-Through (Hirschsprung's and Anorectal Malformation)

1. Overview: the laparoscopic pull-through has revolutionized the treatment of Hirschsprung's disease and portions of the procedure have now been extrapolated to children with imperforate anus. Both entities are considered in this section.

2. About 80% of patients with Hirschsprung's will have their transition zone in the rectosigmoid region. While controversial, a transanal primary pull-through can be considered if the preoperative workup confidently displays a low transition zone. Patients with questionable transition zones or suspected intermediate or long segment disease will need intraoperative biopsies at the beginning of the procedure in order to define the level of aganglionosis.

3. The patient is supine in steep Trendelenberg. Access to the perineum will be needed, so the legs and entire lower half of the abdomen should be included in the prep.

4. A Foley catheter is helpful in this procedure and is particularly useful for helping to identify the fistula in patients with imperforate anus. Cystoscopy may be indicated in cases where the anatomy is difficult to define or catheter placement challenging.

5. A Pena nerve stimulator is used to mark the extent of the anal muscular complex. Skin sutures can be placed to mark the limits if desired.

6. Port placement is demonstrated in Fig. 35.9.

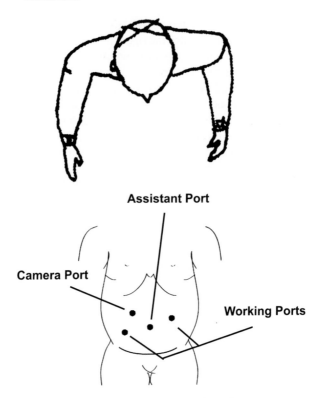

Fig. 35.9.  Port placement for laparoscopic pull-through.

7.  For Hirschsprung's, take colon biopsies immediately after trocar placement to determine extent of aganglionosis. Mark the bowel 5 cm proximal to the first region which shows abundance of ganglion cells. This will be the level of bowel transaction and the eventual anastamosis.

8.  Take down the retroperitoneal attachments with electrocautery and mobilize the bowel well enough proximal to the marked area of ganglionosis so that the pull-through can be achieved tension free.

9.  Sequentially take down the mesentery in a proximal to distal direction until the peritoneal reflection is reached.

10.  Circumferentially enter the pelvis by staying close to the rectum as the peritoneal reflection is opened.

11. For patients with imperforate anus, mobilization begins at the peritoneal reflection. Care should be taken anteriorly while searching for the fistula.

12. After adequate mobilization of the colon, attention is placed back on the perineum and the anal muscular complex is confirmed once again with the Pena nerve stimulator.

13. For Hirschsprung's, transanal dissection should be done in the typical fashion of the surgeons preferred procedure (Swenson vs. Soave).

14. A Veress needle with a Step (Covidien) sleeve is a good method to mark the center of the anal complex and penetrate into the pelvis percutaneously using the laparoscope to confirm the trajectory.

15. Dilate the Step sleeve with a 10-mm Step blunt tip trocar.

16. Pass a Babcock grasper through the open tract and pull the bowel through the anus being sure to keep the orientation proper.

17. Complete the anastomosis in an interrupted fashion to the perineum.

# H. Meckel's Diverticulum

1. Painless GI bleeding is the most commonly presenting symptom for a patient with a Meckel's diverticulum. Other presentations include obstruction, volvulus from Meckel's band to the anterior abdominal wall, or perforated viscus from an ulceration created by ectopic tissue within the Meckel's.

2. The patient is placed supine in a slight Trendelenberg position with the table rolled slightly to the left.

3. Port placement is similar to an appendectomy according to Fig. 35.1.
   a. While a 5 or 12 mm port at the umbilicus may be selected for an appendectomy, a 12-mm port is a better choice for a Meckel's diverticulectomy with plans to use a stapler for the resection.

4. Locate the Meckel's diverticulum by starting at the ileocecal valve and running the bowel proximally.

5. Identify the omphalomesenteric vessel. This vessel will dive directly into the mesentery and may be tethered at the tip of the Meckel's or perhaps even to the anterior abdominal wall.

6.  The omphalomesenteric vessel can be taken down with hook cautery, the harmonic scalpel, or the LigaSure.
7.  The Meckel's is then amputated from the ileum by using a stapler. Care should be taken to avoid narrowing the lumen of the ileum. It is not essential to have the offending bleeding ulcer within the resected specimen. If the heterotopic tissue is present in the specimen, then any ulcer in the nearby ileum will usually completely heal in a matter of days.
8.  If a perforation from the ulcer is suspected, careful exploration is required.

# I.  Intussusception

## 1. Overview

a.  Intussusception refractory to radiographic reduction is now gaining momentum in MIS. In open surgery, the classic teaching was to squeeze on the distal intussuscipians and slowly push the intussusceptum back out the way it came, much like squeezing a tube of toothpaste. Pulling on the intussuscpetum was considered a dangerous move as compromised bowel may tear. Intussusception was an early contraindication for MIS because it is very difficult to reduce an intussusception in this manner laparoscopically. However, one key reasons the recommendation to push and not pull was probably related to the often delayed presentation of many of these patients. The diagnosis of this condition is being made earlier now and the bowel may not be as fragile as it was many years ago when the classic teaching was defined. Recent data suggests that intussusception reduction can be accomplished using MIS safely and effectively by teasing and pulling the intussusceptum out rather than squeezing. This should be reserved for selected candidates

## 2. Description of procedure

a.  The patient is placed supine in a slight Trendelenberg position with the table rolled slightly to the left.
b.  Port locations are often similar to an appendectomy according

to Fig. 35.1 but may need to be adjusted on a case-by-case basis depending on how far down the bowel has been enveloped.

c.   All ports can be 5-mm ports as long as a resection is not required.

d.   Locate the intussuscepted bowel at the point of insertion.

e.   Begin gentle traction on the intussusceptum with instruments that have a broad grasp while holding the intussuscipians in place. The broad grasping instruments with larger surface area for point of contact distribute the pressure more evenly over the bowel. Avoid instruments with a small surface area. Apply sustained and even traction.

f.   Conversion to open may be necessary if there is failure of progression or any bowel tearing.

g.   Once reduced, inspect the bowel for viability as well as a potential lead point.

h.   Consider a resection of the any bowel that has questionable viability or if a lead point is discovered. The appendix or a Meckel's could be the lead point which may require resection. More often, a lead point is not identified.

# Section II: Thoracoscopy

## A.  Empyema

Thoracoscopy has dramatically changed our treatment of empyema in the past 10 years. Children seemingly languished in hospitals for weeks while trying to recover from pneumonias that were complicated by an empyema. The previous strategy of waiting to see whether these fluid collections would resolve, reserving operations for only the worst collections, has been replaced with early intervention and drainage at the first sign of collection. However this approach has also been recently disputed and fibrinolytics through small drains has been advocated. To date, the ideal management has not been proven.

The pleural fluid that develops from a parapneumonic process is thin early and becomes more viscous with each passing day. Chest-tube or catheter drainage alone is often ineffective. Thoracoscopy with irrigation and drainage is a very effective way of reexpanding a trapped lung and the procedure is described herein.

1. Single-lung ventilation is usually not necessary, as a carbon dioxide ($CO_2$) insufflation pressure of just 5–6 cm is adequate to keep the lung down for adequate visualization.

2. Place the first trocar along the midaxillary line, usually through the fifth or sixth intercostal space.

3. If the fluid is very thin with no significant loculations, irrigation and drainage may be accomplished through the same trocar by removing the camera and inserting a suction-irrigator.

4. When loculations are thick, we prefer to use at least two trocars. Additional trocars can be placed 2–3 rib spaces away from the camera.

   a. Although it is important to break down as many loculations as possible, it is not necessary to peel off all the fibropurlent material on the chest wall or pleural surface.

   b. Copious irrigation and drainage usually suffice for complete lung reexpansion once the adhesions have been taken down completely, and the majority of the rind can be left behind.

   c. Excessive rind removal may lead to an air leak from the lung.

5. Leave a small chest tube in place postoperatively through one of the trocar sites. Suction for 24 h followed by another 24 h on water seal is usually all that is required. Removal of the tube after this point is usually safe, and recurrences are rare.

## B. Blebectomy for Spontaneous Pneumothorax

1. Spontaneous pneumothorax is common among adolescents and young adults. Patients are often thin and can be active athletes. Controversy of timing of surgical management has plagued pediatric surgeons for years. Three occurrences treated with chest tubes prior to operative intervention had been the traditional teaching. However, MIS has significantly changed the timing of this intervention. Many surgeons now advocate earlier surgical intervention.

2. If the patient is significantly compromised on presentation, a chest tube or pigtail catheter should placed as soon as possible.

3. At the time of surgery, the patient is paced in a lateral decubitus position. Usually three trocars are all that is required: one 5-mm camera trocar, one 5-mm trocar for a grasper, and a 12-mm port for stapling and specimen extraction.

4.  A blebectomy is performed by stapling across the apex of the affected lung as the apex is the most common region where blebs are found. Preoperative CT scans may or may not show these blebs. A vascular load stapler is ideal.
5.  Another area of controversy centers on whether or not pleurodesis is warranted. While occasionally done for patients on their first occurrence, it should be strongly considered in patients who have had multiple spontaneous pneumothoraces.
6.  A small chest tube should be placed postoperatively through one of the trocar sites. Suction for 24 h followed by another 24 h on water seal is usually all that is required. Removal of the tube can be done after any air leak has resolved.

# C. Pectus Excavatum (Nuss Procedure)

Pectus excavatum is a chest wall anomaly that has come under increasing scrutiny in recent years. Long assumed to be cosmetic only, recent data suggests that the exercise induced shortness of breath frequently seen in pectus excavatum patients may have true physiological origins directly related to the mechanical deformity. Many experts feel that this may be due to a compromise in the preload of the right atrium and shifting of the mediastinum from the inward sterna protrusion. Thoracoscopy is a critical component of the Nuss procedure which adds a much higher level of safety in this potentially hazardous operation. The goal is to secure a custom designed bar behind the sternum which causes anteriorly forced tension on the encroaching sternum. Thoracoscopy aids in this procedure by providing a view of the dangerous segments of this procedure. The repair is done as follows:

1.  Place the patient supine with arms extended at 90° to the torso.
2.  The patient is measured and a bar selected. Generally, the size of the bar is determined by the patient's partial circumference measured at the point of maximal sternal depression.
    a.  Measure from mid axillary line to mid axillary line and subtracting 1 in. to account for the soft tissues. The resulting length is the size of the ideal pectus bar.
3.  Bend the bar into the desired shape. Chest wall templates can be used to assist with the shaping.
4.  The patient is marked for incisions on the lateral chest walls followed by delineating the desired location for entrance and

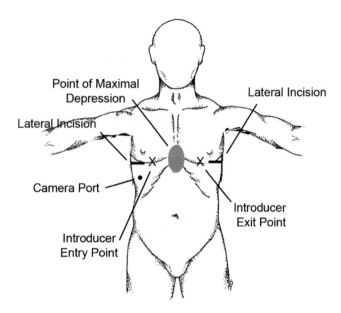

Fig. 35.10. Patient markings, incisions, and trocar placement for the Nuss procedure.

exit of the introducer bar into and out of the chest cavity on each side. The trocar site for a 5-mm thoracoscope is made two rib spaces below the intended bar entry site and offset inferiorly and laterally by a 45° angle. The use of the scope is a critical safety component of this operation which cannot be overstated (Fig. 35.10).

5.    The lateral chest incisions are made at the marked locations and subcutaneous pockets are created circumferentially with the most medial aspect reaching the intended introducer bar entry and exit sites on both sides.

6.    Bluntly enter the chest on the patient's right through the right lateral incision using a large clamp.

7.    Very carefully place the Nuss dissector into the chest and be sure the tip is in view at all times. Visualization and careful control of this instrument is critically important as dissection near the heart can be catastrophic when not performed properly.

8.    Dissect directly behind the sternum by sweeping the introducer from side to side gently. The tip of the introducer should be

pointed at the anterior chest wall at all times and advanced with small moves. The 30° camera should follow the tip as it passes behind the point of maximal depression and beyond the midline. The surgeon passing the introducer or an assistant should have their finger in the contralateral incision palpating for the tip of the dissecting introducer in between the ribs at the intended introducer exit site.

9. The slightly insufflated right chest will extend beyond the midline anteriorly, an advantage which is of crucial help in this dissection. If the tip of the introducer cannot be felt, then placing a contralateral 5-mm port and scope should be considered.

10. When the tip of the introducer can be safely seen by the scope against the anterior chest wall from the right side and simultaneously palpated between the ribs from the left sided incision with the surgeon's or assistant's finger, then the surgeon can pass the introducer out between the ribs on the other side safely.

11. Tie two umbilical tapes to the introducer bar and retreat the introducer back out of the patient taking care to follow the curve of the introducer.

12. One umbilical tape is tied to the preformed pectus bar while the other tape is kept in reserve in case the first tape breaks.

13. The preformed pectus bar is brought through the chest by pulling on the umbilical tape with one hand while guiding the bar with the other hand. The scope is useful for this step to be sure the bar is following along the proper tract.

14. The umbilical tape is removed and the bar flipped into position securing with a stabilizer bar. The bar is sewn into position on both sides.

15. A 16 Fr chest tube will fit in through the 5-mm trocar and placed on suction temporarily. This chest tube can be removed after the skin incisions are closed. A small residual pneumothorax is common but usually of no significance.

## D. Congenital Diaphragmatic Hernia

A congenital diaphragmatic hernia (CDH) can be repaired either thoracoscopically or laparoscopically but most pediatric surgeons prefer the thoracoscopic approach. The advocates of the thoracoscopic technique claim the visualization is better over the laparoscopic approach but reaching the most posterolateral aspect of the defect can be difficult from the chest. Proponents of the laparoscopic approach enjoy a much easier angle to reach the posterolateral diaphragmatic defect at its most lateral location but reduction of the viscera into the abdomen can limit visualization. Robotic surgery performed from the chest has recently been shown to overcome the shortcomings of the standard thoracoscopic approach. However, the long articulating instrument length introduces another set of challenges with lack of workable space if the patient is less than 3 kg. Since both the laparoscopic and thoracoscopic CDH repair has its own advocates and critics, we discuss both options:

## 1. *Laparoscopic CDH repair*

a.  Position the patient supine rolled in a 45° manner to allow the viscera to fall to the contralateral side of the CDH defect.
b.  Trocar placement is at the umbilicus for the camera, the upper midline, and the ipsilateral mid-axillary line (Fig. 35.11).
c.  Keep insufflation pressures low, preferably 7–10 cm $H_2O$. $CO_2$ Insufflation may not be tolerated due to $CO_2$ retention and hypercarbia as a baseline in CDH patients.
d.  A fourth trocar may be necessary for retraction if the bowel or spleen impairs visualization.

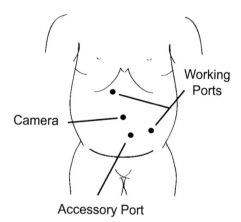

Fig. 35.11. Port placement for a laparoscopic (abdominal approach) to a left congenital diaphragmatic hernia.

e.  Use an atraumatic grasper to gently reduce the viscera back into the abdomen. If the spleen is herniated into the chest, reduce it by grasping attachments near the hilum without grasping the hilar vessels themselves. When the inferior pole of the spleen comes into the abdomen, the rest usually slips in with gentle traction.

f.  Mobilize the diaphragmatic edge of the defect as it fuses with the lateral chest wall. This may enhance primary closure which is preferred over patch closure.

g.  Close the defect using interrupted horizontal mattress sutures. In general, we prefer to work from lateral to medial. Pledgets may be required if undue tension is noted.

h.  Patch closure has also been accomplished using a variety of prosthetic materials. In patients with a tight primary closure, the patch material can be used as a reinforcement sewing it directly over the repair. The material is brought in through a 5-mm trocar rolled up like a carpet. Once inside, it can be easily unrolled and sewn in place preferably in an interrupted fashion.

## 2. Thoracoscopic CDH repair (our preferred approach)

a.  The patient should be placed in a lateral decubitus position.

b.  Port placement for a left thoracoscopic CDH is shown in Fig. 35.12.

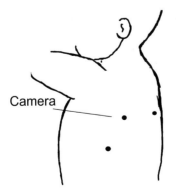

Fig. 35.12.  Port placement for a thoracosocopic left CDH repair.

c. Reduce the viscera by using laparoscopic peanuts and gentle traction.

d. Mobilize the diaphragmatic edge of the defect as it fuses with the lateral chest wall as well as possible. This may enhance primary closure which is preferred over patch closure.

e. Close the defect using interrupted horizontal mattress sutures. Again, we prefer to work from lateral to medial. Pledgets may be required if undue tension is noted. Reaching the most posterolateral aspect can be particularly difficult in thoracoscopy. Consider passing the suture out of the chest and around a rib, making a small skin incision to assist with this maneuver. Usually, only one or two sutures around the rib are required for this section of the defect. The closure then proceeds medially.

f. Patch closure has also been accomplished using a variety of prosthetic materials. The material is brought in through a 5-mm trocar rolled up like a carpet. Once inside, it can be easily unrolled and sewn in place preferably in an interrupted fashion. In patients with a tight primary closure, the patch material can be sewn directly over the repair as reinforcement.

# E. Pulmonary Resections for Sequestration and CCAM

1. Pulmonary lobectomy is now a common MIS pediatric procedure. Typical indications include intralobar pulmonary sequestration and congenital cystic adenomatoid malformation. Extralobar sequestrations are also easily removed thoracoscopically and are usually tethered only by their vascular source. However, the intralobar sequestration and CCAM usually requires a formal lobectomy. Recently, segmentectomies have been proposed for smaller lesions.

2. Place the patient in a lateral decubitus position rotated anteriorly.

3. For a lobectomy, plan the operation as if reading a book from front to back. The surgeon should stand at the patient's front and the dissection proceeds posteriorly.

4. Place the port intended for the camera over the estimated location of the fissure, in the posterior axillary line.

5. Working ports are placed according to the lobe in which the resection is planned to maintain the ergonomic principles outlined earlier.

6. Begin by taking down the inferior pulmonary ligament to aid in mobilization.

    a. If the lobectomy is performed for a sequestration, the aberrant arterial supply is often located in the inferior pulmonary ligament. Great care should be taken in dissecting this large arterial vessel. This vessel can be clipped or sealed with a device such as the LigaSure or harmonic as long as it is less than 6 or 7 mm in diameter. If the vessel is larger, formal suture ligating may be necessary.

7. Complete the fissure. The LigaSure is ideal for this step.

8. Identify the hilar anatomy including the segmental pulmonary artery branches, the pulmonary vein, and the lobar bronchus.

9. Carefully take down the pulmonary artery followed by the vein leaving the bronchus for last, if possible. The vessels may be ligated, clipped, or sealed and divided with the LigaSure or harmonic. The bronchus should be suture ligated.

10. Remove the specimen through one of the trocar sites. It may be necessary to slightly extend the trocar site to extract the specimen.

# F. Repair of Esophageal Atresia with Tracheoesophageal Fistula

Repair of esophageal atresia with tracheoesophageal fistula (TEF) using a minimally invasive approach has become increasingly popular. The initial results are preliminary and long term results are unknown. There are five different types of TEF. We describe repair of the most common variant, the proximal esophageal atresia with distal TEF.

1. The trocar placement is shown in Fig. 35.13, and a transpleural approach is required.

2. The first step is identifying and dividing the azygos vein. The vessel can be taken down and divided using the LigaSure. Alternatively, the vessel can be clipped and divided.

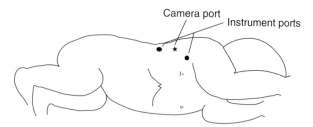

Fig. 35.13. Patient position and trocar placement for repair of tracheoesophageal fistula.

3.   Dissection of the upper mediastinum will demonstrate the proximal esophagus, the distal esophagus, the trachea, and the fistula. The anesthesiologist can assist the surgeon in finding the proximal pouch by manipulating the nasogastric tube.

4.   The fistula takedown can be done in variety of ways. One recently advocated method is to simply clip the fistula close to the origin at the trachea using a 5-mm endoclip. Alternatively, the fistula can be divided in a piecemeal fashion to minimize the leak from the trachea and closed sequentially with interrupted absorbable sutures.

5.   Mobilize the distal and proximal esophagus. Avoid overdissection but mobilization needs to be adequate to bring the two ends together without undue tension. Traction sutures may be necessary to help facilitate the mobilization.

6.   Perform an interrupted anastomosis with 4–0 or 5–0 suture.
    a. Each suture must include mucosa to avoid stricture.
    b. The first suture may not bring the two ends together adequately, but this will be overcome with subsequent suture placement.
    c. Place the knots on the inside of the lumen for the back row.
    d. Have the anesthesiologist gently slide a feeding tube or nasogastric tube past the completed back row of the anastomosis and down into the distal esophagus. The surgeon may have to help guide the tube with a grasper. The nasogastric tube serves as a sizer for the repair. It can be removed at the end of the procedure.
    e. Complete the front row of sutures over the tube with the knots on the outside of the esophagus.

7. A chest tube is left in place following the repair.
8. A swallowing study is suggested about 7 days postoperatively. The chest tube can be removed once there is no evidence of a leak.

# Selected Readings

Fox D, Morrato E, Campagna EJ, Rees DI, Dickinson LM, Partrick DA, Kempe A. Outcomes of laparoscopic versus open fundoplication in children's hospitals: 2005–2008. Pediatrics. 2011;127(5):872–80.

Garey CL, Laituri CA, Ostlie DJ, Snyder CL, Andrews WS, Holcomb GW III, St Peter SD. Single-incision laparoscopic surgery in children: initial single-center experience. J Pediatr Surg. 2011;46(5):904–7.

Holcomb GW III, Rothenberg SS, Bax KM, Martinez-Ferro M, Albanese CT, Ostlie DJ, van Der Zee DC, Yeung CK. Thoracoscopic repair of esophageal atresia and tracheoesophageal fistula: a multi-institutional analysis. Ann Surg. 2005;242(3):422–8; discussion 428–30.

Mattioli G, Pini-Prato A, Barabino A, Gandullia P, Avanzini S, Guida E, Rossi V, Pio L, Disma N, Mameli L, Mirta DR, Montobbio G, Jasonni V. Laparoscopic approach for children with inflammatory bowel diseases. Pediatr Surg Int. 2011;27(8):839–46.

Nakhamiyayev V, Galldin L, Chiarello M, Lumba A, Gorecki PJ. Laparoscopic appendectomy is the preferred approach for appendicitis: a retrospective review of two practice patterns. Surg Endosc. 2010;24(4):859–64.

Saad S, Mansson J, Saad A, Goldfarb MA. Ten-year review of groin laparoscopy in 1001 pediatric patients with clinical unilateral inguinal hernia: an improved technique with transhernia multiple-channel scope. J Pediatr Surg. 2011;46(5):1011–4.

Slater BJ, Chan FP, Davis K, Dutta S. Institutional experience with laparoscopic partial splenectomy for hereditary spherocytosis. J Pediatr Surg. 2010;45(8):1682–6.

Vick LR, Gosche JR, Boulanger SC, Islam S. Primary laparoscopic repair of high imperforate anus in neonatal males. J Pediatr Surg. 2007;42(11):1877–81.

Wood JH, Partrick DA, Hays T, Sauaia A, Karrer FM, Ziegler MM. Contemporary pediatric splenectomy: continuing controversies. Pediatr Surg Int. 2011;27(11):1165–71.

# 36. Complications in Pediatric MIS

*John J. Meehan, M.D.*

## A. General Complications Related to Minimally Invasive Surgery

### 1. Veress needle injuries

The Veress needle technique is a safe and effective method for starting a pneumoperitoneum. It also has the advantage of avoiding the problematic continual loss of pneumoperitoneum which may occur from a Hasson technique with an incision that is too generous. However, vascular and visceral injuries can occur as a result of Veress needle placement. Here are some keys to help reduce that possibility:

a.  After making the skin incision, bluntly dissect the subcutaneous tissue away until the fascial layer is well visualized.

b.  Use a clamp on the fascia such as a Kocher clamp in order to hold upward traction on the abdominal wall. A small nick in the fascia with an 11 blade or cautery will facilitate Veress needle placement without apply significant force.

c.  Upon passing the Veress needle into the abdominal cavity, a "click" sound should be audible, indicating that the sharp needle tip has retracted and the blunt tip is now protruding from the tip of the device.

d.  Confirm location of the needle by sweeping the needle in a plane parallel to the operating room table. It should sweep around unimpeded and be easily visible distending the abdominal wall. Keep upward traction on the abdominal wall while performing this check.

e.  A second confirmation test can be performed by injecting saline through the Veress needle. It should flow easily without resistance. Upon releasing the syringe from the needle injection port, the remaining fluid in the Veress needle clear plastic hub should fall freely into the abdomen by gravity.

f.   After the abdomen has been insufflated with $CO_2$, the camera is inserted and careful inspection of the entire abdomen should be performed particularly just underneath the port site. Any injuries or suspected injuries should be treated immediately.

g.   Because of the thinner anterior posterior diameter, pediatric patients are potentially at a higher risk of Veress needle injuries than adult patients. Careful introduction of this device is crucial in small patients.

## 2.   Trocar Injuries

a.   Despite manufacturer claims that one trocar may be safer than another, bladed and non bladed trocars can both cause significant injury. Bladed trocars have the danger of the sharp object on the end of the device yet non bladed trocars often require additional force for placement.

b.   Pediatric patients are at increased risk due to the smaller cavity size and thinner abdominal or chest walls.

c.   The aorta and bifurcation of the iliacs is almost directly below the level of the umbilicus making this a common region for trocar related vascular injuries. Vascular injuries can be quite devastating if not dealt with promptly, particularly in children. Immediate laparotomy should be performed if this injury is suspected as time is of the essence.

d.   Visceral injuries also occur and can have devastating consequences if not realized at the time of the initial surgery. The first trocar is often the offending projectile but any trocar, even those watched under direct vision, can cause injuries.

e.   Careful inspection of all possible trocar trajectories immediately after placement is an important safety routine all MIS surgeons should follow.

## 3.   Trocar site hernias

a.   As stated above, a pediatric patient will generally have a much thinner abdominal wall than an adult patient. This makes trocar site hernias more likely. These complications may show up weeks, months, or even years after a minimally invasive case.

b.  The risk of this complication may be reduced by closing fascia on all pediatric trocar incisions greater than 5 mm. Some 5-mm incisions also require closure when the patient is thin. A good rule of thumb: if the patient is thin enough that you can see the fascia by exploring the wound, then the fascia should be closed. Most incisions 3 mm or less do not require closure.

c.  Due to the risk of incarceration, trocar site hernias should be repaired.

## 4.  Abdominal wall hemorrhage

a.  This complication is rare in children. The inferior epigastric vessels are commonly associated with this complication, often occurring at the camera port in a laparoscopic appendectomy.

b.  Most abdominal wall hemorrhages are self limited and tamponade in the soft tissues requiring no further intervention. Occasionally, a trocar site will need to be reopened, the hematoma drained, and the offending vessel cauterized or ligated. Rarely, a bleeding trocar site may bleed intra-abdominally and may also need either exploration and ligation or interventional radiology and embolization.

## 5.  Abdominal wall crepitus

a.  This occurs as a result of leakage of $CO_2$ into the preperitoneal or subcutaneous space. It is often alarming to families and floor nursing staff but requires no intervention. It should dissipate in 24–36 h.

b.  If abdominal wall erythema and fever coincide with the crepitus, the possibility of necrotizing fasciitis must be entertained and may require emergent debridement and broad-spectrum antibiotics. Fortunately, this is exceedingly rare.

## 6.  Hypercarbia

a.  Hypercarbia is more common in smaller children. It is particularly problematic for patients with $CO_2$ retention as baseline such as babies with congenital diaphragmatic hernia (CDH).

b. Good communication with the anesthesiologist is crucial, especially in children with CDH. If temporary desufflation or reduction of $CO_2$ pressure does not resolve the problem, abandoning the MIS approach may be required.

## 7. Abdominal compartment syndrome and tension pneumothorax

a. Overinsufflation of the abdomen or chest may cause significant hemodynamic compromise and the pneumoperitoneum or pneumothorax may need to be reduced or outright released.

b. The exact value which results in an abdominal compartment syndrome or a pneumothorax that causes cardiovascular compromise is not definable. Each patient must be considered on a case by case basis.

c. If a patient cannot tolerate the minimum insufflation pressures, abandoning the MIS approach may be required.

d. Recommended starting points for insufflation pressures:

| Weight | Abdomen ($cmH_2O$) | Chest ($cmH_2O$) |
|---|---|---|
| Less than 10 kg | 8–10 | 0–3 |
| 10–20 kg | 11–13 | 3–5 |
| Greater than 20 kg | 15 | 5 |

# B. Complications of Specific Surgical Procedures

## 1. Laparoscopic Appendectomy

a. **Wound infection**. Even in open operations, postappendectomy wound infections are less common in children than in adults. However, wound infections still occur and may require drainage. Antibiotics may be necessary if cellulitis develops, but simply opening the wound may suffice. The use of an endoscopic specimen bag at the time of the initial procedure may help reduce this complication but not entirely.

b. **Intra-abdominal abscess**. This common complication occurs in both the open and laparoscopic appendectomy. It is markedly more common in perforated appendicitis than nonperforated, but either preceding condition is possible. Patients may present with, fever, ileus, depressed appetite, diarrhea, constipation, or continued vomiting. Ultrasound or computed tomography (CT) scan is used to identify a fluid collection but may be of limited value early in the postoperative course. It may take at least 5–7 days following the initial procedure before either of these tests is of any value, as most patients will have some normal postoperative fluid present immediately following the primary appendectomy. Due to the new concerns regarding radiation exposure from CT scans, most pediatric hospitals are trending toward ultrasound as a preferable evaluation method over CT scans. However, CT scan is still used at alarmingly high rates. Our hospital is actively trying to phase out its use of CT scans and ultrasonographers have become more and more adept at using the standard ultrasound to define these postoperative collections. Small collections may not be amenable to percutaneous drainage and often resolve with continued antibiotic coverage. Large collections can be handled with percutaneous drainage under radiological guidance by a skilled interventional radiologist. Reexploration is rarely required.

c. **Appendiceal stump leak**. Fortunately, this complication is rare. Some of these children present with a picture that is similar to a postoperative abscess. More often, however, the patient is significantly more compromised with overwhelming sepsis. The exact cause of this complication may be related to patient disease but is often a technical issue such as an improperly secured endoloop or an inadequate staple line. Placing two endoloops on the patient side of the appendix and one on the specimen side during the initial procedure may help reduce the risk of this complication. If the appendiceal stump has questionable viability after the appendix is amputated, the surgeon should consider oversewing the stump using viable cecal tissue similar to the pursestring method used in the classic open approach.

## 2. *Cholecystecomy*

a. **Bile duct injury**. The common bile duct or common hepatic duct could be injured as a result of over dissection, direct injury, or an errant application of an endoclip. Careful identification of all pertinent structures will reduce this complication. An intra-operative cholangiogram should be taken in any cases where the anatomy is questionable or a suspected injury may have occurred. Primary repair may be acceptable with a small incomplete injury. A Roux-en-Y choledochojejunostomy via an open technique is recommended for transaction or significant injury.

b.  **Bile duct leak**. Post operative leaks from the cystic duct stump may occur as a result of a direct injury or an inadequately ligated cystic duct. Depending on the size of the patient, the rate and volume of the leak, and the skill of an available interventional pediatric gastroenterologist, a stent may be placed which may avoid any operative intervention. Many of these leaks will seal in 6–8 weeks at which time the stent can be safely removed. A temporary percutaneously placed drain may be needed.

## 3. Splenectomy

a.  **Bleeding**. Bleeding may occur from a number of sources including the splenic artery, splenic vein, or short gastrics. Embolization may be possible if the source is arterial. Serial hematocrit checks may be useful to monitor the rate of bleeding. Reexploration is mandatory if significant bleeding is suspected or conservative measures fail.

b.  **Retained accessory spleen**. Thoroughly inspect the left upper quadrant tissues during a splenectomy including the splenic hilar bed and the omentum. All accessory spleens should be removed at the initial operation. Missing an accessory spleen may result in reexploration.

c.  **Pancreatic injury**. The distal pancreas may be injured during dissection or ligation of the splenic vessels. If this injury is identified at the initial surgery, one may need to consider stapling across the tail of the pancreas if the injury is thought to be significant. A drain may be required which can be placed at the same time. Delayed recognition may result in a pseuodocyst. Drainage may be accomplished either percutaneously or via a cystgastrostomy performed endoscopically or laparoscopically.

d.  **Gastric injury**. This injury may occur during cauterization of the short gastrics. Recognition at the time of the initial procedure is important and primary repair will often suffice by simply oversewing the injury. Unrecognized injuries may present with sepsis or large volumes of free intra-abdominal air. If necessary, an upper gastrointestinal (GI) series with Gastrografin will confirm the injury. Exploration and repair is required.

e.   **Colon injury**. Although exceedingly rare, this complication can be repaired primarily if recognized at the time of surgery. Contamination can be handled with irrigation and suctioning. A colostomy should be considered in delayed injuries when the contamination or injury is extensive.

f.   **Problems related to specimen retrieval**. Surgeons often find that the most challenging part of a laparoscopic splenectomy is removing the specimen, especially in cases where the spleen is quite large. Inadvertent spilling of the splenic specimen may occur due to the bag ripping or damage to the specimen itself during manipulation. This can result in a retained section of specimen. Planning the retrieval and having flexibility to alter plans is paramount to avoid this complication. Extending the trocar incision an extra centimeter or two is a valuable trade for many minutes of frustrating "berry picking." Irrigation and repeated suctioning of the right upper quadrant is important if any splenic elements are spilled during the attempted removal.

g.   **Postsplenectomy sepsis**. This overwhelming and potentially fatal complication is more likely to occur in younger patients, particularly those less than 5 years of age. Preoperative immunizations for *Pneumococcus* and *Hemophilus influenzae* should be given whenever possible, and soon after surgery if it cannot be given ahead of time. These vaccinations have been instrumental in markedly reducing this complication. Patients with postsplenectomy sepsis may present with a rapid onset of fever and full-blown sepsis. Broad-spectrum antibiotics and fluid resuscitation should be started immediately. Daily prophylactic penicillin should also be given for young patients until the age of 18.

h.   **Diaphragmatic irritation and injury**. This injury is also uncommon but may present at shoulder pain which may be difficult to distinguish from the benign diaphragmatic irritation also commonly noted following splenectomy. In cases where the diaphragm is irritated but not injured, a fluid collection and abscess may be the cause and may be visible with either ultrasound or CT. A fever will often accompany the latter. Most of these symptoms resolve within a few days, however large collections may require drainage. If an injury to the diaphragm is suspected, chest X-ray with a PA and lateral view can help demonstrate the injury. Fluoroscopy may be helpful as well.

## 4. Pyloromyotomy

a. **Mucosal tear**. This complication is more likely to occur near the pyloroduodenal junction from a myotomy that was carried too far distally. If suspected, the anesthetist can insufflate air through an orogastric tube and the surgeon can inspect the myotomy for bubbling. Although not foolproof, it is a reasonable screening method for leak detection but there is a significant false negative rate. If an injury is detected, repair should then be performed with an absorbable suture and omentum tacked over the repair. Classical teaching states that complete closure of the entire myotomy is necessary and a second myotomy 90–180° away from the first will be required. This may be difficult to reach laparoscopically and opening may be required.

b. **Inadequate pyloromyotomy**. Postoperatively, many infants with hypertrophic pyloric stenosis continue to vomit even if the pyloromyotomy was done properly. Swelling at the pylorus may have a role. Most patients will vomit once or twice but tolerate all of their other feeds and this generally indicates all is well. The majority of these patients go home within 24 h of surgery. However, some patients routinely vomit more persistently for more than the first 24 h. We do not routinely investigate vomiting in the first 36–48 h following a pyloromyotomy. However, patients with persistent vomiting beyond this time should undergo an upper GI series to determine the potential cause. An inadequate pyloromyotomy will require reoperation. Prevention can be achieved by assuring independent movement of the two halves of the pyloric ring during the initial surgery.

## 5. Fundoplication

a. **Gastric volvulus**. This can occur from a gastrostomy placed too close to the pylorus. Patients will present with gastric distention and shock. This requires fluid resuscitation, antibiotics, and emergent exploration. The stomach should be detorsed and the gastrostomy site relocated.

b. **Esophageal tear**. This may occur from either a bougie that is too large or from overdissection at the hiatus. Repair is required and mediastinal drainage may be necessary in cases of significant contamination or those discovered in a delayed manner.

c. **Gastric perforation**. This complication can occur by several methods. The first is the bougie insertion or manipulation. Hurst bougie dilators may be more likely to cause this perforation while the tapered Maloney bougie dilator may have a slightly lower risk. Perforations may also occur as a result of collateral damage in taking down short gastric vessels. The risk from this step can be reduced by minimizing the distance along the greater curve that the short gastric are taken to the absolute minimum while still adequately mobilizing the stomach. Perforations also occur as a result of difficulties while placing gastrostomy tubes, a common adjunct procedure for fundoplications in children.

d. **Slipped wrap**. This complication may occur from many possibilities including overdissection of the hiatus, wrap breakdown, and poor healing. Recurrent reflux, upper GI obstruction, pain, or any combination of these symptoms may occur and reexploration and repair is often necessary.

e. **Gas-bloat syndrome**. Many pediatric patients who require a fundoplication are neurologically impaired and often have significant aerophagia. Regardless of the type of repair, significant volumes of air may be swallowed with no release of the gastric air volume. Usually, this problem is self-limited but is more pronounced in complete wraps such as the Nissen fundoplication. This can be overcome by "burping" the stomach by venting a gastrostomy tube if present. If a gastrostomy tube is not present, one should be considered. Another cause may be related to poor gastric emptying which can be demonstrated with a radionuclide gastric emptying study. Pyloromyotomy or pyloroplasty has been advocated in patients with severe delayed gastric emptying or persistent feeding intolerance, but this is controversial. Another option is abandoning the use of the stomach as a means for enterally feeding and placing a G–J tube.

## 6. Undescended testicle

a. **Atrophic testis**. The risk of testis atrophy after testicular vessel ligation is well known regardless of the approach. An orchiectomy may be required.

## 7. Contralateral Hernia Exploration

a.   **Hernia sac tear**. Care should be taken when placing or removing the trocar or scope through the ipsilateral hernia sac when exploring the contralateral inguinal canal. When the inspection is complete, close inspection of the sac to look for any tears should be performed. If a tear is discovered, the hernia sac must be ligated proximal to the site of injury.

## 8. Meckel's Resection

a.   **Leak**. Patients with a leak from a Meckel's resection may present with fever, abdominal pain, lethargy, and sepsis. Emergent exploration and repair is required.

b.   **Obstruction**. An errant staple line which narrows the lumen of the small bowel at a Meckel's resection site can cause an obstruction. Conservative measures with a nasogastric tube and fasting the patient are acceptable to see whether a partial obstruction will resolve on its own. Those that cannot resolve by conservative measures require reexploration.

c.   **Bleeding**. The most common presenting symptom of Meckel's diverticulum is painless bleeding. The bleeding often comes from the small bowel lumen just beyond the Meckel's as the secretions from the aberrant gastric tissue in the Meckel's create an ulcer. These ulcers are often not within the Meckel's themselves and are often not included in the resection nor do they need to be included in all cases. Although these ulcers may still bleed for a short time after Meckel's resection, they usually heal completely on their own and often require no intervention. Many patients pass bloody stools for several days following a resection even if the ulcer is no longer bleeding as they are simply evacuating the blood that had already accumulated intraluminally before the initial resection. Rarely, a bleed may persist and require a reexploration, but this is exceedingly uncommon.

## 9. Pull-Through Procedures

a.   **Hirschprung's Enterocolitis. Unique to patients with Hirschprung's disease**, enterocolitis is a common preoperative and postoperative problem for children with Hirschsprung's disease. An appropriate pull-through will certainly markedly reduce the risk of enterocolitis but these episodes can still occur even in the perfect pullthrough. Enterocolitis, anastomotic stricture, ischemic bowel, cuff abscess or stricture, and simple gastroenteritis may all appear with similar symptoms and sorting out the etiology may be difficult. Abdominal distention, fever, sepsis, and inability to pass stool are more indicative of enterocolitis. Explosive passage of stool is often found on rectal examination. Rectal irrigations up to three or four times a day will improve these patients dramatically. Antibiotic coverage is recommended until normal bowel diameter is reestablished on plain film. Repeated bouts of enterocolitis may necessitate a biopsy of the pullthrough specimen to confirm the presence of ganglion cells.

b.  **Ischemic bowel**. Ischemia may occur from excessive tension on the pull-through bowel or overmobilization of the mesentery. These patients can present with a wide variety of symptoms including diarrhea, bloody stool, or overt sepsis. If the symptoms are mild, a colonoscopy can be performed to evaluate the mucosa of the pull-through segment. Patients who present with severe symptoms may have a necrotic section and will require exploration.

c.  **Anastomotic stricture**. These patients might present with symptoms similar to enterocolitis. The diagnosis is usually obvious on rectal examination and dilatation with Hegar dilators (to about 12 or 13 for infants) may be sufficient. Rectal dilatations can be performed by the family at home for several weeks if necessary.

d.  **Cuff abscess/cuff stricture**. The cuff created during a Soave endorectal pull-through should be divided at the time of the initial operation to avoid this complication from occurring. Abscesses can be drained transrectally or percutaneously.

e.  Urethral diverticulum (for males following imperforate anus repair). A urethral diverticulm may present as difficulty voiding or with recurrent urinary tract infections. Large diverticulums may require revision.

# C. Complications of Specific Surgical Thoracic Procedures

## 10. Empyema

a. **Wound infection**. This common complication often is largely dues to the underlying pathology of the infected lung. Local wound care is all that is generally required.

b. **Retained loculated abscess**. Occasionally, a repeat thoracoscopic evaluation and drainage may be needed for patients with reaccumulation of their fluid collection. Aggressive takedown of all loculations with irrigation and suctioning may help reduce the possibility of this occurring.

c. **Bronchopleural fistula**. This devastating complication is fortunately relatively uncommon but can be problematic as the diseased lung may not have the capacity to heal. Depending on the stability of the patient and the size of the leak, conservative management of a prolonged air leak that is phasic with respirations may eventually seal. However, continuous air leaks are less likely to seal on their own and often require reexploration with closure of the fistula.

## 11. Blebectomy for Spontaneous Pneumothorax

a. **Recurrent pneumothorax**. A recurrent pneumothorax is a well recognized common complication following blebectomy for spontaneous pneumothorax. This most often occurs as a result of retained pathology which may not have been visually apparent at the first exploration. Reexploration with stapling across the apex of the lung and any new blebs usually suffices. However, sclerotherapy with talc or another sclerosing agent should also be entertained if it was not done previously. Even if it had been done at the first procedure, a repeat application of the sclerosing agent is also reasonable even if it failed the first time.

## 12. Nuss Procedure

a. **Infection**: A wound infection is perhaps one of the most frustrating complications following Nuss repair of Pectus excavatum. An infected bar can lead to mediastinitis, empyema, or sepsis. Even for suspected minor infections of the soft tissues, aggressive antibiotic coverage should be considered. If the tract that the bar traverses becomes infected, dealing with the infection aggressively will require opening the wound and aggressively washing out the wound daily or every other day until the wound is as clean as possible. The bar tract should be irrigated during these explorations as completely as possible. Multiple trips to the operating room may be required. IV antibiotic therapy needs to be tailored as specifically as possible to the underlying pathogen. Ultimately, bar removal may be required. Bar salvage may be accomplished with aggressive wound care, IV antibiotics, wound vac therapy, and even antibiotic impregnated absorbable calcium beads.

b. **Retained pneumothorax**: A small retained pneumothorax is almost universal in all patients following a Nuss procedure. As long as the pneumothorax is small (less than two rib spaces) and asymptomatic, no further therapy is required as the almost certainly resolve. Symptomatic or larger pneumothoraces should be treated with tube thoracostomy, often easily placed at the bedside through the port site that had been used during the bar placement procedure.

c. **Late intrathoracic bleed**: A handful of case reports have shown patients who were several months out from having the pectus bar placed when they suddenly developed an unexplained intrathoracic bleed. The inferior mammary artery is often the bleeding vessel although an intercostals is another possibility. Embolization of the offending vessel should be considered.

d. **Cardiac perforation**: This life threatening complication must be dealt with promptly. Avoidance is the key with careful visualization of the introducer bar under direct vision from a thoracoscopically placed camera will help reduce the risk of this from occurring. Even with the camera properly placed and the technique done in even the most experienced hands, this complication is still a possibility on every single case. In the unfortunate event that this devastating complication occurs, patient survival will depend on the quick recognition and prompt response. Preparedness is the key and includes having a sternal saw ready and open on the back table for all Nuss procedures. A median sternotomy should be done expeditiously gaining control and repairing as quickly as possible.

## 13. *Congenital Diaphragmatic Hernia (CDH) Repair*

a. **Recurrence**. One of the biggest criticisms of the MIS CDH repair is an unacceptably high recurrence rate. Early reports showed poor results using an MIS approach but these results have improved somewhat in recent years. The problem stems from an inability to effectively reach the most posterolateral aspect of the Bochdalek defect. This region is often deep in the sulcus and minimal to no diaphragm exists. Creative repairs include suturing around the rib passing the suture extracorporeally and tying over the rib by making a small skin incision and then closing the skin over the knot. Recurrences also can occur if defects are large or patch closure is required.

b. **Intra-abdominal visceral or solid organ injury**. This complication may occur if sutures are not clearly seen as they are passed from the thoracic domain and into the abdominal domain. Careful visualization of needle trajectory is paramount.

## 14. *Pulmonary Lobectomies and Segmentectomies (CCAM and Intralobar Sequestration)*

a. **Bleeding**. A thorough understanding of the pulmonary vessels is paramount to avoiding this potentially life threatening complication. Bleeding should be dealt with promptly using clip applier, suture ligature, or a thermal sealing device such a LigaSure.

b. **Bronchopleural fistula**. Same as the section above (see Sect. 11).

## 15. **Tracheoesophageal Fistula Repair**

a. **Reflux**. Gastroesophageal reflux is a common complication following TEF repair no matter how the repair was done. Prophylactic use of antireflux medications may help treat this problem but many patients go on to need a fundoplication.

b. **Stricture**. Stricture is also a common complication following TEF repair and seems to have a higher rate among the MIS TEF repair in early series. Repeated dilatations usually suffice for most patients although a revision may be required in extreme cases.

c. **Esophageal leak**. This is another complication that is somewhat higher than the open method in some initial series. This complication is often discovered on the initial swallowing study before feeds are initiated and feeds should be held if found. Many of these leaks will go on to seal themselves spontaneously but the mediastinum needs to have a drainage tube present until this issue is resolved. Leaks that do not respond to conservative measures will require another operative repair.

d. **Recurrent fistula**. Recurrent fistulas may present with aspiration pneumonia or perhaps even a life-threatening aspiration event at anytime following a TEF repair. The most common time is within the first few days or weeks after feeds are initiated but these may not show up for several weeks or even months. A reexploration is required.

## Selected Readings

Adam LA, Meehan JJ. Erosion of the Nuss bar into the internal mammary artery 4 months after minimally invasive repair of pectus excavatum. J Pediatr Surg. 2008;43(2): 394–7.

Alam S, Lawal TA, Peña A, Sheldon C, Levitt MA. Acquired posterior urethral diverticulum following surgery for anorectal malformations. J Pediatr Surg. 2011;46(6): 1231–5.

Bailez MM, Cuenca ES, Di Benedetto V, Solana J. Laparoscopic treatment of rectovaginal fistulas. Feasibility, technical details, and functional results of a rare anorectal malformation. J Pediatr Surg. 2010;45(9):1837–42.

Fox D, Morrato E, Campagna EJ, Rees DI, Dickinson LM, Partrick DA, Kempe A. Outcomes of laparoscopic versus open fundoplication in children's hospitals: 2005–2008. Pediatrics. 2011;127(5):872–80.

Holcomb GW III, Rothenberg SS, Bax KM, Martinez-Ferro M, Albanese CT, Ostlie DJ, van Der Zee DC, Yeung CK. Thoracoscopic repair of esophageal atresia and tracheoesophageal fistula: a multi-institutional analysis. Ann Surg. 2005;242(3):422–8; discussion 428–30.

Krickhahn A, Petersen C, Ure B. Transvesical resection of a mucocele after laparoscopically assisted anorectal pull-through for imperforate anus with rectobulbar urethral fistula. J Pediatr Surg. 2011;46(1):e29–31.

Singh R, Cameron BH, Walton JM, Farrokhyar F, Borenstein SH, Fitzgerald PG. Postoperative Hirschsprung's enterocolitis after minimally invasive Swenson's procedure. J Pediatr Surg. 2007;42(5):885–9.

Part VIII
# Flexible Endoscopy: General Principles

# 37. Flexible Endoscopes: Characteristics, Troubleshooting, and Equipment Care*

*Gary C. Vitale, M.D.*
*Brian R. Davis, M.D.*

## A. Characteristics of Flexible Endoscopes

Flexible endoscopy provides a quantum leap in the area of diagnosis and therapy of the aerodigestive tract.

1.  **Optical properties**: Four types of flexible endoscopes are currently in use. They transmit images differently.
    a.  **Fiberoptic endoscopes** are based upon fiberoptic light transmission technology. Light is conveyed through a bundle of fine glass fibers, each smaller than a human hair (6,070 μm in diameter), packed tightly together.
        i.  Each individual fiber is clad in a wrapping of greater optical density, creating a reflective layer that causes light to bounce back and forth within the fiber with little loss of light. This cladding does not transmit light itself creating a dark rim around the portion of the image produced by each fiber and accounting for the characteristic newsprint-like image produced by fiberoptic endoscopes.
        ii. Thousands of fibers are packed tightly together in a bundle each carrying a small parcel of light to or from a portion of the viewing area.

---

*This chapter was contributed by Bipan Chand, MD and Jeffrey L. Ponsky, MD in the previous edition.

    iii.  One bundle of fibers carries light into the examined organ, and a second bundle transmits the image from the organ interior to the viewing optic.

    iv.  The latter bundle must have all the fibers arranged in a "coherent bundle" (i.e., in the same spatial arrangement at both ends of the fiber, causing the portion of the total image that each carried to be in its proper position).

    v.  Major disadvantages with flexible fiberoptic endoscopes include fragility. When individual fibers break, light transmission is decreased and the visual image develops dark spots (corresponding to the broken fibers).

    vi.  These endoscopes are generally direct-viewing endoscopes, thus the endoscopist looks directly into an eyepiece. An optical beam splitter allows a second observer to view the image. Alternatively, a small video camera may be placed on the end of the endoscope and the image viewed on a video screen. These additional sidearms and external video screens introduce optical interference, which reduces visual clarity.

b.  **Videoendoscopy** applies video technology to endoscopy, with significant improvements in image quality and endoscope durability. An increasing number of endoscopes in use today are videoendoscopes.

    i.  Light is transmitted to the tip of the endoscope through a fiberoptic bundle as in the endoscopes described earlier.

    ii.  However, the viewing fiberoptic bundle is replaced with a charge-coupled device (CCD) chip camera, placed at the tip of the endoscope. This chip carries a digital image back to a video processor which displays an image on a color monitor.

    iii.  The CCD chip camera uses a dense grid of photocell receptors, each of which generates a single pixel on the monitor. Resolution depends on the density of the receptor packing on the chip camera.

    iv.  Some videoendoscopes use a single color (e.g., black–white) CCD chip which can create color images by rapidly cycling through a color wheel.

Newer videoendoscopes use three color CCD chips and provide the most accurate color resolution.

v.   Most videoendoscopes incorporate an automatic iris in the system to decrease the problem of glare due to tissue reflection.

vi.  Videoendoscopes have the advantage of allowing everyone involved in the procedure to view the field. The CCD chip also allows smaller scope diameters to transmit the same quality image.

c.   **Narrow Band and Multiband Imaging**

a.   Filters restrict tissue illumination to two different spectral ranges with shallow depth penetration of short-wavelengths into tissues to emphasize mucosal microvasculature indicative of pathologic conditions.

b.   Filters adjusted to two peak absorption spectrums for hemoglobin separate the blue (415 nm) wavelength to detect superficial capillaries, which appear brown, and green (540 nm) wavelengths for deeper vessels, which are displayed in cyan.

c.   Multiband imaging (MBI) is marketed as Fuji Intelligent Color Enhancement (FICE, Fujinon, Saitama, Japan). Image processing enhances mucosal surface structures by using selected wavelengths in reconstituted virtual images.

d.   MBI is driven by an image-processing algorithm based on spectral estimation methods. Reflectance spectra of corresponding pixels are mathematically estimated to reconstruct a virtual image of a single wavelength.

e.   MBI single wavelength images can be assigned to the red, green, blue monitor inputs to display a composite, color-enhanced image.

f.   Narrow band imaging (NBI) and MBI can also be coupled with electronic or optical zoom magnification.

g.   Classification of NBI and MBI mucosal patterns has been described for various conditions, including Barrett's esophagus and colon polyps.

d.   **Endomicroscopy**

a.   High-resolution endoscopes are capable of discriminating objects 10–71 microns in diameter, compared with the naked eye discriminating 125–165 microns.

b. Conventional endoscopes use CCDs with pixel densities of 100,000–200,000. There are commercially available endoscopes with pixel densities of 850,000.

c. Viewing from baseline to magnification is done with use of a rotary dial, a thumb lever or a foot pedal for magnification from ×1.5 to ×105.

d. Surface patterns of vascular and crypt architecture may characterize Barrett's esophagus, early gastric cancer, villous atrophy, and differentiate benign from malignant colon polyps (Table 37.1).

2. **Endoscope Categories:**

a. Esophagogastroduodenoscope (Gastroscope) can reach the proximal jejunum, has a defined working length (925–1,100 mm) and one or two instrument channels (2.0–6.0 mm).

b. Enteroscopes allow evaluation of the proximal two thirds of the jejunum. The working length is longer (21,800–2,800 mm) and instrument channels slightly smaller (1.0–3.5 mm).

c. Duodenoscopes are side-viewing instruments designed for ampullary biopsy and ERCP. Working length (1,030–1,250 mm), diameter (7.4–12.6 mm), and channel size (2.0–4.8 mm) are all standard.

  i. Olympus V-Scope employs a V-shaped distal scope tip-based elevator which can be locked in place to maintain wire and instrument position.

  ii. Multilumen scopes and therapeutic scopes with large diameter channels allow for passage of choledochoscopes and complex therapeutic maneuvers.

d. Choledochoscopes are thin caliber endoscopes passed through the instrument channel of a duodenoscope for direct visualization of the bile and pancreatic ducts.

  i. Conventional mother–daughter coupling involves a narrow diameter choledochoscope advanced through the therapeutic channel of an ERCP scope with two independent endoscopists required for effective visualization and sampling.

  ii. SpyGlass® (Boston Scientific) technology is a single operator-driven scope that can be advanced through the therapeutic channel of a side-viewing ERCP scope

Table 37.1. Indications for advanced imaging technology.

Chromoendoscopy
  Diagnosis of Barrett's metaplasia, early esophageal squamous cell cancer/
    adenocarcinoma
  Differentiates between benign and malignant lesions of the stomach and
    colon
  Diagnosis of Helicobacter pylori and ectopic gastric mucosa
Endomicroscopy
  Diagnosis of Barrett's metaplasia, early esophageal squamous cell cancer/
    adenocarcinoma
  Diagnosis of Helicobacter pylori as the cause of gastritis
  Diagnosis of early gastric and colorectal cancer
  Diagnosis of ulcerative colitis
  Narrow and multiband imaging
  Diagnosis of Barrett's metaplasia, early esophageal squamous cell cancer/
    adenocarcinoma
  Diagnosis of ulcerative colitis
  Diagnosis of gastrointestinal adenomas
Narrow and Multiband Imaging
  Diagnosis of Barrett's metaplasia, early esophageal squamous cell cancer/
    adenocarcinoma
  Diagnosis of ulcerative colitis
  Diagnosis of gastrointestinal adenomas
Endoscopic Ultrasound
  Staging and FNA biopsy of esophageal cancer
  Staging and biopsy of early gastric cancers
  Identifies gastric and esophageal tumors suitable for endoscopic mucosal
    resection
  Detection of peritoneal carcinomatosis and local ascites
  Diagnosis of chronic pancreatitis
  Diagnosis and staging of pancreatic adenocarcinoma
  Drainage of pancreatic pseudocysts
  Neurolysis of celiac plexus for pain control in pancreatic cancer
  Diagnosis of microlithiasis, common bile duct stones, cholangiocarcinoma/
    gallbladder cancer

to directly cannulate the bile and pancreatic ducts. Biopsy forceps and electrohydraulic lithotrypsy probes can be advanced through the SpyGlass® for determination of visualized pathology and destruction of impacted stones.

iii.   Peroral choledochoscopy (Cook) is a developmental product which deploys an anchoring tube per routine ERCP in the intra-hepatic biliary tract. The ERCP scope is removed and the choledochoscope then can be advanced over the anchoring tube into the proximal bile duct for direct visualization and sampling.

e.   Echoendoscopes are hybrid instruments that allow for high resolution ultrasound imaging of the luminal digestive tract and adjacent organs. Standards include a working length (975–1,325 mm), diameter (7.9–13.7 mm), instrument channel size (2.2–3.7 mm), and orientation of optical (forward or oblique) and US (longitudinal or radial) images.

f.   Colonoscopes are designed to evaluate the colon and distal terminal ileum. Working length (1,330–1,700 mm), diameter (11.1–13.7 mm), and instrument channel size (2.8–4.2 mm) are standard.

g.   Sigmoidoscopes are shorter versions of the colonoscope for evaluation of the sigmoid colon and rectum. Standards include working length (630–790 mm), diameter 12.2–13.3 mm), and instrument channel size (3.2–4.2 mm).

h.   NOTES Scopes:

   a.   Shape-Lock Cobra™ (USGI Medical) is an overtube designed for transluminal surgery which locks in a rigid configuration allowing three separate movable channels to be deployed and operate independently allowing triangulation and independent movement.

   b.   Spider Surgical System™ (TransEnterix, Inc.) has been designed for single incision surgery but can also be deployed through intraluminal access to allow two arms to be manipulated by cables that interact with a handle as well as allowing passage of long wire-guided instruments for therapeutic intervention.

i.   **Endoscopic Ablative Therapies**

   i.   Endoscopic mucosal resection (EMR) involves the use of variceal banding technology which suctions the mucosal layer into a variceal banding cap for banding and subsequent removal.

   ii.   Endoscopic submucosal dissection(ESD) involves the use of injection and elevation of tissue planes with subsequent submucosal dissection using a needle knife or insulation tip protected knife with provision of a near full thickness enteric wall specimen for resection of early esophageal and gastric cancers.

iii. Photodynamic therapy (PDT) for Barrett's esophagus involves systemic injection of porfimer sodium followed by mucosal ablation by a KTP/dye laser (Laserscope, San Jose,Calif.) delivered by using a cylindrical diffuser inserted in a 20-mm diameter reflective esophageal balloon.

iv. Radiofrequency ablation (RFA)(BARRX™) involves measurement of the zone of Barrett's esophagus followed by deployment of the Halo 360 System™ balloon-based catheter which doses adjustable radiofrequency energy circumferentially to ablate the mucosal surface.

j. **Endoscopic Antireflux Therapy**

a. Stretta™ involves application of a radio frequency ablation probe at three consecutive levels surrounding the gastroesophageal junction to produce a submucosal fibrosis which reduces compliance of this region to relieve reflux not associated with a hiatal hernia or Barrett's esophagus.

b. Esophyx™ is an endoscopically deployed stapling technology which recreates the Angle of His by firing pledgeted sutures between a folding cartridge deployed in the fundus and the endoscope arm in the esophageal lumen at the region of the gastroesophageal junction.

c. NDO Plicator™ functions to create full-thickness pledgeted plications at the gastroesophageal junction which function to narrow the lumen at the gastroesophageal junction and attempt to recreate the Angle of His.

k. **Bariatric Endoscopic Therapies**

a. Bard Endocinch™ has effectively decreased the stoma size in gastrojejunostomy revision for gastric bypass patients, reducing stomas from 25 to 10 mm producing weight loss in patients with dilated gastric pouches.

b. Endoscopic balloon therapy involves placement of a double lumen silastic balloon in the body of the stomach to promote early satiety.

c. Endoscopic deployed sleeves involve placement of a wire basket in the gastric antrum with a silastic sleeve which is opened as the endoscope is advanced through the duodenum into the distal small bowel that serves to divert nutritional flow from the proximal jejunum.

3. **Channels**: Flexible endoscopes provide one or more instrument channels (2–3 mm) for passage of diagnostic and therapuetic instruments as well as for suctioning. Air and water insufflation channels permit distention of the bowel and cleaning of the lens.

4. **Instrument tip control**: Tip deflection is controlled by stacked angulation control knobs on the headpiece. The larger wheel allows for 12 and 6 o'clock manipulation while the smaller wheel allows for 3 and 9 o'clock maneuvering. The shaft of the instrument may also be torqued in a clockwise or counterclockwise manner to change direction. Locks are provided, but for most purposes wheels should be allowed to move freely. ERCP-capable side-viewing endoscope also has an elevator lever which can be used to advance instruments from a 30° to a 90° angle with the deflecting scope tip.

5. **Illumination and image capturing**: Illumination is provided by an external source, either a xenon arc or a halogen-filled tungsten filament lamp. Modern endoscopes also include electronic systems to capture still images and record video footage. Air/water and suction valves are located on the upper front portion of the headpiece to aid visualization. The headpiece also houses remote switches to modify or capture the video image.

# B. Equipment Setup

The endoscopic equipment is generally arranged on a multiple level cart which allows mobility and easy access. The cart generally includes a monitor, video processor, light source, water bottle, and image printer.

1. A fiberoptic cable connects the endoscope to the light source. This umbilical cable also contains connectors for suction, water, and insufflation gas.

2. Air and water are introduced through a common channel by depression of a trumpet-like valve on the control head of the scope.

   a. Partial depression of the valve insufflates air and distends the viewed lumen.

b.   Complete depression of the valve forces air backward into the attached water bottle, forcing a stream of water to the tip of the instrument. This washes the lens.

c.   Depression of an adjacent trumpet valve enables suctioning of air or fluid at the tip of the instrument.

d.   Insufflation, irrigation, and suction should be tested prior to each use of the endoscope.

3.   Common problems include sticky valves, lack of water in the water bottle, failure to secure all connections, or leaks in the valve apparatus.

4.   To avoid pitfalls during the procedure, become well versed in the construction and function of the particular endoscopic system in use. All endoscopes are not constructed in the same manner. Accurate assessment of problems arising during a procedure often allows rapid resolution.

5.   Adopt a **standard approach to equipment setup**. Problems commonly arise when one or another step is forgotten.

a.   Choose the appropriate size (length and diameter) and type of endoscope for the intended purpose. Both pediatric and adult upper gastrointestinal endoscopes are available.

b.   Connect the umbilical cable of the endoscope to the light source.

c.   Turn on all electric equipment on the cart, even if use of a particular item (e.g., videocassette recorder) is not planned. The connections of the various pieces of equipment may require that all be on for any to work properly.

d.   Ensure that the water bottle is filled with clean water.

e.   Connect the hose from the water bottle to the side of the umbilical cable, near where it enters the light box. Generally, the fittings are arranged with a Luer-Lok or other mating set of connectors so that the hose can only connect to one place.

f.   Connect suction to the remaining site on the umbilical cord.

g.   Obtain a cup or basin of water and test insufflation (by insufflating air under water and observing bubbles), water irrigation (with the tip of the endoscope out of the water), and suction (by aspirating the water from the cup). If any of these functions are sluggish or nonfunctional, first check the connections. (See Section C, Troubleshooting, for additional tips).

h.  Take the light source off standby and aim the tip of the endoscope into the cupped fingers of one hand. A sharp image of the fingers should be seen on the monitor.

i.  Check the tip deflection controls and verify that any locking devices are "off" so that the tip is free to move.

j.  Verify that any additional items that may be required (such as biopsy forceps, polypectomy snares) are available, of appropriate size, and in good working order.

## C. Troubleshooting

A systematic approach to identifying the problem, followed by creative measures to circumvent or repair the difficulty will usually permit satisfactory completion of the examination. As mentioned previously, attention to detail during the setup phase can help minimize problems during the examination. Common problems and solutions are listed in Table 37.2.

## D. Equipment Care

Flexible endoscopes are expensive and relatively fragile. Attention to care is important.

1.  The light fibers are fragile and easily broken. Coil the endoscope into gentle curves, rather than folding it in acute angles. Do not drop the endoscope, allow a wheeled cart to roll over it, or allow the patient to bite down on the endoscope.

2.  Avoid extreme angulation of the tip wherever possible. Do not force biopsy forceps or other instruments down the channel when the tip is sharply angulated, as damage to the biopsy channel may result.

3.  Ensure that polypectomy snares and sclerosing needles are fully withdrawn into the sheath before passing through the channel. Lubricate instruments with a suitable lubricant to facilitate passage.

4.  The outer coating of the endoscope is delicate, particularly in the region near the tip. A rubber sheath, designed to flex as the tip bends, covers this region of the endoscope.

Table 37.2. Common problems with flexible endoscopes and suggested solutions.

| Problem | Check the following |
|---------|---------------------|
| No light at distal end | 1. Light source plugged in and turned on<br>2. Light source ignited<br>3. Not in "standby" mode<br>4. Lens at distal tip is dirty<br>5. Bulb is burned out |
| Out of focus | 1. Adjust focus ring<br>2. Fiberoptic scope clean lens |
| No irrigation | 1. Water bottle contains water<br>2. Water bottle connected to umbilical cord<br>3. Connection tight<br>4. Lid of water bottle screwed on tightly<br>5. Power turned on<br>6. Valve stuck or occluded |
| No insufflations | 1. Umbilical cord firmly seated into light source and screwed in if necessary.<br>2. Power turned on<br>3. Valve stuck or occluded |
| Clogged valve or nozzle | 1. Take valve apart and clean<br>2. Flush channel of endoscope with cleaning solution, followed by clear water. |
| Difficulty passing instrument | 1. Check tip angulation; decrease angulation and try again<br>2. Ensure that the instrument is fully closed<br>3. Check size of instrument relative to instrument channel; try smaller diameter instrument |

5. After each use, wash off any gross contamination and suction water through the endoscope. Do not allow blood, mucus, stool, or other foreign matter to dry on the endoscope or in the channels or valves.

6. Endoscopes are rarely actually sterilized. Generally, high-level disinfection with a chemical agent (such as glutaraldehyde) is used. Disinfection does not work well when foreign matter (mucus, blood, enteric contents) are present. Therefore, the endoscope must be mechanically cleaned before disinfection. Many endoscopy suites use automated cleaners that rapidly wash, disinfect, and rinse the endoscope. Ultrasonic cleaners are available in some units.

7. Ethylene oxide gas sterilization is an option, but it requires an overnight cycle. Newer methods of sterilization and newer

endoscopes that are more tolerant of sterilizing conditions are being developed. Be careful to follow the manufacturer's instructions for sterilization to avoid potentially severe damage to the endoscope.

# Selected References

Chiu HM, Chang CY, Chen CC, et al. A prospective comparative study of narrow-band imaging, chromoendoscopy, and conventional colonoscopy in the diagnosis of colorectal neoplasia. Gut. 2007;56:373–9.

Harewood GC, Gostout CJ, Farrell MA, et al. Prospective controlled assessment of variable stiffness enteroscopy. Gastrointest Endosc. 2003;58:267–71.

Konishi K, Kaneko K, Kurahashi T, et al. A comparison of magnifying and nonmagnifying colonoscopy for diagnosis of colorectal polyps: a prospective study. Gastrointest Endosc. 2003;57:48–53.

Louis H, Deviere J. Endoscopic-endoluminal therapies: a critical appraisal. Best Pract Res Clin Gastroenterol. 2010;4:969–79.

Maluf-Filho F, Dotti CM, Halwan B, Quieros AF, Kupski C, Chaves DM, Nakao FS, Kumar A. An evidence based consensus statement on the role and application of endosonography in clinical practice. Endoscopy. 2009;41:979–87.

Teoh AY, Chiu PW, NG EK. Current developments in natural orifice transluminal endoscopic surgery: an evidence based review. World J Gastroenterol. 2010;16:4792–9.

Vassiliou MC, von Rentein D, Wiener DC, Gordon SR, Rothstein RI. Treatment of ultralong-segment Barrett's using focal and balloon-based radiofrequency ablation. Surg Endosc. 2010;24:786–91.

Vitale GC, Davis BR, Tran TC. The advancing art and science of endoscopy. Am J Surg. 2005;190:228–33.

# 38. Endoscopy Handling*

*Kevin El-Hayek, M.D.*
*John Rodriguez, M.D.*
*Bipan Chand, M.D., F.A.C.S.*

## A. Room Characteristics and Setup

In order to perform any endoscopic procedure comfortably and effectively, the room must be set up appropriately. Most medical centers have dedicated rooms or suites which include endoscopic equipment with video monitors, oxygen, suction, and noninvasive monitoring devices. Other characteristics of the endoscopy suite include sufficient space for necessary equipment, personnel, and ease of movement of the patient on a gurney or bed. The majority of dedicated endoscopy suites have an additional monitor behind the endoscopist to allow the assistant(s) to view the procedure. Take a few minutes to consider the room layout and the proposed endoscopic examination prior to bringing the patient into the room and setting up the equipment (see Fig. 38.1).

Whenever possible, it is preferable to have patients transported to such an environment, where often a dedicated and trained endoscopy team is available to assist. In some instances, it is necessary to perform endoscopy in an operating room, at the patient's bedside, or in another location—particularly in an intensive care setting when patients are too ill for transport. While the location may be different, the principles of room setup remain. Access to patients in an intensive care unit can be quite challenging due to the presence of multiple

---

*This chapter was contributed in the previous edition by Bipan Chand, MD, and Jeffrey L. Ponsky, MD, FACS.

N.J. Soper and C.E.H. Scott-Conner (eds.), *The SAGES Manual: Volume 1 Basic Laparoscopy and Endoscopy*, DOI 10.1007/978-1-4614-2344-7_38, © Springer Science+Business Media, LLC 2012

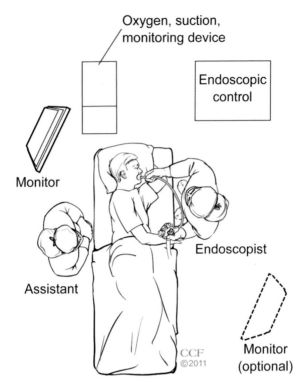

Fig. 38.1. Components and room setup of a standard endoscopy suite (reprinted with permission, Cleveland Clinic Center for Medical Art and Photography © 2011).

intravenous lines, invasive monitors, or ventilator attachments. These extra appendages can hinder the ability of an endoscopist to perform an effective exam. Therefore, it is important to remove extraneous tables and chairs and to move all attachments to allow access to the patient prior to the arrival of endoscopy equipment. A "travel cart" should be organized to include a video monitor tower and additional equipment, including bite blocks, anesthetic spray, lubrication, sponges, irrigation, and therapeutic tools as indicated. Whenever possible, the video monitor should be positioned directly across from the endoscopist, in direct line of sight. The endoscopy cart should also be positioned close to the intended working area.

# B.  Patient and Endoscopist Position

The position of the patient and endoscopist are dictated by the type of exam to be performed. An assistant should stand on the opposite side of the endoscopist to allow for access to the airway and intravenous lines. Both the assistant and endoscopist should also have monitoring data in view at all times. Adjust the height of the gurney or bed so that the endoscopist can stand comfortably with good posture throughout the entire exam. Details of specific positioning are included in the following chapters, but below are some key highlights.

1.  For **upper gastrointestinal endoscopy**, position the patient left side slightly down with the head of the bed slightly tilted up. The endoscopist faces the patient near the head of the bed on the left side, providing easy access to the oropharynx (see Fig. 38.2).

2.  For **lower gastrointestinal endoscopy**, the patient is typically placed in a left lateral decubitus position with hips flexed and both knees brought up toward the chest. The endoscopist stands

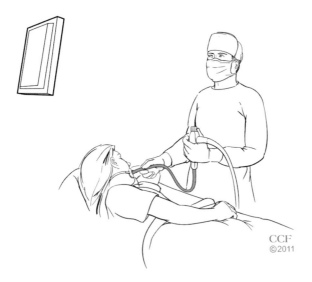

Fig. 38.2.  Position of endoscopist and patient for upper gastrointestinal endoscopy. Stand comfortably, facing the patient and the video monitor. Generally, the video monitor will be across from the endoscopist in direct line of site (reprinted with permission, Cleveland Clinic Center for Medical Art and Photography © 2011).

facing the back of the patient just below the patient's buttocks. An inverse room set up is generally required for this procedure with the video monitor directly across from the endoscopist. It is sometimes necessary to have the patient in a supine position to allow for access to the abdomen during a challenging colonoscopy. In this instance, the patient's legs can be placed in either a "frog leg" configuration or with both knees upright (see Fig. 38.3).

3.  When **both upper and lower gastrointestinal endoscopy** is indicated, begin with the upper exam. During the exchange of endoscopes, the patient's orientation (head to foot) in the room should be reversed either by moving the gurney or repositioning the patient on gurney or bed. Taking the time to perform this maneuver helps avoid a suboptimal exam.

4.  For **advanced endoscopic procedures**, such as endoscopic retrograde pancreaticocholangiography (ERCP), patients are often placed in a prone position to allow for easier access to the ampulla.

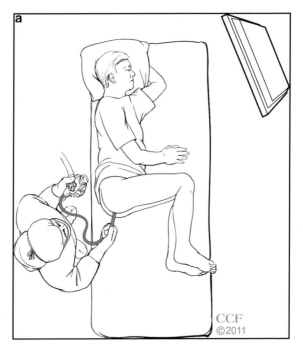

Fig. 38.3. Position of endoscopist and patient for lower gastrointestinal endoscopy. (**a**) Patient is positioned in left lateral decubitus position. (**b**) Patient is positioned supine in "frog leg" configuration (reprinted with permission, Cleveland Clinic Center for Medical Art and Photography © 2011).

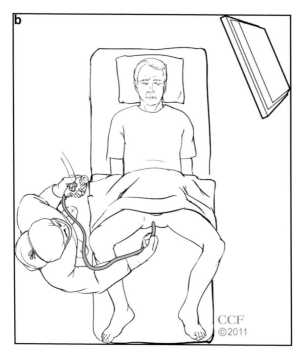

Fig. 38.3. (continued)

## C. Endoscope Manipulation

There are two main components of the endoscope—the headpiece and the shaft. In order to breakdown the actual manipulation of the endoscope, it is helpful to focus on the tasks of each hand of the endoscopist. Some endoscopists use both hands at all times to control the various aspects of the headpiece while an assistant advances and withdraws the shaft. However, significantly greater control can be attained if the endoscopist manipulates the controls with the left hand and advances or withdraws the shaft with the right hand. This is the method described here. There are no left-handed endoscopes, and this method is used by both right-handed and left-handed endoscopists. Specific techniques useful for performing various endoscopic examinations are given in the sections that follow.

## 1. Left Hand

a. The endoscope headpiece should fit comfortably in the **palm** of the endoscopist's left hand. The control buttons should lie between the thumb and forefinger. Endoscopists with small hands may need to experiment to find a comfortable position that will allow access to all controls. The key is to keep the hand rotated so that the thumb can manipulate the large control wheel.

b. The **thumb** of the left hand manipulates the large control wheel of the endoscope headpiece, deflecting the tip of the endoscope up and down. It is important to note that the movement on the big wheel appears inversely to what is seen on the monitor. That is, turning the big wheel downward deflects the tip of the endoscope upwards and vice versa (see Fig. 38.4). Newer endoscopes also have up to four buttons which control various aspects of the endoscope image and documentation. Each of these buttons can be programmed to control video aspects, such as still photography, videography, and narrow band imaging based on the technology available. When performing brisk movements with the big wheel, endoscopists may inadvertently depress these buttons.

c. The **index finger** rests on one of the upper of two trumpet valves on the front aspect of the headpiece. When the upper valve is fully depressed, suction is applied from the endoscope tip. It is important to note that suction occurs from the lower hemisphere of the endoscope tip which corresponds to the 5 o'clock position on the video monitor. Therefore, the endoscopist must position the endoscope tip above a pool of fluid when performing a suctioning maneuver; otherwise, the effect will be to desufflate the lumen or capture the mucosa. Also, since the suction port corresponds to the working channel, the presence of instruments within this channel decreases the power of the suction (see Fig. 38.5). Some endoscopists also control the lower of the two trumpet valves with the index finger, which is described below.

d. The **long finger** rests on the lower trumpet valve on the front aspect of the headpiece. On this valve, there is a central hole that emits a continuous stream of air when the endoscope is secured to the control tower. The endoscopist should ensure that air is present from this valve prior to starting the exam. When there is no stream of air present, the endoscope base is often not

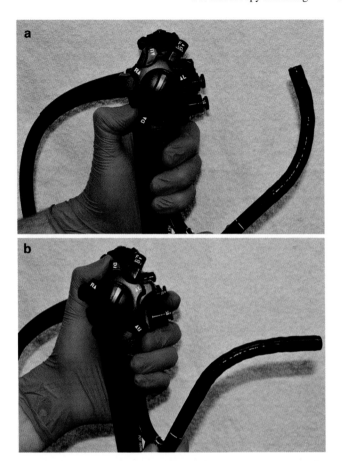

Fig. 38.4. Manipulation of the large wheel with the left thumb. (**a**) Rotation of the large wheel downward creates upward deflection of the endoscope tip. (**b**) Rotation of the large wheel upward creates downward deflection of the endoscope tip.

fully secured to the control tower. When this hole is occluded, insufflation is achieved. The amount of insufflation delivered can be modulated both on the control tower with low, medium, and high settings, as well as with varying finger pressure. Complete occlusion of the hole emits the maximum amount of insufflation while complete release allows for no insufflation. **When the trumpet is depressed fully, the endoscope tip is irrigated for better visualization.**

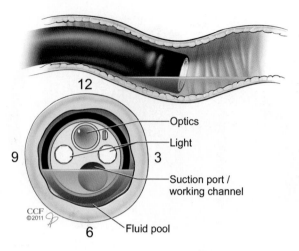

Fig. 38.5. Appropriate positioning of endoscope to perform suctioning of a fluid pool (reprinted with permission, Cleveland Clinic Center for Medical Art and Photography © 2011).

e.   The **ring and little fingers** are generally used to secure the headpiece handle firmly within the left hand.

## 2. Right Hand

a.   The endoscopist's right hand primarily controls the shaft, performing advancement and withdrawal of the endoscope, as well as various torque maneuvers.

b.   When the endoscope can be left in a fixed position, the right hand is free to access the small wheel, which is located on the endoscope headpiece. Rotating the small wheel downward deflects the endoscope tip to the right while rotating the wheel upward deflects the endoscope to the left.

c.   The right hand is also useful to access the working channel, typically located below the headpiece handle. This channel normally has a cap and an access port through which biopsy forceps, sclerotherapy devices, and

d.   Other instruments can pass (see Fig. 38.6). If tissue is caught within the suction port, removing this cap allows for the tissue to fall away from the endoscope—this maneuver can help avoid mucosal trauma. Depending on the manufacturer, the working

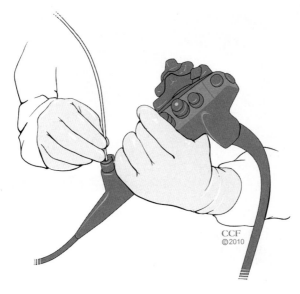

Fig. 38.6. The location of the working channel on most endoscopes with corresponding access via the right hand (reprinted with permission, Cleveland Clinic Center for Medical Art and Photography © 2011).

channel output corresponds to the 5 o'clock position on the video monitor. While diagnostic endoscopes have one working channel, therapeutic endoscopes often have dual channels for multiple instruments.

e. The **ring or little fingers** of the right hand can also be used to steady the shaft while manipulating the small control wheel, giving the endoscopist a "third hand" to perform more complex maneuvers (see Fig. 38.7).

## D.  Basic Maneuvers

### 1.  Insertion

a. When inserting the endoscope into an orifice, it is helpful to "choke up" with the right hand on the shaft to allow for better tip control.

b. When performing an upper endoscopy, a gentle downward deflection of the tip allows for better clearance of the posterior aspect of the tongue.

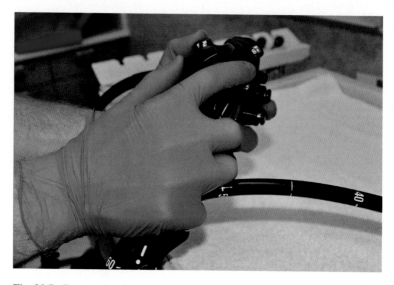

Fig. 38.7. By grasping the endoscope shaft with the fifth finger of the right hand, the first three fingers are liberated to control the small wheel, which deflects the endoscope tip to the right and left.

    c.    Anesthetic spray administered to the back of the patient's throat prior to beginning an upper endoscopic procedure allows for less gagging during insertion.

    d.    For lower endoscopy, position the tip in a straight line with the endoscopist's hand to avoid injury to the anal canal on insertion.

    e.    A generous amount of lubrication can help with endoscope insertion;however, this may interfere with endoscope visualization. To avoid this pitfall, apply lubrication directly to the endoscope shaft, at least a few centimeters from the tip.

## 2. Advancement

    f.    When advancing the endoscope, an important factor is to keep all walls of the lumen in plain view. Provide enough insufflation to allow for distension of the bowel and passage of the endoscope. Keeping a circumferential view of the lumen will help avoid bowel injury.

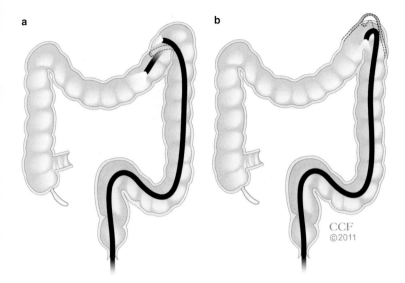

Fig. 38.8. (**a**) Minor tip deflection with gentle advancement and mild torsion allows the endoscope to traverse bends while maintaining a gentle curve. (**b**) Sharp angulation of the tip (like a candy cane) hinders advancement and may result in paradoxical motion, where the target gets further away rather than closer and can contribute to perforation (reprinted with permission, Cleveland Clinic Center for Medical Art and Photography © 2011).

g.  Use gentle tip deflection, especially when navigating turns. Sharp tip angulation may result in an apparent paradoxical motion on the video monitor (see Fig. 38.8).

## 3. Torque

h.  Grasping the shaft and rotating it clockwise or counterclockwise is referred to as torque. This maneuver is critical in many endoscopic exams, especially early in the procedure when the right hand may not be available to access the small wheel. It is also helpful during difficult aspects of an exam when meeting resistance due to bowel tortuosity. It is common to use a torque maneuver during a lower gastrointestinal exam while navigating the sigmoid colon, the splenic flexure, and the hepatic flexure.

i.  Just below the headpiece of most endoscopes, there is a mechanism to stiffen the endoscope shaft. Stiffening the endoscope

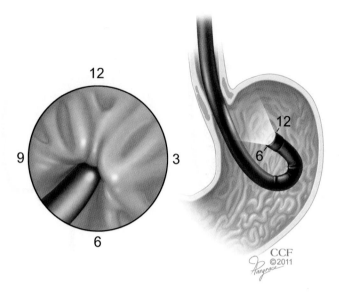

Fig. 38.9. Retroflexed view of the endoscope within the stomach and corresponding monitor image (reprinted with permission, Cleveland Clinic Center for Medical Art and Photography © 2011).

reduces its flexibility, which can aid the endoscopist when performing a torquing maneuver in a redundant portion of bowel. There are usually up to three levels of stiffening commonly found on lower gastrointestinal endoscopes.

## 4. Retroflexion

j.  Turning the endoscope tip to look back upon the shaft is termed retroflexion. To perform this maneuver, the endoscopist performs a firm torque maneuver either clockwise or counterclockwise while maximally rotating the large wheel. The corresponding image on the monitor is therefore reversed. Therefore, when the endoscopist withdraws the endoscope, the image appears closer and vice versa. Two common procedures where retroflexion is helpful is in viewing the gastric cardia and fundus on upper gastrointestinal endoscopy, as well as the lower rectum and upper anal canal on lower gastrointestinal endoscopy (see Fig. 38.9).

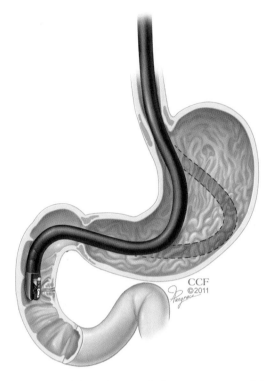

Fig. 38.10. Shortening of the endoscope during an upper gastrointestinal exam (reprinted with permission, Cleveland Clinic Center for Medical Art and Photography © 2011).

## 5. Shortening the endoscope

k.  Following significant advancement of the endoscope, it is not uncommon for it to loop within the bowel. Withdrawing the endoscope in this instance does not correspond with any movement of the tip. When this scenario occurs, it is helpful to shorten the endoscope by pulling back the shaft until the tip begins to move in reverse or does not move at all. Performing this maneuver increases the amount of control the endoscopist has with the shaft. It also allows for the endoscope to travel a farther distance within the bowel (see Fig. 38.10).

## 6. Withdrawing

l. After completion of the exam, the endoscopist must withdraw the endoscope in a controlled manner. Performing withdrawal in this fashion allows for closer examination of the mucosa, as pathology is frequently diagnosed during this time. It is important to have a circumferential view of the bowel lumen while performing this maneuver. Grasping the shaft with the ring or little finger of the right hand will free up the first three fingers to manipulate the small wheel.

## 7. Other considerations

m. Most endoscopes have locking mechanisms for both the large and small wheels, which allows an endoscopist to freeze a certain configuration of the endoscope. Performing this maneuver allows the endoscopist freedom to perform more complex navigation and tool manipulation within the working channel.

n. Residual lubrication on the endoscope or the endoscopist's hand can hinder movements, such as advancement, torque, and withdrawal. It is helpful to have towels readily available to remove lubrication from these areas.

The basic maneuvers outlined above are by no means all inclusive, and there are times when an endoscopist will deviate from the basics to complete difficult procedures. Experienced endoscopists know that equal if not more vital directional control is provided by rotation and elevation of the endoscope's headpiece in concert with gentle torsion of the shaft. These often imperceptible maneuvers occur throughout the procedure, and in combination with tip control allow complex manipulations to be performed. An accomplished endoscopist is rarely motionless during a procedure, but continually performs an "endoscopic dance."

## E. Training

The standardized concept of endoscopic training for surgical residents was first introduced by the American Board of Surgery in the early 1980s. Over the last 3 decades, endoscopy has become a very important diagnostic and therapeutic tool for general surgeons. The Resident Review Committee (RRC) recently increased the requirements to 35 upper gastrointestinal endoscopies and 50 colonoscopies from 29 previously. This requirement was first implemented for surgical residents graduating in 2009.

Proficiency in endoscopic techniques is only achieved through practice and experience. The most common criteria used to determine competency in colonoscopy is completion rate. The number of procedures required to be considered competent is still an area of debate, and there is wide variation among different organizations. Early studies in colonoscopy training consistently showed that more than 100 procedures were required for trainees to achieve a completion rate close to 90%. The caveat to these studies is that completion rate is not always associated with recognition of pathology. Teaching trainees endoscopic skills in the clinical setting remains a challenge. Virtual reality (VR) simulators are playing an important role in helping residents develop their basic endoscopic skills without jeopardizing patient safety. Simulators allow trainees to become familiar with the equipment as well as common maneuvers in a nonthreatening environment. Several studies have shown a benefit in trainees undergoing VR training prior to performing procedures on patients. The most commonly used simulator is the GI Mentor I/II developed by Simbionix (Cleveland, OH). VR trainers will likely become universally accessible and become an essential part of endoscopic training.

The Fundamentals of Endoscopic Surgery (FES) is a program being developed by SAGES as a test of knowledge and skills in gastrointestinal endoscopy. This test is intended to assess competency among surgical residents. Trainees are required to complete a Web-based didactic curriculum and are later examined through a multiple choice exam and a hands-on skills test. This design allows a thorough assessment on cognitive knowledge as well as the technical skills required for basic endoscopy.

# Selected References

The fundamentals of endoscopic surgery. 2011. http://www.fesprogram.org. Accessed on 20 Jan 2011.

Ponsky J. Atlas of surgical endoscopy. St. Louis, MO: Mosby Year Book; 1992.

Cooper GS. Indications and contraindications for upper gastrointestinal endoscopy. Gastrointest Endosc Clin N Am. 1994;4(3):439–54.

Jaffe PE. Technique of upper gastrointestinal endoscopy. Gastrointest Endosc Clin N Am. 1994;4(3):501–21.

Mellinger JD, Ponsky JL. Endoscopic evaluation of the postoperative stomach. Gastrointest Endosc Clin N Am. 1996;6(3):621–39.

Van Dam J, Brugge WR. Endoscopy of the upper gastrointestinal tract. N Engl J Med. 1999;341(23):1738–48.

Sivak MV. Gastroenterologic Endoscopy. 2nd ed. Philadelphia: WB Saunders; 2000.

Accreditation Council for Graduate Medical Education. Memorandum regarding changes in minimum requirements for laparoscopy and endoscopy. 2006. http://www.acgme.org/acWebsite/RRC_440/440_minReqLaparoscopy.asp. Accessed on 20 Jan 2011.

Bittner 4th JG, Marks JM, Dunkin BJ, Richards WO, Onders RP, Mellinger JD. Resident training in flexible gastrointestinal endoscopy: a review of current issues and options. J Surg Educ. 2007;64(6):399–409.

Cotton PB, Williams CB, Hawes RH, Saunders BP. Practical Gastrointestinal Endoscopy: The Fundamentals. 6th ed. Hoboken: Blackwell; 2008.

Morales MP, Mancini GJ, Miedema BW, Rangnekar NJ, Koivunen DG, Ramshaw BJ, Eubanks WS, Stephenson HE. Integrated flexible endoscopy training during surgical residency. Surg Endosc. 2008;22(9):2013–7.

Vassiliou MC, Dunkin BJ, Marks JM, Fried GM. FLS and FES: comprehensive models of training and assessment. Surg Clin North Am. 2010;90(3):535–58.

# 39. Monitoring, Sedation, and Recovery*

*Jennifer Hrabe, M.D.*
*Joseph J. Cullen, M.D., F.A.C.S.*

## A. Introduction

Sedation is an integral part of upper and lower endoscopy and serves to alleviate patient discomfort, reduce risk of injury to the patient, and facilitate optimal examination during the procedure. For the purposes of this chapter, we use the term endoscopy to include all forms of endoscopy including colonoscopy. The majority of patients undergoing endoscopy have sedation provided by the endoscopist. An understanding of commonly used medications and an awareness of appropriate patient monitoring is important to safely provide sedation for patients undergoing these procedures.

## B. Monitoring

1. Pre-Procedure

   Prior to embarking on the procedure, adequately evaluate the patient. Perform a thorough assessment, taking care to note the following:

   a. Major organ system pathologies, particularly cardiac or pulmonary. Pay special attention to snoring, stridor, sleep apnea;

---

*This chapter was contributed by Bipan Chand, M.D. and Jeffrey L. Ponsky, M.D. in the previous edition.

b.   Current medications, drug allergies, and previous adverse reactions with sedation or anesthesia;

c.   Time of last meal;

d.   Use/abuse of alcohol or drugs;

e.   Physical examination should include determination of vital signs, heart and lung auscultation, and assessment of airway anatomy. Females of childbearing age should have a pregnancy test;

f.   The patient's condition should be classified according to the American Society for Anesthesiology (ASA) physical status classification. Generally, patients with ASA I-III are acceptable candidates for sedation by the proceduralist; strong consideration should be given to sedation by an anesthesiologist for ASA IV-V patients.

2.   Emergency equipment and medications should be immediately available. This includes airway and cardiac equipment (oxygen, suction machine, oxygen delivery systems such as nasal cannulas and face masks, oral and nasal airways, laryngoscopes and endotracheal tubes, defibrillators).

3.   During the procedure

a.   Heart rate, blood pressure, respiratory rate, oxygen saturation, and level of consciousness should be evaluated throughout the procedure. These parameters should be checked prior to administration of sedation and at 3- to 5-min intervals thereafter.

b.   Consider cardiac monitoring in patients with significant cardiac disease or history of arrhythmias. These parameters do not supplant evaluation of the patient by clinical observation. Always remember that hypercapnia may develop despite normal oxygen saturation.

c.   It is advisable to have a nurse or assistant trained in endoscopic sedation present throughout the procedure.

4.   Post-Procedure

Continue to monitor the patient during recovery. There are various scales designed to determine whether a patient is ready for discharge. One such scale is the Aldrete scale, which includes examination of ventilation and oxygenation, circulation, and consciousness.

# C. Sedation

Endoscopy is generally performed under moderate sedation, commonly referred to as "conscious sedation." At this level, the patient responds meaningfully to verbal and physical stimuli and does not require airway support. Patients who require lengthier or more complex procedures and those who are anticipated to be difficult to sedate secondary to long-standing narcotic, benzodiazepine, or alcohol use may require deeper sedation. In these cases, it may be prudent for sedation to be provided by an anesthesiologist.

Medications commonly used for endoscopic sedation are benzodiazepines and opiates. Droperidol, diphenhydramine, and promethazine are occasionally used to augment sedation. Endoscopist-administered propofol is receiving increased attention and interest, though is not yet standard practice and should be performed only by those who have received appropriate credentialing and training.

## 1. Topical anesthetics

a. For upper endoscopy, sprays commonly used to anesthetize the pharynx include lidocaine, tetracaine, and benzocaine.

## 2. Intravenous sedation

a. Benzodiazepines—Commonly used benzodiazepines include midazolam and diazepam (Table 39.1). Their effects include sedation, amnesia, anxiolysis, and muscle relaxation; adverse effects include respiratory depression. Respiratory depression is dose-dependent. The elderly, those with underlying respiratory disorders, and patients also receiving opiates are at increased risk for clinically significant respiratory depression.

b. Opiates—Fentanyl, meperidine, and morphine are among the more commonly used opiates for endoscopy (Table 39.1). Their primary effects are analgesia and sedation. Side effects include hypotension and respiratory depression.

c. Propofol—Use of propofol for endoscopic procedures has grown secondary to its fast onset and rapid recovery. It produces sedation and amnesia but offers no analgesia. Side effects include decreased cardiac output and hypotension. Propofol adminis-

Table 39.1. Commonly used medications during endoscopic procedures.

| Medication | Pharmaceutical class | Dosing[a] | Onset | Duration | Common adverse effects |
|---|---|---|---|---|---|
| Diazepam | Benzodiazepine | Initial: 2.5–10 mg<br>Bolus: 5 mg every 5 min | 1–5 min | 20–60 min | Respiratory depression |
| Midazolam | Benzodiazepine | Initial: 1–2 mg<br>Bolus: 0.5–1 mg every 2 min | 1–2 min | 15–80 min | Respiratory depression |
| Fentanyl | Opioid | Initial: 50–100 mcg<br>Bolus: 25–50 mcg | 1 min | 30–60 min | Respiratory depression, hypotension |
| Meperidine | Opioid | Initial: 25 mg<br>Bolus: 25 mg | 5 min | 1–4 h | Respiratory depression, hypotension |
| Flumazenil | Benzodiazepine antagonist | 0.1–0.3 mg bolus, or infusion of 0.3–0.5 mg/h | 1–2 min | 40–80 min | Precipitation of benzodiazepine withdrawal |
| Nalaxone | Opiod antagonist | 0.2–0.4 mg, repeat as needed | 1–2 min | 30–45 min | Precipitation of narcotic withdrawal |

[a]Dose reduction recommended in elderly or debilitated patients

tration has historically been restricted to anesthesiologists, though several gastroenterology organizations have endorsed administration by appropriately trained nonanesthesiology personnel.

d.   Flumazenil, naloxone—Occasionally, patients can become over-sedated and will require reversal of their sedation. Flumazenil competitively antagonizes benzodiazepines while naloxone competitively antagonizes opioids (Table 39.1). Of note, the duration of the sedation may outlast that of the reversal, so patients must be monitored carefully and re-dosed with flumazenil or naloxone as needed.

# Selected References

Cohen LB. Patient monitoring during gastrointestinal endoscopy: why, when, and how? Gastrointest Endosc Clin N Am. 2008;18(4):651–63. vii.

Cohen LB, Delegge MH, Aisenberg J, Brill JV, Inadomi JM, Kochman ML, Piorkowski Jr JD, AGA Institute. AGA Institute review of endoscopic sedation. Gastroenterology. 2007;133(2):675–701.

Lubarsky DA, Candiotti K, Harris E. Understanding modes of moderate sedation during gastrointestinal procedures: a current review of the literature. J Clin Anesth. 2007;19(5):397–404.

Thomson A, Andrew G, Jones DB. Optimal sedation for gastrointestinal endoscopy: review and recommendations. J Gastroenterol Hepatol. 2010;25(3):469–78.

Waring JP, Baron TH, Hirota WK, Goldstein JL, Jacobson BC, Leighton JA, Mallery JS, Faigel DO. Guidelines for conscious sedation and monitoring during gastrointestinal endoscopy. Gastrointest Endosc. 2003;58(3):317–22.

# 40. Flexible Endoscopy: Principles of Documentation

*Raphael Sun, M.D.*
*Joseph J. Cullen, M.D., F.A.C.S.*

## A. Introduction

Fiberoptic endoscopy and colonoscopy have been increasingly employed and expanded for the diagnosis and treatment of various gastrointestinal diseases. For the purposes of this chapter, we use the term endoscopy to include all forms of endoscopy including colonoscopy. The use of endoscopy has become an important development to the gastrointestinal surgeon and allows the surgeons to make their own visual observations rather than rely on the description of another physician's endoscopic findings. It is important for the gastrointestinal surgeon–endoscopist to accurately document endoscopic techniques used and findings. This chapter focuses on the pre-procedure, procedural, and post-procedure principles of documentation for endoscopic procedures.

## B. Purpose of Documentation

Providing an accurate visual and written record of findings is critically important in order to:

1. Facilitate continuity of care either within the same health system or when a patient transfers their care.
2. Demonstrate accountability. With proper documentation, records can help clarify any concerns, questions, disputes, or legal proceedings.
3. Provide quality assurance.

N.J. Soper and C.E.H. Scott-Conner (eds.), *The SAGES Manual: Volume 1 Basic Laparoscopy and Endoscopy*, DOI 10.1007/978-1-4614-2344-7_40, © Springer Science+Business Media, LLC 2012

4. Facilitate research. Procedural records can be used to track valuable data. Accurate documentation can provide accurate data for quality improvement programs or for future clinical studies.

## C. Informed Consent

Each institution has its own consent for procedure or operation. Prior to any procedure, the physician and patient must briefly discuss the procedure along with its risk, benefits, and alternatives. Informed consent is considered a process, and the signed written document (the "consent") is the documentation of that process. The most important preparation is an adequate explanation and good rapport with the patient. The written informed consent must include the following:

1. The proper patient name, physician and team members, and the procedure.
2. The nature and purpose of the procedure. This must be explained to the patient and documented on the written form in easily understandable language.
3. Any anticipated benefits, possible alternative methods of treatment, risks involved, and possible consequences and complications are explained to the patient at a level where they can fully understand.
4. Both the patient and the physician must sign the informed consent and the consent must be placed in the chart or in the electronic medical record prior to the procedure.

## D. Nursing Documentation

Excellent nursing staff can greatly facilitate the performance of endoscopic procedures. Oftentimes, these endoscopic procedures are performed with a nurse or nursing assistant in the endoscopic suite for monitoring including:

1. Monitoring the patients' vital signs
2. Assisting in the procedure
3. Administrating medications for sedation

It is important for nursing staff to develop and perform pre-procedural assessments. In addition, flow sheets are commonly used to document data including:

1.  The initiation and completion of a proper "timeout"
2.  Patient identification
3.  Administration of pre-procedural antibiotics
4.  Administration of initial and ongoing sedation medication
5.  Vital signs including assessment of adequate oxygenation during the procedure

These flow sheets that are filled out by nursing staff do not exclude the need for other documentation. These documents need to be filled out in chronological order and should be filled out as close to the actual event for increased accuracy and credibility.

# E.  Procedure Note

Similar to any operation and/or procedure note, the following must be documented in any endoscopic procedure.

1.  Pre-procedure diagnosis and post-procedure diagnosis
2.  Procedure performed
3.  Endoscopist performing the procedure
4.  Assistants to the endoscopist
5.  Anesthesia
    a.  This is an important part of documentation. Most endoscopic procedures are performed under conscious sedation. This means there is not a separate anesthesia record as many endoscopists will administer medications for conscious sedation.
    b.  Document which medications were given to the patient, including specific medication and doses, timing, and route of administration.
6.  Instruments used
    a.  Document the type of scope used.
    b.  Document any additional instruments, such as snares, forceps for biopsy, electrocautery, etc.
7.  Indications
    a.  Provide a brief explanation regarding any pertinent past medical history and the indications for the procedure.

8. Extent of examination. Document the anatomical landmarks to define which portion of the gastrointestinal tract was examined. For example, during colonoscopy it is important to document visualizing the cecum by noting the appendiceal orifice or ileo-cecal valve. For upper procedures, it is important to document the location of the lower esophageal sphincter or second and third portion of the duodenum.

9. Description of the procedure
   a. Adequate visualization during the procedure is important for completion and for documentation. Documenting an adequate prep for colonoscopy or removal of gastric blood to visualize a potential bleeding source for upper endoscopy should be clearly documented.
   b. Document which portions of the gastrointestinal tract was passed and visualized.
   c. Document any interventions, such as biopsy and location, electrocautery, ligation, insertion of PEG tube, embolization, etc.

10. Diagnostic impression

## F. Findings

It is important that the endoscopist record any findings that will allow the entire healthcare team to be informed of the patient's pathology. Accurate documentation of findings allows comparison to any previous or future studies. With advancements in technology, modern endoscopes allow recording and documenting in video or digital format which can be stored in CD, hard drives, or the hospital electronic records. Many endoscopes also have the ability to print images during the examination.

## G. Future Technology for Documentation

As noted above, modern endoscopes facilitate acquisition of still and video images for documentation. New technologies that provide an alternative to traditional flexible endoscopy present unique documentation opportunities and challenges.

1.  Capsule endoscopy
    This small ingestible camera takes images of the mucosa of the gastrointestinal tract as it passes through. The images are transmitted by radiofrequency and are captured and stored onto a computer. Currently, capsule endoscopy is mainly used to evaluate small bowel disease and has not been proven to be useful for colorectal diseases. This emerging technology will eliminate the details of documentation as the procedure is simplified and the images are directly visualized and stored.

2.  Virtual colonoscopy is an emerging technique that may prove to be useful in the future and could potentially change the principles of documentation for endoscopy.

## Selected References

http://www.csgna.com/en/guidelines/endoscopy.html from the Canadian Society of Gastroenterology Nurses and Associates.

Indman PD. Documentation in endoscopy. Obstet Gynecol Clin North Am. 1995; 22(3):605–16.

Preminger GM, Delvecchio FC, Birnbach JM. Digital image recording: an integral aspect of video endoscopy. Stud Health Technol Inform. 1999;62:268–74.

Stettin J. Electronic documentation in endoscopy: present status and future perspectives from a company standpoint. Endoscopy. 2001;33(3):276–9.

# 41. Diagnostic Upper Gastrointestinal Endoscopy

*Jarrod Wall, M.B., B.Ch., Ph.D.*
*John D. Mellinger, M.D., F.A.C.S.*

## A. Indications

1. Diagnostic upper gastrointestinal endoscopy, or esophagogas-troduodenoscopy (EGD), may be indicated for symptom evaluation, malignancy surveillance, and in several special circumstances (Table 41.1).
2. Therapeutic EGD is appropriate for acute upper gastrointestinal bleeding, foreign body ingestion, polyp removal, dilation of stenoses, placement of feeding or drainage catheters, eradication of esophageal varices, and palliative therapy of obstructing neoplasms.

## B. Patient Preparation

1. Do not permit the patient to eat or drink for 6–8 h before routine elective EGD. This minimizes aspiration risks associated with a sedated procedure and facilitates a complete and unhampered examination.
   a. Consider a **longer period of preparation** (NPO, and/or liquid diet) if gastric outlet obstruction or impaired gastric motility is anticipated.
   b. If retained ingested material, secretions, or blood are likely, consider **preprocedural gastric aspiration or lavage**.

N.J. Soper and C.E.H. Scott-Conner (eds.), *The SAGES Manual: Volume 1 Basic Laparoscopy and Endoscopy*, DOI 10.1007/978-1-4614-2344-7_41, © Springer Science+Business Media, LLC 2012

Table 41.1. Indications for EGD.

| Indication | Specific examples |
|---|---|
| Symptoms | • Dyspepsia[a] |
| | • Dysphagia |
| | • Odynophagia |
| | • Pyrosis[a] |
| | • Nausea and vomiting |
| Malignancy surveillance | • Barrett's epithelium |
| | • Gastric polyps |
| | • Familiar polyposis syndromes |
| | • Gastric ulcer |
| | • Esophageal ulcer |
| | • Marginal (postgastrectomy) ulcer |
| Other circumstances | • Occult gastrointestinal bleeding |
| | • Cirrhosis (to evaluate varices) |
| | • Malabsorption (for small intestine biopsy) |

[a] If persistent, recurrent despite medical management, or associated with other gastrointestinal symptoms or signs such as weight loss

2. **Obtain informed consent** for the procedure. This includes a discussion of specific complications as well as anticipated outcomes and their general frequency. Review alternative therapies, the information to be gained from the proposed study, and anticipated practical impact on the patient's care. If a new technique is likely to be employed, frank discussion of experience with the new method is in order.

3. Prior to performing upper gastrointestinal endoscopy, it may be necessary to manipulate a patient's chronic anticoagulation and antiplatelet agents. This will be more important in situations when therapeutic interventions are planned. If the procedure planned is low risk, as is the case in diagnostic upper endoscopy, then it is likely that anticoagulation and antiplatelet agents can be continued without interruption. Guidelines are available to help with management of anticoagulation and antiplatelet medications before and after upper endoscopy.

4. Consideration should be given to the need for antibiotic prophylaxis prior to endoscopy. Whether they are indicated or not is related to patient factors, in concert with the type of procedure planned. A useful set of consensus guidelines has been compiled by the American Society for Gastrointestinal Endoscopy.

5. Apply monitoring devices (see Chap. 49) and ensure that a secure intravenous line is in place. Use of ultrathin endoscopes (5-mm diameter), which may be passed transorally or transnasally, may facilitate performance without sedation and decrease or eliminate the need for advanced monitoring and intravenous access.

6. Have the patient **remove dentures**.

7. **Topical anesthesia** is usually employed prior to EGD. Effective topical anesthesia facilitates intubation and comfort of the otherwise neurologically intact patient (especially when sedation is not employed) and may allow a smaller amount of sedation to be used.

   a. Deliver the topical agents to the posterior pharynx by spray or gargle, rather than to the oral cavity and tongue only.

   b. Topical anesthetics take a few minutes to work. Use this time to check the endoscope (see Chap. 47) and verify that all items that might be needed (such as biopsy forceps) are available.

   c. Test the patient's gag response before attempting endoscopy. This is a good indicator of patient tolerance.

   d. Several applications of topical anesthesia may be required.

   e. Topical agents are probably of marginal importance when deeper conscious sedation is required.

# C. Performance of Diagnostic Upper Gastrointestinal Endoscopy: Normal Anatomy

1. Place the patient in the left lateral decubitus position with a pillow under the head.

2. Place a bite block between the teeth.

3. Lubricate the endoscope with water-soluble lubricant and hold it in front of the patient's mouth. The initial insertion is best done under visual guidance.

   a. Hold the endoscope in the right hand, approximately 20–30 cm from the tip.

   b. This facilitates passage through the upper esophageal sphincter without the need to release and regrasp the instrument. If the endoscope is held farther back, it may buckle.

c.   Position the endoscope in front of the mouth in such a way that a simple deflection of the large (up/down) control wheel with the thumb of the left hand moves the tip to the desired curve (inferiorly in the axis of the patient's midline).

d.   Rotate the instrument with the right hand to orient this downward deflection in the appropriate axis.

e.   Next, straighten the instrument, pass it through the bite block, and insert it to the level of the posterior pharynx.

f.   Maintain the endoscope in the midline of the pharynx, and deflect the tip inferiorly by repeating the maneuver as just rehearsed. Attention should now shift to the video monitor. The base of the tongue and epiglottis will be seen anteriorly.

g.   Advance the endoscope slowly and smoothly to minimize gagging, using torque with the right hand to accomplish right/left movements and left thumb deflections to make anterior/posterior adjustments. Visualize the laryngeal cartilages and vocal cords, and advance the scope in the midline immediately posterior to the arytenoid cartilages (Fig. 41.1).

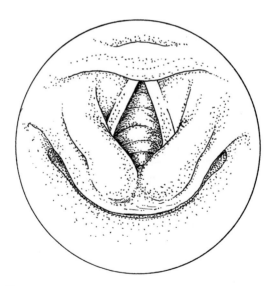

Fig. 41.1. The esophageal opening is recognized as a simple slit at the base of the triangle formed by the glottis, just behind the arytenoid cartilages. The two piriform sinuses lie on each side of the esophageal opening.

h. Passage through the upper esophageal sphincter is facilitated by having the patient swallow, which relaxes the sphincter.

   i. Often the simple presence of the instrument in this area will initiate a swallow and allow passage through the upper esophageal sphincter.

   ii. If the patient is not too deeply sedated, asking him or her to perform a swallow may achieve the same.

   iii. If gentle pressure in the appropriate midline position does not achieve the desired result, withdraw the scope and repeat the maneuver; lateral deflection into the piriform sinus area can easily occur and lead to injury if increasing pressure is applied.

i. Alternative techniques, such as placing two fingers in the patient's mouth to guide the endoscope and keep it in the midline, are especially useful for patients who are under anesthesia.

j. If an endotracheal tube is in place, it is crucial that someone hold the endotracheal tube to prevent accidental dislodgment. It may be necessary to deflate the balloon to allow the endoscope to pass.

4. Advance the endoscope slowly down the length of the esophagus, again using torque and limited deflection of the up/down control wheel to allow preservation of a luminal view at all times. Never advance the endoscope without a visible lumen (Fig. 41.2).

5. Watch for peristaltic activity, distensibility, and mucosal appearance. Measure the distance from the incisors to the squamocolumnar junction (where the white esophageal epithelium abruptly gives way to pink gastric mucosa). Identify the location of the diaphragm by asking the patient to sniff. Visible contraction of the diaphragm will produce extrinsic compression of the esophagus.

6. As soon as the endoscope enters the stomach, step back from the table and allow the instrument to assume an unrestrained, straightened posture. This is often best accomplished by completely letting go of the scope with the right hand as one steps back.

7. With the patient on the left side, this will typically orient the instrument in the stomach such that the greater curve will be at the 6 o'clock position, the lesser curve at 12 o'clock, and the anterior and posterior walls to the left and right, respectively

b                          a

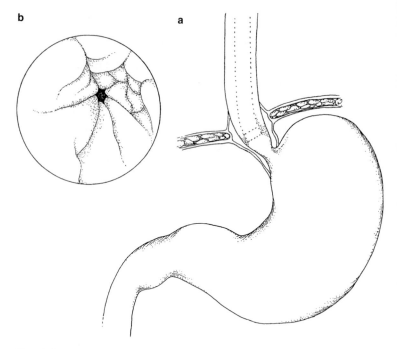

Fig. 41.2 (**a**) The endoscope is advanced down the relatively straight esophagus until the lower esophageal sphincter is identified. (**b**) The lower esophageal sphincter often coincides with the transition from squamous epithelium (*white*) of the esophagus to mucosa (*pink*) of the stomach.

(Fig. 41.3). Insufflate sufficient air to obtain a good view, and note rugal folds, peristaltic activity, and distensibility. Avoid overdistention, as this may trigger pylorospasm.

8. Continue to advance the endoscope down the length of the stomach, maintaining upward deflection of the tip in a gentle curve to preserve an antegrade view and hug the lesser curvature (Fig. 41.4).

9. Advance the endoscope to the pylorus and carefully note the pyloric channel and duodenal bulb. Often, some of the best views of the bulb are achieved prior to pyloric intubation via such an antegrade view. Make very fine maneuvers of the deflection wheels to hold the pylorus in the center of the visual field as gentle continued advancement of the scope allows it to pass into the proximal duodenum (Fig. 41.5).

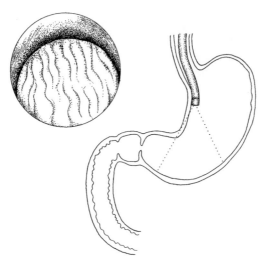

Fig. 41.3.  With the patient in the left lateral decubitus position, the endoscopist facing the patient, and the scope relaxed as described in the text, entry into the stomach will generally give a view oriented with the lesser curvature at 12 o'clock, the greater curvature at 6 o'clock, anterior at 9 o'clock, and posterior at 3 o'clock.

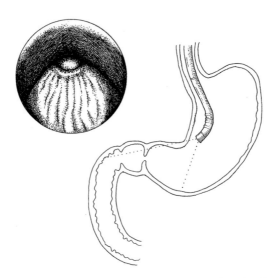

Fig. 41.4.  As the endoscope is advanced, the lumen is kept in view. A gentle upward deflection of the tip helps the endoscope hug the lesser curvature.

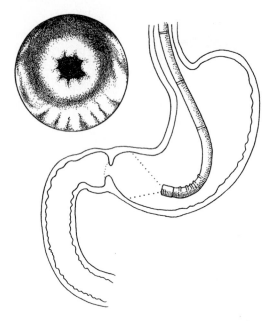

Fig. 41.5. The pylorus is viewed from the gastric antrum. The endoscope is gently advanced while keeping the pylorus directly in the center of the visual field. Sometimes the pylorus will be observed to open and close. Position the endoscope ready to pass through the pylorus when it opens.

10.  Rarely, application of a brief period of suction will allow the pylorus to be drawn over the scope if it seems unwilling to otherwise admit the same, provided the suction is applied as the tip of the scope sits immediately in front of the opening of the pyloric channel.

11.  Carefully visualize the duodenal bulb before advancing the instrument further. The posterior bulb is often the most challenging area to visualize well. Inspection of this area can be achieved by withdrawing the endoscope and using torque and fine deflections of the tip to achieve an adequate view (Fig. 41.6).

12.  Advance the endoscope as far into the second portion of the duodenum as luminal visualization permits (Fig. 41.7).

  a.  In some cases, full introduction into the second and third portion of the duodenum is easily achieved in this fashion.

  b.  More commonly, the posterior sweep of the duodenum requires some further maneuvering. In such settings, the

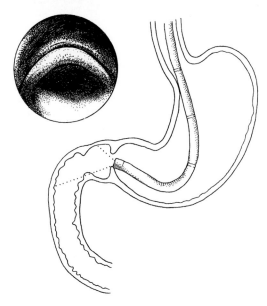

Fig. 41.6.   The duodenal bulb lacks folds. At the distal and superior aspect is the superior duodenal fold, which marks the entrance to the second portion of the duodenum.

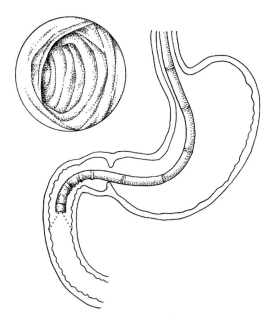

Fig. 41.7.   The second portion of the duodenum is recognized by its concentric semicircular folds.

luminal view is lost as the duodenum turns posteriorly near the junction of its first and second portions.

c.  Deflect the tip of the instrument slightly upward with the left thumb on the larger control wheel and simultaneously rotate the left wrist 90° clockwise. This is best accomplished with the right hand completely off the endoscope.

d.  Next, pull back on the endoscope to straighten it and achieve further advancement of the tip. This "paradoxic motion" occurs as the instrument moves from the looped, greater curvature position in the stomach (which usually follows initial antegrade intubation), to a lesser curve or "short stick" position.

e.  Further antegrade intubation can also be accomplished after this maneuver, if deeper duodenal entry is desired.

13. As the endoscope is withdrawn, carefully inspect all areas.

14. Position the endoscope with its tip in the gastric antrum and retroflex it.

a.  Deflect the tip of the instrument upward, using the left thumb on the larger control wheel, while simultaneously rotating the left wrist 90° counterclockwise. Frequently an "owl's eye" view of both pylorus and cardia may be seen as the tip crosses the incisura to look directly back at the cardia (Fig. 41.8).

b.  This maneuver is easily accomplished with the right hand off the endoscope.

c.  Manipulate the endoscope with the right hand (torque, advancement, withdrawal) to obtain optimal visualization of the incisura, cardia, fundus, and remaining proximal stomach. Grasp the endoscope 10–20 cm from the patient's mouth to allow a wide range of movements to be done with fluid motions.

d.  Often the "gastric lake" of dependent fundic fluid is seen from this vantage point, and should be suctioned to allow complete inspection. Suction of fluid is most efficient when the meniscus of the fluid surface is oriented transversely across the endoscopic field of visualization. In this position, the suction port (at 6 o'clock in the visual field) is located completely under the fluid, while a luminal view is preserved above the same. Short bursts of suction at a lower setting minimize capturing of the gastric mucosa in the port, which requires repositioning before continuing

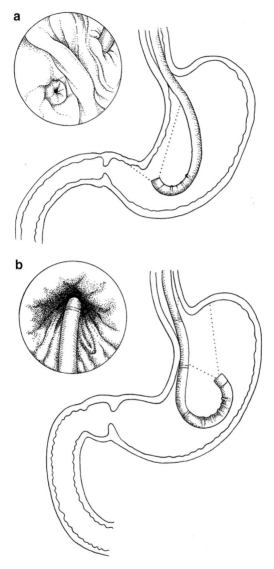

Fig. 41.8. Retroflex the endoscope to visualize the cardia. (a) Perform this maneuver by deflecting the tip sharply back. An owl's eye view of both pylorus and cardia may be seen as the tip crosses over the incisura. (b) As the cardia is identified, move the tip in a circular manner to inspect the entire cardia. Pull the endoscope back to bring the tip (now sharply retroflexed) closer to the area of interest.

the suction process. By proceeding in this fashion, fluid evacuation can be accomplished efficiently while continuing dynamic inspection of the lumen.

15. Return the endoscope to its normal (straight, antegrade) position and gradually remove it, reinspecting all areas as the instrument is removed.

16. Suction excess air after the stomach is reinspected during withdrawal. Carefully inspect the esophagus, hypopharynx, and larynx during removal.

## D. The Postoperative Stomach

The postoperative stomach offers some special challenges worthy of brief mention. Foregut disease states, which may prompt surgical intervention and the associated anatomic changes, are listed in Table 41.2. As a general rule, the endoscopist does not need to change the technique of the examination because of these alterations, other than being sensitive to, and able to recognize and identify specific problems related to, their presence. Preendoscopic review of prior operative reports or contrast studies can be invaluable, particularly in patients with multiple previous operations.

Table 41.2.   Anatomic alterations associated with specific surgical interventions.

| Disease category | Anatomic changes | Surgical procedures |
|---|---|---|
| Gastroesophageal reflux | • Augmentation of the cardia | • Fundoplication |
| Peptic ulcer disease | • Gastric outlet alteration<br>• Partial absence of stomach | • Pyloroplasty<br>• Gastroduodenostomy<br>• Gastrojejunostomy<br>• Antrectomy with Billroth I, Billroth II, or Roux-en-Y reconstruction |
| Neoplasia | • Partial or complete absence of stomach | • Subtotal or total gastrectomy, varying reconstructions |
| Morbid obesity | • Gastric partitioning<br>• Gastric bypass | • Vertical banded gastroplasty<br>• Gastric bypass |

A few additional techniques assist the endoscopist in these special situations. These techniques, in conjunction with a sound understanding of anatomy and the basic maneuvers described in Sect. C, will enable the endoscopist to conduct the postoperative exam with the same facility as in the normal anatomic setting. When difficulty is encountered or anticipated, consider one or more of these special techniques:

1.  **Longer but small caliber instruments**, such as a pediatric colonoscope, are useful for accessing the jejunal limbs after gastrojejunostomy (Fig. 41.9).
2.  A **side-viewing duodenoscope** may facilitate visualization of the proximal stomach when a small, surgically reduced pouch precludes normal retroflexion.
3.  **Vital staining** or other special tests are used to visualize subtle mucosal changes (Lugol's solution, methylene blue), or to monitor posvagotomy parietal cell function (pH indicators).
4.  Change the **position of the patient** to avoid retained material (bezoars), or to place the area being intubated in a more dependent location.

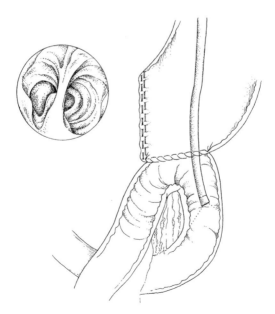

Fig. 41.9.  A pediatric colonoscope facilitates intubation of the jejunal limbs, particularly the afferent limb, after gastrojejunostomy.

# E.  Tissue-Sampling Techniques

**Biopsy and brushing techniques** are an important adjunct to endoscopic visualization in the conduct of upper gastrointestinal endoscopy. Brush cytology, forceps biopsy, large-particle biopsy, and chromoscopic techniques enhance the diagnostic yield beyond that provided by endoscopic inspection alone.

**Cytology** is particularly useful in the evaluation of fungal and viral infections of the foregut and is also an acceptable way to evaluate for *Helicobacter pylori* infection. It can add 10% to the diagnostic yield of biopsy alone in the evaluation of upper gastrointestinal malignancy. Brush cytology for malignancy is 85–90% sensitive and close to 100% specific in the foregut setting. In touch cytology, a standard biopsy sample is processed by rolling it on a slide and then fixing and staining the same for cytologic review. This technique has been shown to be a useful adjunct to biopsy alone when evaluating for infectious organisms including *Candida*, *Helicobacter*, and *Giardia*.

**Standard biopsy** techniques offer high diagnostic yields for a number of foregut pathologies, provided the disease is manifested at the mucosal level. Appropriate targeting of the tissue being sampled can be important in optimizing diagnostic yield. In the setting of evaluation for *H. pylori*, it has been shown that diagnostic yields are comparable from all areas of the stomach, and virtually all infected patients can be identified by a combination of three biopsy samples, obtained from the prepyloric antrum, lesser curve near the incisura, and greater curve body. With malignant ulcers, yields are highest with multiple biopsies (7–10), obtained from the rim of the ulcer as well as its base. Such approaches, particularly when combined with brush cytology and salvage cytology of material retained in the endoscope biopsy channel following forceps biopsy, allow documented diagnostic accuracies of 100% with malignant gastric ulcers.

1.  Perform **brush cytology** by passing a sheathed brush through the endoscope biopsy channel.

    a.  Position the sheath adjacent to the area to be sampled and extend the brush.

    b.  Vigorously move the sheath–brush complex to and fro across the area being evaluated. This dislodges cells onto the brush.

    c.  Retract the brush back into the sheath to prevent sample loss while the sheath is being withdrawn through the endoscope biopsy channel.

    d.   The material obtained is then processed onto slides for cytologic evaluation.

    e.   Washing the brush itself in balanced salt solution may allow recovery of additional material for pathology review.

2.  **Forceps biopsy** provides sufficient tissue (generally limited to the mucosa) for histologic examination. Several kinds of biopsy forceps are available, and it is important to choose the proper type for the intended purpose.

    a.   **Spiked forceps** have a tiny needle like projection between the jaws of the forceps to facilitate obtaining multiple samples on a single pass of the forceps. The endoscopist's ability to grasp tissue that is oriented tangentially to the endoscope may be enhanced by helping the forceps to firmly engage the tissue to be sampled.

    b.   **Large cupped forceps**, or jumbo forceps as they are often called, require a therapeutic-size endoscope with a 3.7-mm biopsy channel. These instruments typically provide a larger mucosal specimen but do not usually allow submucosal sampling.

3.  **Endoscopic mucosal resection** is sometimes useful when larger areas of mucosa are to be sampled or excised. This allows more complete removal of areas of suspicious mucosal pathology. It is particularly applicable in the setting of early gastric cancer, where it is used in concert with endoscopic ultrasound evaluation.

    a.   **Inject saline** underneath the target lesion to elevate the mucosa and produce an easier target to snare. Hypertonic saline prolongs the effect.

    b.   Resect the target lesion with a **standard snare technique**.

    c.   The technique may be modified by using two small-caliber endoscopes simultaneously. This allows the first endoscope to provide forceps traction after injection, while the second endoscope applies the snare around the base of the lesion.

    d.   Another modification utilizes a single cap-fitted endoscope capable of applying suction to the tissue, which is snared after being drawn into the cap.

4.  **Large-particle biopsy** allows submucosal tissue sampling in the setting of infiltrative submucosal pathology not amenable to standard mucosal biopsy techniques. The risk of perforation is higher with such techniques, and other alternatives for submucosal evaluation and sampling are becoming available via endoscopic ultrasound (see Sect. F).

a. Use a **therapeutic, two-channel endoscope**. Pass a snare down one channel and a biopsy forceps down the second.

b. **Open the snare** and place it over the area to be sampled.

c. **Pass the biopsy forceps** through the snare. Pick up and elevate both mucosa and submucosa, thus allowing the snare to incorporate a deeper level of tissue than would otherwise be possible.

5. **Chromoscopic techniques** are briefly mentioned because of their particular utility in the postoperative setting. Probably underutilized in the USA, chromoscopy can be employed along with magnification video endoscopy to enhance detection of neoplastic and preneoplastic mucosal abnormalities.

a. **Lugol's solution** (typically 20 mL of a 1–2% solution applied directly via an endoscopic catheter) stains glycogen-containing tissue, which is present in normal esophageal squamous mucosa. Areas of intestinal metaplasia, carcinoma, and inflammation stain negatively with this agent and may thus be more apparent for biopsy sampling after its application.

b. **Methylene blue** is usually applied as a 0.5–1% solution in similar volume following application of a mucolytic agent and is taken up selectively by absorptive epithelium, such as intestinal metaplasia.

# F. Endoscopic Ultrasound

Endoscopic ultrasound (EUS) is an area of expanding significance in diagnostic upper gastrointestinal endoscopy. Current **areas of application** include the diagnosis and staging of upper aerodigestive tract neoplasia, diagnosis of submucosal pathology, and diagnosis of choledocholithiasis. A specially designed endoscope is required.

EUS-guided **fine-needle aspiration cytology** offers great promise in adding to the diagnostic potential of this modality and may make it a diagnostic procedure of choice in the setting of esophageal, gastric, pancreatic, and even pulmonary neoplasia. Its staging potential in these settings, particularly in view of this tissue-sampling capability, is increasingly being shown to be superior to radiologic methods such as computed tomography. EUS is also showing promise in the diagnosis and monitoring of submucosal pathology such as stromal and neuroendocrine lesions, and varices.

With continuing technologic improvements, including the availability of instruments capable of combined luminal visualization and EUS, through the scope's high-frequency/high-resolution probes, Doppler capability, therapeutic echoendoscopes with elevator-equipped biopsy channels, and improved tissue-sampling instrumentation, EUS is poised for increasing importance and utilization in the years ahead. Factors that may limit its application include instrument cost, a steep learning curve required for meaningful interpretation (50–100 cases), and the need for further studies documenting significant and cost-effective changes in patient management based on its use. References in Section give further information on this emerging diagnostic tool.

## Selected References

Cooper GS. Indications and contraindications for upper gastrointestinal endoscopy. Gastrointest Endosc Clin North Am. 1994;4:439–54.

Hirota WK, Peterson K, Baron T, Goldstein JL, Jacobson BC, Leighton JA, Mallery JS, Waring JP, Fanelli JD, Wheeler-Harbough J, Faigel DO. Standard of practice committee of the American society for gastrointestinal endoscopy. Gastrointest Endosc. 2003;58:475–82.

Jane PK. Technique of upper gastrointestinal endoscopy. Gastrointest Endosc Clin North Am. 1994;4:501–21.

Kwok A, Faigel DO. Management of anticoagulation before and after gastrointestinal endoscopy. Am J Gastroenterol. 2009;104:3085–97.

Lightdale CJ (ed.) Advances in endoscopic ultrasound. Gastrointest Endosc 2002;56: S1–97

Mellinger JD, Ponsky JL. Endoscopic evaluation of the postoperative stomach. Gastrointest Endosc Clin North Am. 1996;6:621–39.

Van Dam J, Brugge WR. Endoscopy of the upper gastrointestinal tract. N Engl J Med. 1999;341:1738–48.

Van Dam J, Chak A, Sivak MV. Technique of upper gastrointestinal endoscopy. In: Sivak MV, editor. Gastroenterologic endoscopy. 2nd ed. Philadelphia: WB Saunders; 2000.

Zaman A, Hahn M, Hapke R, Knigge K, Fennerty MB, Katon RM. A randomized trial of peroral versus transnasal unsedated endoscopy using an ultrathin videoendoscope. Gastrointest Endosc. 1999;49:279–84.

# 42. Percutaneous Endoscopic Feeding Tube Placement

*Melissa S. Phillips, M.D.*
*Bipan Chand, M.D., F.A.C.S.*
*Jeffrey L. Ponsky, M.D., F.A.C.S.*

## A. Indications

Adequate nutrition has been shown to improve wound healing, decrease complications, and lower overall mortality following surgery. Nutrition provided as enteral alimentation is safer and more cost-effective than parenteral nutrition in patients with a functioning gastrointestinal tract. Enteral nutrition results in less infectious complications and may offer immune and metabolic related advantages. Gastrostomy placement is the most common way to gain enteral access and is indicated as a route for enteral feedings in patients with functioning gastrointestinal tracts who are unable to take adequate oral nutrition. Neurologic diseases, including cerebrovascular events, severe dementia, progressive neurological processes, and severe psychomotor retardation constitute the most frequent indication for gastrostomy tube placement. Neoplastic processes of the head, neck, and esophagus may require feeding tube placement secondary to dysphagia from their primary lesion or to maintain adequate nutrition during chemotherapy treatment. Patients with multisystem trauma or severe facial trauma may also be candidates for gastrostomy tube placement. An alternative indication for gastrostomy tube placement is decompression of the GI tract, such as in patients with obstruction from unresectable malignancies, carcinomatosis, or severe radiation enteritis.

When enteral access is being used for nutrition, patients should demonstrate a potential for extended survival, usually accepted as greater than 4 weeks life expectancy with nutritional support. Critically ill

N.J. Soper and C.E.H. Scott-Conner (eds.), *The SAGES Manual: Volume 1
Basic Laparoscopy and Endoscopy*, DOI 10.1007/978-1-4614-2344-7_42,
© Springer Science+Business Media, LLC 2012

patients with a low probability of survival are not appropriate candidates for percutaneous endoscopic gastrostomy (PEG) or other invasive methods of feeding tube placement. If a patient's clinical status is uncertain, nutritional support should be started though a nasoenteric feeding tube and continued until it is likely that the patient will tolerate an invasive procedure and demonstrates a potential for extended survival.

A nonfunctioning GI tract (with the exception of PEG placement for decompression) or the presence of peritonitis are absolute contraindications for PEG placement. Relative contraindications to gastrostomy tube placement include massive ascites, severe malnutrition that would prevent mature formation of the gastrocutaneous tract, and overall clinical decompensation including fever of unknown etiology or sepsis. Patients with psychologically based eating disorders, such as anorexia nervosa, must be fully evaluated including an ethics consult before undertaking permanent access. Specific consideration must be given to patients with coagulopathy, morbid obesity, previous abdominal surgeries, hiatal hernia, and a history of peritoneal dialysis. Many of these relative contraindications can be overcome, allowing for successful placement of percutaneous enteral access.

There are multiple methods for placing enteral access tubes. Broad categories may be created based on the discipline performing the procedure. These are divided primarily into surgical approaches, including both open and laparoscopic techniques, and percutaneous endoscopic approaches. Each approach has advantages and disadvantages that are detailed below (Table 42.1). This chapter focuses on the endoscopic pathways most frequently employed by the surgeon for enteral access. When considering gastrostomy placement, two methods of PEG placement are commonly used. These include the oral introduction ("pull" or "push" approach) and the abdominal wall introduction ("introducer" approach) of the gastrostomy tube. The placement of jejunal access for feeding tubes is also discussed in Section D.

# B. The Oral Insertion Technique for PEG Placement

The oral insertion technique is the most common approach for endoscopic gastrostomy tube placement. Variations on this approach include the "pull" and "push" method of placement. Multiple commercially prepared kits are available for the oral introduction method. Two trained

Table 42.1. Advantages and disadvantages of methods of gastrostomy formation.

| Method | Advantages | Disadvantages |
|---|---|---|
| Surgical gastrostomy | • Secure fixation of stomach to anterior abdominal wall<br>• Permanent tract may be created | • Requires laparotomy<br>• May require general anesthesia |
| Laparoscopic gastrostomy | • Less invasive<br>• May achieve secure fixation of stomach to abdominal wall<br>• Visual selection of site of entry onto the stomach | • Requires laparoscopic access<br>• Requires general anesthesia |
| PEG | • May be performed under local anesthesia<br>• May be done in the endoscopy suite<br>• Single puncture, no incision | • Requires patent upper gastrointestinal tract<br>• Early dislodgement of tube may require laparotomy<br>• Potential for injury to adjacent viscera unless technique carefully followed |

individuals are needed for this approach: one to perform the endoscopy and the other to perform the PEG insertion.

Insertion of an orally introduced "pull" PEG:

1. Keep the patient fasting for 8 h.
2. Obtain intravenous access for the administration of sedation and systemic pain relief. All patients must have appropriate monitoring during this sedation, including blood pressure monitoring and pulse oximetry. Dedicated capnography may be available in many endoscopy units. A dedicated member of the team should monitor for adverse events and be able to provide rescue measures if required. Intravenous antibiotics, aimed at coverage of skin flora, should be administered within 1 h of the procedure to decrease the associated wound infection rate.
3. Place the patient supine on the endoscopy table.
4. Prepare the upper abdomen by clipping hair and prepping with chlorhexidine.
5. Topical anesthesia of the oropharynx may be supplemented with intravenous sedation although this may increase the risk for aspiration in the supine position. Local anesthesia will be infiltrated at the PEG site.
6. After adequate sedation, introduce the endoscope into the stomach. Perform a full upper endoscopy to evaluate for pathology

and rule out gastric outlet obstruction. The stomach is then fully insufflated.

7. The anterior abdominal wall is then examined for evidence of transillumination which indicates that the inflated stomach is closely apposed to the anterior abdominal wall without intervening viscera. It may be necessary to turn off the room lights and use the X-illumination function of the videoendoscope to see this. The initial site chosen should be between the greater and the lesser curve of the stomach (to avoid major vasculature) and between the junction of the body and stomach. Avoid the costal margin to prevent pain.

8. Gently depress the abdominal wall with one finger. The endoscopist should see the wall indent in a one-to-one fashion with palpation of the abdominal wall (Fig. 42.1). This maneuver allows for ideal communication between the endoscopist and the individual performing the abdominal access.

9. The "safe-tract" method is then used to confirm that no intervening organs, specifically loops of bowel, are between the stomach and the anterior abdominal wall (Fig. 42.2). Pass a small-caliber needle attached to a syringe filled with local anesthetic through the abdominal way while negative pressure is applied to the plunger. The endoscopist should see the needle enter the stomach at the same instance the assistant sees air within the syringe. If air is seen before the needle is visualized in the gastric lumen, the needle has passed through another organ, likely the colon. Once confirmation that no other hollow viscus is between the stomach and abdominal wall, the selected site is infiltrated with local anesthesia. The authors believe the "safe-tract" technique, above transillumination and direct palpation, to be the most reliable method for identifying the best site for introduction.

10. Make a skin incision, generally around 1 cm in length, using a #11-blade. A larger incision appears to decrease the incidence of infection around the tube site, allowing efflux of bacteria that were introduced during the passage of the gastrostomy through the oropharynx.

11. The endoscopist should position an open snare against the anterior stomach wall at the expected entry site. The needle–catheter combination is then introduced through the anterior abdominal wall and into the stomach. The snare is then used to grasp the catheter and subsequently the wire.

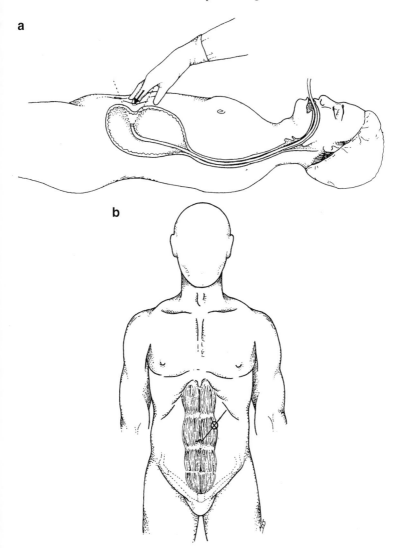

Fig. 42.1. (**a**) Transillumination and finger depression of the abdominal wall confirm juxtaposition of the inflated stomach and the anterior abdominal wall. (**b**) The site selected will generally be approximately halfway between costal margin and umbilicus.

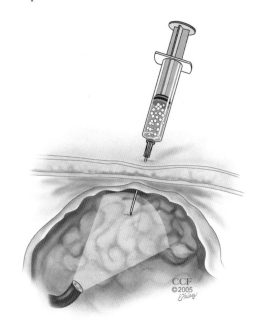

Fig. 42.2. The "safe-tract" technique is used to confirm intragastric location by insertion of a small syringe through the anterior abdominal wall while visualizing this endoscopically. If air is seen in the syringe before the needle is seen in the lumen, the endoscopist must be concerned about intervening viscera. (Reprinted with permission, Cleveland Clinic Center for Medical Art & Photography (C) 2005–2001. All Rights Reserved).

12. In the "pull" technique, the looped guide wire is passed by the assistant through the catheter on the abdominal wall and the endoscopist uses the snare to grasp the wire. The endoscopist then withdraws the endoscope, snare, and guide wire through the patient's mouth (Fig. 42.3). Care must be taken to avoid pulling the guide wire through the abdominal wall, and loosing access to the stomach.

13. The PEG tube contains an all-in-one apparatus that has a long flexible tube with internal bumper and a short stiff dilating end attached to a small prelooped wire. By passing the loop of the PEG through the looped guide wire, the PEG tube is secured outside the patient's mouth. Water-soluble lubricant is applied

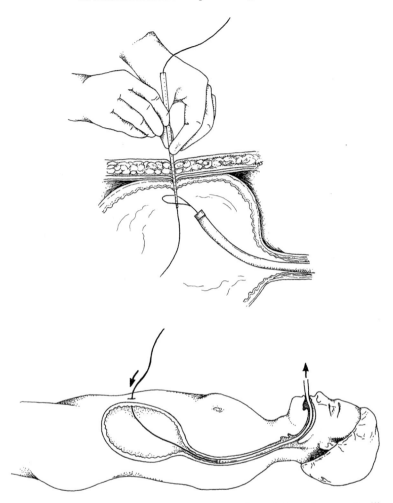

Fig. 42.3.   The guide wire is grasped using a snare through the endoscope. It will then be withdrawn through the esophagus and out the mouth.

to the stiff short dilating end to facilitate passage. The endoscopist may use the snare to hold the flange of the PEG, allowing the endoscope to follow the PEG into the stomach. Reinsertion of the endoscope allows one to assess the gastrostomy site for hemostasis and ideal length of the tube in relationship to the subcutaneous tissue; however, studies have not shown this to be an absolute requirement when performing the procedure.

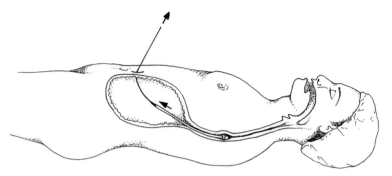

Fig. 42.4. The PEG tube is pulled back into the stomach and the endoscope reintroduced.

14. Apply gentle pressure to the abdominal side of the guide wire, advancing the tapered PEG tube and endoscope to enter the mouth and then the esophagus (Fig. 42.4). If the endoscope is being reintroduced, when the endoscope reaches the 30-cm mark, discontinue the pressure and open the snare to release the flange. Remove the snare. Use gentle traction on the guide wire to advance the PEG into the body of the stomach under direct endoscopic visualization.

15. After the tapered portion has exited the anterior abdominal wall, the flexible portion of PEG will be seen. Use gentle pressure to confirm that the internal bumper of the PEG tube is engaged on the stomach wall. Avoid overt traction of the tube (and more importantly the bumper) against the anterior portion of the abdominal stomach so as to prevent a "buried bumper" syndrome.

16. The endoscopist, having followed the PEG into the stomach, visualizes the entry site and confirms hemostasis. Visual confirmation of adequate position of the external bumper, which should be snug but not tight against the gastric wall, is the final maneuver prior to securing the catheter (Fig. 42.5).

The "push" technique is very similar to the technique described above with one main exception. Instead of "pulling" the guide wire to advance the orally introduced PEG, both ends of a nonlooped guide wire are held under tension and the PEG is advanced or "pushed" over that wire from the mouth side until the PEG exits the abdominal wall.

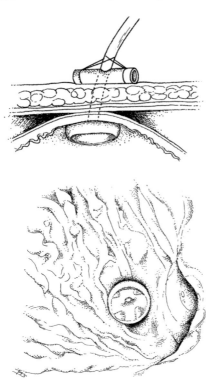

Fig. 42.5. The position of the bumper can be verified endoscopically. The bumper should be snug but not tight against the gastric wall.

## C. The Abdominal Wall Introducer Technique for PEG Placement

In some patients, the ability to introduce the PEG orally may be limited, such as those with a near obstructing oropharyngeal cancer or severe benign esophageal stricture. In these patients, introduction of the PEG through the abdominal wall has the advantage of avoiding these obstructions. This approach may also decrease seeding of aerodigestive malignancies to the anterior abdominal wall. The "introducer" method utilizes the Seldinger technique to place a balloon-tip catheter in the stomach under endoscopic guidance. This approach is less common than the oral introduction methods but is advantageous in that it requires only a single passage of the endoscope, and the endoscope can be of a much smaller diameter to allow ease of passage. Disadvantages include dislodgment of the tube if the balloon is inadvertently deflated and smaller diameter tubes in commercially available kits.

Insertion of an "introducer" technique PEG:

1.  Prepare the patient as above. Use transillumination, finger indentation, and most importantly the "safe-tract" technique to obtain proper location as described in Section B, items 1–7.
2.  Make a skin incision 4 mm in diameter using #11-blade.
3.  Under endoscopic visualization, pass the needle–catheter combination through the anterior abdominal wall into the gastric lumen and advance a guide wire into the stomach. Remove the needle.
4.  Using Seldinger technique, pass the dilator and then the introducer sheath over the guide wire. This is facilitated by a twisting motion and firm but gentle pressure.
5.  Endoscopic visualization of this entire process is essential to assuring the safety of this approach. If the dilator or sheath has difficulty with entry and tents the mucosa of the stomach rather than entering smoothly, the endoscopist can apply counterpressure with the closed tip of a biopsy forceps or increase the insufflation of the stomach to facilitate entry.
6.  Once the sheath as entered the stomach, test the balloon tip of the catheter to assure patency. After lubrication with water-soluble lubricant, the balloon-tipped gastrostomy tube is introduced through the sheath into the stomach.
7.  The sheath is peeled away and the balloon tip is inflated with saline. The tube is then secured with the balloon just touching the gastric wall to allow for mature tract formation.

## D.  Endoscopic Placement of Jejunal Feeding Tubes

Patients with certain conditions may benefit from feeding jejunostomy tubes rather than gastrostomy tubes. These include the need for long-term enteral support with one of the following: gastric dysmotility with paresis or pulmonary aspiration, severe gastric reflux, or prior gastric resections precluding the placement of a PEG. Small-caliber feeding tubes may be placed through the pylorus under endoscopic or fluoroscopic guidance. This tube may be a nasoenteric tube for short-term access or a jejunal extension tube placed adjacent to or through a previously placed PEG. Periprocedural fluoroscopy may supplement the placement of jejunal feeding tubes.

For placement of a jejunal extension through or adjacent to a preexisting PEG:

1. With the patient in the lateral decubitus position, advance the endoscope into the stomach and perform a full upper endoscopy to rule out gastric outlet obstruction or duodenal problems.

2. Pass the jejunal extension through or beside the PEG tube under endoscopic visualization. The distal end of the tube should have a suture, which is grasped using the working channel of the endoscope.

3. Advance the endoscope, thus delivering the feeding tube through the pylorus under direct vision. Advance the endoscope and feeding tube as far as possible into the small bowel.

4. Clip the suture to the wall of the small bowel using a commercially available endoscopic clip. The purpose of this is to prevent dislodgement upon removal of the endoscope. The clip will release and migrate over the next week or two.

5. Withdraw the endoscope into the stomach, taking care not to dislodge the jejunal extension.

For placement of a nasoenteric feeding tube:

1. Introduce a standard endoscope through the mouth and a complete upper endoscopy is performed. Advance the gastroscope into the small bowel as far as possible.

2. Advance a nasoenteric feeding tube with manufacturer-placed guide wire through the working channel of the gastroscope into the small bowel.

3. Advance the feeding tube–guide wire combination as the scope is withdrawn through the mouth, keeping the tip of the wire in a static position (this can be monitored by fluoroscopy).

4. Once the scope has been removed completely, a soft plastic tube (available in the kit) is passed nasally and exits through the mouth. The nasoenteric tube is passed in a retrograde fashion through this tube, allowing the nasoenteric tube to exit through the nare.

5. Fluoroscopy can be used to confirm placement. Once placement is confirmed, remove the guide wire from the nasoenteric tube and secure the tube in place.

The direct percutaneous endoscopic jejunostomy (DPEJ) is another method of placing a feeding jejunal tube. This method has been shown to reduce gastrointestinal reflux related aspiration although there is no difference in aspiration of oropharyngeal secretions. Disadvantages of DPEJ are higher rates of bleeding, leakage, and inadvertent visceral injury. Placement is similar to the oral introduction technique of a pull PEG described in Section B with a few exceptions.

1. Use a longer endoscope, such as a pediatric colonoscope, to assure passage beyond the Ligament of Trietz into the small bowel for placement.
2. Fluoroscopy should be available to help with localization of the chosen loop of small bowel, often in the early or midjejunum. As the most challenging aspect of a DPEJ is the identification of the small bowel site, the use of transillumination and one-to-one palpation visualized endoscopically may aid with the fluoroscopic identification.
3. Once the site has been identified, the "safe-tract" technique (described in Section B, number 9) is a critical and mandatory part of avoiding unintended viscus injury.
4. After the DPEJ has been introduced, it is important to confirm appropriate positioning of the internal bumper using endoscopic visualization. Water-soluble contrast may also be injected through the DPEJ to confirm placement in the small bowel.

# E. Complications of Percutaneous Feeding Tube Placement

Overall, endoscopically placed feeding tubes are safe, effective ways to provide enteral nutrition. Not unlike other procedures, however, these procedures do carry an associated risk. Dislodgement of the tube is a feared complication, as most endoscopically placed tubes are not secured to the anterior abdominal wall. Although not routine in the author's practice, the use of T-fasteners during the original procedure (see Chap. 26) may help secure the gastric wall to the anterior abdominal wall if inadvertent early tube dislodgement occurs. In the early postprocedural period, this may lead to spillage of gastric contents and require laparotomy for repair. In patients with a reliable abdominal exam and no evidence of peritonitis, conservative management can be attempted with nasogastric decompression, bowel rest, and broad spectrum antibiotics.

If successful, a repeat PEG can be placed 5–7 days later. Any patient with increasing abdominal pain, signs of an acute abdomen, or clinical decompensation require immediate laparotomy. In patients with a mature tract, such as those with a tube in place for more than 2 weeks, the tube may be reinserted and a water-soluble contrast study can be used to confirm intragastric placement before use.

Clogging of the tube is a common complication and is associated with smaller diameter tubes and medication administration. Prevention, through routine water flushes, is the best treatment. Soda or commercially available enzymatic treatments may be required to restore patency of the lumen. In worst case scenarios, a clogged tube may require removal and replacement using the guidelines above.

Superficial wound problems, most commonly leaking around the tube, are not unusual after endoscopic feeding tube placement. These are best treated by minimizing mobility and ensuring lack of tension on the feeding tube as well as cleaning the area with soap and water. True wound infections, such as peritubal abscesses, are rare and require incision and drainage. Fungal infections are treated with topical antifungal medications.

Benign pneumoperitoneum may be present in up to 20% of patients undergoing feeding tube placement, but can be managed conservatively if the patient has a benign clinical examination without abdominal pain, fever, leukocytosis, or peritonitis. Neoplastic seeding of aerodigestive malignancies has been described but is infrequent and the abdominal wall introducer method attempts to avoid this. Other rare complications include esophageal perforations, unintentional visceral injury, hemorrhage, and aspiration can be reduced by good technique.

# F.  Summary

Percutaneous access is a safe and reliable way to provide enteral nutrition to patients, decreasing the risk of infectious complications and improving overall mortality. Indications for endoscopic feeding access include neurologic disease, trauma, neoplastic processes, and decompression for unresectable obstruction. Endoscopic options involve the oral introduction technique, including "push" and "pull" approaches, and the abdominal wall introducer technique. Safety should be assessed during placement using transillumination, one-to-one palpation, and the "safe-tract" method. Jejunal access, either as an extension through a PEG or as direct access to the small bowel offer additional treatment options in patients with poor gastric emptying. The complication profile includes tube dislodgement, wound problems, clogging of the tube, pneumoperitneum, and rare instances of inadvertent visceral injury. Having a broad knowledge of the endoscopic and surgical treatment options available allows the surgeon to choose the tailor the technique to fit the specific needs of his or her patient.

## Selected References

Eisen GM, Baron TH, Dominitz JA, et al. American society for gastrointestinal endoscopy: role of endoscopy in enteral feeding. Gastrointest Endosc. 2002a;55(7):794–7.

Eisen GM, Baron TH, Dominitz JA, et al. American society for gastrointestinal endoscopy: complications in upper GI endoscopy. Gastrointest Endosc. 2002b;55(7):784–93.

Gauderer MWL, Ponsky JL, Izant R. Gastrostomy without laparotomy: a percutaneous endoscopic technique. J Pediatr Surg. 1980;15:872–5.

Herman LL, Hoskins WJ, Shike M. Percutaneous endoscopic gastrostomy for decompression of the stomach and small bowel. Gastrointest Endosc. 1992;38:314–8.

Ljungdahl M, Sundbom M. Complication rate lower after percutaneous endoscopic gastrostomy than after surgical gastrostomy: a prospective, randomized trial. Surg Endosc. 2006;20:1248–51.

MacFadyen Jr BV, Catalano MF, Raijman I, et al. Percutaneous endoscopic gastrostomy with jejunal extension: a new technique. Am J Gastroenterol. 1992;87:725–8.

Ponsky JL, Aszodi A. Percutaneous endoscopic jejunostomy. Am J Gastroenterol. 1984;79:113–6.

Ponsky JL, Gauderer MWL. Percutaneous endoscopic gastrostomy: a nonoperative technique for feeding gastrostomy. Gastrointest Endosc. 1981;27:9–11.

Russell T, Brotman M, Norris F. Percutaneous endoscopic gastrostomy: a new simplified and cost effective technique. Amer J Surg. 1984;148:132–7.

Shike M, Latkany L. Direct percutaneous endoscopic jejunostomy. Gastrointest Endosc Clin N Am. 1998;8:569–80.

Stellato TA, Gauderer MWL, Ponsky JL. Percutaneous endoscopic gastrostomy following previous abdominal surgery. Ann Surg. 1984;200:46–50.

Zopf Y, Rabe C, Bruckmoser T, et al. Percutaneous endoscopic jejunostomy and jejunal extension tube through percutaneous endoscopic gastrostomy: a retrospective analysis of success, complications and outcome. Digestion. 2009;79:92–7.

# 43. Capsule Enteroscopy

*Jeremy A. Warren, M.D.*
*Bruce V. MacFadyen Jr., M.D., F.A.C.S.*

## A. Background

Evaluation of the small intestine is difficult. Standard endoscopic techniques have very limited ability to assess the small bowel and radiographic techniques have low diagnostic yield for most diseases in the small intestine. Since its introduction in 2000, capsule endoscopy (CE) has rapidly become an important diagnostic step in the evaluation of patients with a variety of small bowel pathology. More than a million capsule endoscopies have been performed worldwide, with over a thousand publications on the subject. Though primarily used for identification of obscure gastrointestinal bleeding (OGIB), indications have continued to expand for the diagnosis of a variety of pathologic entities in the small bowel as well as the esophagus and colon and even bladder.

## B. Device

1. Multiple devices are now on the market, including PillCam SB, ESO, and COLON 2 (Given Imaging), MicroCam (Intromedic), EndoCapsule (Olympus), and OMOM (Jinshan Science & Technology Co.) with specific designs targeting small bowel evaluation, esophagoscopy and colon imaging, and variations in imaging technology and data transmission.
2. Typical size: $11 \times 26$ mm, weighing 4–6 g.
3. Powered by two silver oxide batteries.

N.J. Soper and C.E.H. Scott-Conner (eds.), *The SAGES Manual: Volume 1 Basic Laparoscopy and Endoscopy*, DOI 10.1007/978-1-4614-2344-7_43,
© Springer Science+Business Media, LLC 2012

4.  Small bowel is illuminated by light emitting diodes. Newest generation capsules feature auto-brightness similar to standard endoscopes, auto or manual exposure compensation and white balance control.

5.  Images are captured by camera chips, typically complementary metal oxide semiconductor (CMOS) camera or charge coupled device (CCD). The CMOS camera is more energy efficient.

6.  Image capture rate is usually two frames per second (fps) for small bowel evaluation. Esophageal evaluation (PillCam ESO, Given Imaging) uses 7 fps during a 20 min exam. Capsule colonoscopy devices feature a 2 h delay in activation, then transmit images at 4 fps. One device alters its frame rate from 0.5 fps in the stomach to 2 fps post-pyloric to increase energy efficiency and improve rate of exam completion (OMOM, Jinshan Scientific). Some newer generation devices have adaptive frame rate technology, allowing variable capture rate depending on the rate of movement in the intestine (PillCam COLON 2, Given Imaging).

7.  Field of view ranges from 140 to 172° with a depth of field from 1 to 30 mm and a resolution of 0.1 mm.

8.  Images are transmitted via radiofrequency modulation to sensors located in a belt or vest worn by the patient. Data is then sent to a workstation for image analysis. The MicroCam device (Intromedic) uses a selective spread spectrum technology (the so-called human body communication) rather than radiofrequency modulation for image transfer, reportedly decreasing power consumption and improving image quality by transmitting noncompressed images.

9.  Future development is focusing on utility of the capsule to perform more advanced diagnostics, such as optical biopsy, pH monitoring and serologic testing. Specific directional manipulation with self-propelled capsules and the use of external magnets are also being studied in order to better target the device to the site of pathology. The Versatile Endoscopic capsule for gastrointestinal Tumor Recognition and therapy (VECTOR) and Nano-based capsule-Endoscopy with Molecular imaging and Optical biopsy (NEMO) are two ongoing European studies evaluating these possibilities.

## C. Indications

1. Most common and best studied indication for CE is the evaluation of OGIB, accounting for over 60% of CE studies. Obscure GI bleeding is defined as bleeding of unknown origin that recurs or persists and which cannot be identified by standard upper and lower endoscopy. It may be classified as overt in patients with clinically obvious bleeding of unknown source, or occult in those with recurring self-limited episodes and chronic iron-deficiency anemia. Obscure GIB accounts for up to 5% of all GI bleeds.

2. Crohn's disease (CD) is increasingly evaluated with CE for both confirmation of diagnosis, evaluation of patients with otherwise undiagnosed symptoms, and to grade the severity of disease. Patients typically require other radiographic small bowel imaging to rule out stricture prior to CE evaluation.

3. Diagnosis of suspected small bowel malignancy.

4. Evaluation of otherwise unexplained abdominal symptoms, such as pain, diarrhea, or weight loss.

5. Surveillance of polyposis syndromes, such as Lynch syndrome, Peutz–Jeghers syndrome or familial adenomatous polyposis.

6. Evaluation of celiac disease.

7. Monitoring of patients following small bowel transplantation.

## D. Contraindications

1. Known small bowel stricture is the only absolute contraindication to CE, though some have proposed its utility in localizing stenotic disease as a marker for patient with disease requiring surgical intervention.

2. Relative contraindications include presence of cardiac pacemaker, previous major abdominal surgery, and inability to swallow the capsule. CE has been FDA (Food and Drug Administration) approved for pediatric patients >2 years, though it has been used in younger patients.

## E.  Patient Preparation

1.  Eight to twelve hours fast prior to the procedure.
2.  Clear liquid diet for 24 h prior to exam.
3.  Purgatory prep with various agents has been shown to provide superior image quality versus clear liquid and overnight fasting alone. Polyethylene glycol, sodium phosphate, and other prokinetic agents have been studied, with no clear evidence of the superiority of any particular agent.

## F.  Procedure

1.  Capsules are typically swallowed with small amount of water.
2.  The capsule may be endoscopically delivered through working channel of a standard endoscope. This is particularly beneficial in patients with gastric motility disorders and may improve the rate of exam completion.
3.  A sensor array is worn by the patient as a belt or vest, depending on the device used. Transmission occurs over the battery life of the device, stored in a portable unit, and analyzed upon completion of the exam. Typical exam time is 6–8 h and generates over 50,000 images.
4.  A complete exam requires visualization of the cecum.
5.  Advancing technology is making outpatient procedures more feasible.
6.  Device is passed in the stool 1–7 days after administration.

## G.  Results

1.  CE results are typically reported as diagnostic yield, diagnostic accuracy or detection rate with no absolute standard for reporting. True sensitivity and specificity are difficult to obtain because of the lack of a gold standard for evaluation of the small bowel for control comparison. This is further complicated in the Crohn's disease population where there is no diagnostic gold standard for the disease.

2. Detection rate varies according to the pathologic etiology. Overall diagnostic yield is around 60%.

   a. Pathology most often found is angiodysplasia (50%), followed by inflammatory mucosal lesions (26%) and neoplasms (8.8%).

   b. Yield is higher in patients with overt OGIB than occult OGIB (88% vs. 48%).

   c. CE is 2–5 times more likely to identify pathology than push enteroscopy, colonoscopy with ileoscopy or barium enterography.

3. Several other imaging modalities, including push enteroscopy, double-balloon enteroscopy (DBE), intraoperative endoscopy, enteroclysis (barium, computed tomography, or magnetic resonance imaging), and mesenteric angiography have been compared with CE. Studies comparing CE with these other techniques consistently show higher diagnostic yield with CE, with the exception of DBE.

   a. DBE has very similar yield, but is more invasive and requires sedation or anesthesia, though does have the significant advantage of allowing therapeutic intervention and biopsy. Up to 50% of DBEs involve some intervention. Several studies indicate the complementary role of DBE and CE, most using CE as the initial study to guide DBE and improve its diagnostic and therapeutic yield.

   b. CE is 3–4 times more likely to identify small bowel pathology than push enteroscopy.

   c. CE is 5.4 times more likely than enteroclysis and 13 times more likely than small bowel follow through in identifying abnormalities in CD.

   d. Emerging radiographic techniques, such as CT and MR enteroclysis, CT (virtual) colonoscopy have only been compared to CE in a few small studies. Higher diagnostic yield was seen with CE in all cases.

   e. No study has directly correlated CE with intraoperative enteroscopy findings, which is clearly a much more invasive procedure, though it is the best and most complete method of evaluating small bowel mucosa.

4. Capsule endoscopy structured terminology (CEST) reporting system, the Lewis Score, and Capsule Endoscopy Crohn's Disease Activity Index (CECDAI) are methods of interpreting

CE findings and correlate visualized lesions with clinical disease activity and therapeutic strategy. These incorporate mucosal appearance, extent of lesions and the presence of ulcerations and stenosis.

5. In the case of capsule colonoscopy and esophagoscopy, a direct comparison with upper GI endoscopy and colonoscopy allow a true calculation of the sensitivity and specificity of this technology.

   a. Capsule esophagoscopy has demonstrated sensitivity of 67–100% with 80–95% specificity in the evaluation of Barrett's esophagus when compared directly to standard esophagoscopy. Sensitivity and specificity for the detection of esophageal varices are 85% and 80%, respectively.

   b. Capsule colonoscopy has a reported sensitivity from 50 to 70% with 73 to 100% specificity in the detection of colorectal polyps. These results are encouraging in the diagnosis of colorectal disease in patients with incomplete or contraindication to standard colonoscopy.

6. The cost of CE is greater than $30,000 for software and hardware and just under $500 per capsule. Cost for inpatient CE per exam is around $2,000 per patient, with outpatient procedures costing less than half that amount. Comparative cost-effectiveness is difficult: Patients with OGIB often undergo multiple upper and lower endoscopies, and radiographic and angiography studies, which may cost in excess of $30,000 per patient, lending to the cost-effectiveness of CE. The choice of DBE versus CE as the initial study is more debatable given the therapeutic interventions possible with DBE. These procedures are often complimentary, using CE to guide DBE.

## H. Adverse Outcomes

1. CE is limited to image capture. Current technology does not allow intervention or advanced diagnostic maneuvers, such as biopsy, pH monitoring, or serologic testing.

2. Capsule endoscopy fails to complete small bowel examination in 10–15% of studies.

3. Capsule retention is the most significant complication, typically occurring in <5% of cases. This is significantly higher in the CD population with greater than four times the risk of retention.

   a. Of retained capsules, nearly 60% require surgical removal. DBE is the next most successful extraction technique.

   b. Patency capsules are dissolvable pills with identical size and shape as capsule endoscopes containing a radiofrequency identification chip to assess passage of the capsule if the patient does not observe its passing. Clinical results have varied, but are likely a useful screening tool to assess patients at risk for capsule retention as newer generation capsules evolve.

4. Up to 1.5% of patients cannot swallow the capsule.

5. Technical failures in data transmission or reception, battery failure or failure of capsule activation occur in around 8% of exams.

# I. Summary

Capsule endoscopy has continued to rapidly become a standard modality for evaluation of small bowel disease. It is minimally invasive with superior diagnostic yield compared to most other endoscopic or radiologic modalities. The primary limitations to this technology at this time are the lack of ability to perform advanced diagnostics or therapeutic intervention and the relatively high rate of incomplete studies. With continued technological advances, improved capsule energy efficiency, image quality, propelling mechanisms, biopsy capability, serologic testing, and drug delivery systems for targeted pharmacotherapy or topical procoagulants, CE will likely play an increasingly important role in evaluation and possible treatment of gastrointestinal disease.

## Selected References

Chen X, Ran ZH, Tong JL. A meta-analysis of the yield of capsule endoscopy compared to double-balloon enteroscopy in patients with small bowel diseases. World J Gastroenterol. 2007;13(32):4372–8.

Chong AK, Taylor A, Miller A, et al. Capsule endoscopy vs. push enteroscopy and enteroclysis in suspected small-bowel Crohn's disease. Gastrointest Endosc. 2005;61:255–61.

Eliakim R. Video capsule colonoscopy: where will we be in 2015? Gastroenterology. 2010;139:1468–80.

Fireman Z. Capsule endoscopy: future horizons. World J Gastrointest Endosc. 2010; 2(9):305–7.

Hadithi M, Heine DN, Jacobs MAJM, et al. A prospective study comparing video capsule endoscopy with double balloon enteroscopy in patients with obscure gastrointestinal bleeding. Am J Gastroenterol. 2006;101:52–7.

Koornstra JJ. Bowel preparation before small bowel capsule endoscopy: what is the optimal approach? Eur J Gastroenterol Hepatol. 2009;21:1107–9.

Liao Z, Gao R, Xu C, et al. Indications and detection, completion, and retention rates of small-bowel capsule endoscopy: a systematic review. Gastrointest Endosc. 2010; 71:280–6.

Marmo R, Rotondano G, Pscopos R, et al. Meta-analysis: capsule enteroscopy vs. conventional modalities in diagnosis of small bowel diseases. Aliment Pharmacol Ther. 2005;22:595–604.

Moglia A, Pietrabissa A, Cuschieri A. Capsule endoscopy. BMJ. 2009;339:796–9.

Rondonotti E, Soncini M, Girelli C, et al. Cost estimation of small bowel capsule endoscopy based on "real world" data: inpatient or outpatient procedure? Dig Liver Dis. 2010;42(11):798–802.

Swaminath A, Legnani P, Kornbluth A. Video capsule endoscopy in inflammatory bowel disease: past, present and future redux. Inflamm Bowel Dis. 2010;16(7):1254–62.

Triantafyllou K. Can we improve the diagnostic yield of small bowel video-capsule endoscopy? World J Gastrointest Endosc. 2010;2(5):143–6.

Triester SL, Leighton JA, Leontiadis GI, et al. A meta-analysis of the yield of capsule endoscopy compared to other diagnostic modalities in patients with obscure gastrointestinal bleeding. Am J Gastroenterol. 2005;100:2407–18.

Triester SL, Leighton JA, Leonitiadis GI, et al. A meta-analysis of the yield of capsule endoscopy compared to other diagnostic modalities in patients with non-stricturing small bowel Crohn's disease. Am J Gastroenterol. 2006;101:954–64.

Westerhof J, Weersma RK, Koornstra JJ. Investigating obscure gastrointestinal bleeding: capsule endoscopy or double balloon enteroscopy? Neth J Med. 2009;67(7):260–5.

# Part X

# Flexible Endoscopy: Basic Lower Gastrointestinal Endoscopy

# 44. Flexible Sigmoidoscopy

*John A. Coller, M.D.*

## A. Indications

The flexible sigmoidoscope is the standard device for endoscopic examination of the distal large bowel. Flexible sigmoidoscopy is used for screening of asymptomatic patients for neoplastic disease as well as one of the methods of investigation of patients with anorectal symptoms.

## B. Instrumentation

The current typical flexible sigmoidoscope is a 65 cm long video endoscopic instrument that records the view from an electronic charged coupled device (CCD) at the tip of the scope and presents the image on a video screen. This device has a considerably improved image quality as compared to earlier fiberoptic sigmoidoscopes. In addition, the findings can be readily documented and annotated. The output from these instruments can easily be incorporated into an electronic medical record.

It is important to understand that the difference between video sigmoidoscopy and video colonoscopy is more than just the length of the instrument. In general, flexible video sigmoidoscopes have a field of view of 120–140°. This is less than the 170° that exists with current video colonoscopes. In addition, although current video colonoscopes have high-definition and narrow band imaging, video sigmoidoscopes are limited to conventional video imaging. Despite the fact that industry has reserved the best enhancements for the flagship colonoscope instruments, the video sigmoidoscopes are still very high quality and effective instruments.

N.J. Soper and C.E.H. Scott-Conner (eds.), *The SAGES Manual: Volume 1 Basic Laparoscopy and Endoscopy*, DOI 10.1007/978-1-4614-2344-7_44, © Springer Science+Business Media, LLC 2012

Most video sigmoidoscopic instruments have an external diameter of between 11.5 and 12.8 mm in diameter and an internal channel of 3.5–4.2 mm providing for large volume tissue biopsy.

## C. Patient Preparation

Adequate bowel preparation is essential for more reasons than simple accuracy. Any residual material that is more substantive than a thin liquid prolongs the examination, contributes to discomfort by requiring greater manipulation and air insufflation, and adds to the risk of injury. Once adherent to the viewing lens, formed stool can be very tenacious, requiring blind removal of the instrument. Stool coating the mucosa obscures surface morphology and vasculature. A pool of opaque liquid between folds may be much deeper than is apparent and consequently may harbor a significant lesion beneath the surface. Fecal debris has a tendency to adhere to an abraded or demucosalized surface more readily than to the surrounding normal epithelium. Consequently, all stool coated surfaces must be exposed if one is to clear the examined area with confidence.

Either cathartic or enema preparation can be used for flexible sigmoidoscopy preparation. Preparation with a hypertonic sodium phosphate enema (Fleets, CB Fleet, Lynchburg, VA) is simple and safe in the vast majority of patients. However, symptomatic hyperphosphatemia and/or hypocalcemia can occur in children or in patients with renal insufficiency or dehydration. This can be administered prior to the patient coming to the office or in the office immediately before the examination.

## D. Technique of Flexible Sigmoidoscopy

1. The most comfortable position for both the physician and the patient is to have the patient in the left lateral decubitus position.
2. After inspecting the perineum, the first step in the examination is a careful digital examination with a well-lubricated gloved finger. This lubricates the anal canal and confirms that there is no lesion or stricture of the distal rectum. Careful palpation of the prostate and of the posterior ampulla of the rectum should be performed.

3. Grasp the control housing with the left hand so that the thumb can manipulate the deflection controls and the second and third fingers can activate the air and suction channels and assist with deflection. After lubricating the shaft (but not the lens), grasp the distal shaft and deflection tip with the right hand, facilitating introduction into the distal rectum. The right index finger should extend to the tip of the scope to help slide the scope into the rectum. The entire deflection tip, about 10 cm, must be inserted before the dial controls become effective.

4. The initial view of the rectum is usually obtained with deflection in the posterior direction and minimal air insufflation. Bear in mind throughout the examination that air insufflation occurs whenever the air button is covered. A "lazy" finger resting on the air insufflation button will cause excess air to be introduced, causing undue discomfort.

5. After obtaining a view of the rectum, position the right hand on the shaft, about 10–15 cm from the anal verge. Use the right hand to maintain shaft position, manipulating the deflection tip with the left hand. Greater speed and efficiency will be obtained if the endoscopist avoids jumping the right hand back and forth between the shaft and the dial controls.

6. Intubation is performed using a combination of tip deflection, shaft torque, and shaft advancement/withdrawal, along with air insufflation and removal.

    a. The two concentric dials on the control housing manipulate the deflection tip. The larger dial deflects the tip in an up-down direction over 180°. The smaller dial provides similar deflection from side to side. When both dials are maximally applied, the tip of the scope will over-deflect to more than 180°. Judicious use of tip deflection greatly facilitates finding the lumen. However, once deflection reaches more than 90° the ability to advance the instrument is impeded. When there is maximal deflection, the leading edge of the scope is no longer the viewing tip but rather the sharply angulated deflection tip of the scope itself (Fig. 44.1b). Severe tip deflection, when necessary, should be restricted to finding the lumen, flattening the deflection as much as possible before attempting further advancement.

    b. Shaft torquing permits the partially deflected tip to press against a fold and ease the scope into the lumen ahead. This is particularly useful when there is considerable circular

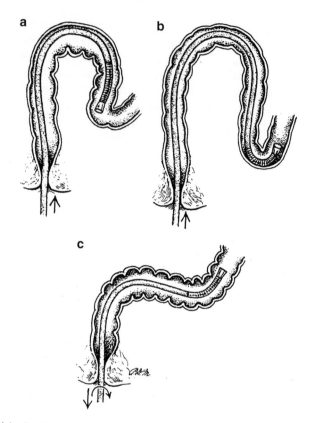

Fig. 44.1. Intubation by elongation. (**a**) The sigmoidoscope is advanced to the proximal sigmoid. (**b**) Severe tip deflection prevents further advancement resulting in sigmoid elongation. (**c**) Clockwise torquing and shaft withdrawal accordionizes the sigmoid.

muscular hypertrophy associated with diverticular disease in the sigmoid. When the full length of the scope has been inserted into a redundant sigmoid, clockwise torque tends to reduce the redundancy, where as counterclockwise torquing usually accentuates the redundancy preventing further intubation. The preferred maneuver at this point is to torque clockwise while retracting the shaft and often performing small amounts of suction. This will help to transition from Fig 44.1b, c. After continued clockwise torquing and flattening of the deflection tip, further intubation can then be accomplished with scope advancement. Finding the lumen by torquing is almost always more effective than simple periscoping with the dials.

c.  Shaft advancement is obviously necessary in order to obtain maximum intubation with the flexible sigmoidoscope. However, it is most important to understand that intermittent scope retraction is an essential element of efficient scope advancement. When the deflection tip is sharply angulated as in Fig. 44.1b, the shaft may be advanced so that the entire shaft is introduced, with a severely distended sigmoid but no further advancement of the tip of the scope. Only by withdrawing the shaft, while flattening the deflection tip and simultaneously torquing clockwise, can the next segment be readily entered and the maximal length of colon examined.

7.  Air insufflation is necessary to distend the lumen and obtain good visualization of the mucosal surface. Avoid unnecessary insufflation, particularly on intubation. If adhesive disease anchors multiple segments of the colon, the excess air will accentuate the acuity of loops making advancement more difficult.

8.  There are three general approaches to the flexible sigmoidoscopic examination: intubation by elongation; intubation by looping; intubation by dither-torquing. Any given examination may use a single approach or a combination of all three.

a.  **Intubation by elongation**: The most basic approach is to simply advance the scope, assuming one has a satisfactory view of the lumen, until all the scope shaft has been inserted. In the case of prior sigmoid resection, it is quite likely that the examination will have extended to the level of the distal transverse colon, which is reasonable for flexible sigmoidoscopy. However, in the non-operated patient, if the sigmoid colon is a very redundant, mobile structure, intubation may proceed unimpeded until there is no scope remaining. One's sense of expeditious accomplishment must be tempered by the fact that only a minimal amount of left colon has been examined. If one is going to get the most out of the sigmoidoscope, the elongated redundancy has to be reduced by evacuating the air that is contributing to the distension and retract on the loop apex in order to negotiate to the sigmoid-descending junction.

    i.    To advance further, direct the deflection tip sharply into the sigmoid-descending junction (Fig.44.1b). If the junction is a sharp deflection, further attempt at advancement will be counterproductive. The severe bend at the deflection tip will be the leading edge of the scope rather than the viewing tip.

    ii.    Reduce the elongated sigmoid by clockwise torquing while slowly withdrawing the scope shaft. At the same time, the severity of tip deflection should be reduced so that further scope advancement can be achieved (Fig. 44.1c).

    iii.    After reduction of the redundant loop, clockwise torque is maintained, with a flattened deflection tip in order to advance the shaft more proximally into the descending colon. On occasion when there is a dolicosigmoid (a long floppy sigmoid colon), often associated with chronic constipation, the flexible sigmoidoscope is simply not long enough to traverse the sigmoid and a colonoscope is required.

    b.    **Intubation by looping**: In general, if the sigmoid has a typical amount of redundancy, one can take advantage of that redundancy to create a loop that will help flatten the sigmoid-descending junction.

    i.    Upon reaching the rectosigmoid, apply counterclockwise torque during shaft advancement. The proximal sigmoid will be directed anteriorly and to the right side of the lower abdomen.

    ii.    This creates an alpha-loop (Fig. 44.2a, b). The sigmoid-descending junction can then be approached in a horizontal direction, thus flattening the angle that has to be negotiated with the deflection tip.

    iii.    Once the deflection tip has been positioned at the mid- or distal-descending colon, the loop can be reduced by simultaneous clockwise torque and shaft withdrawal (Fig. 44.2d). As the loop is removed, the tip of the scope will extend more proximally as the sigmoid colon accordionizes onto the scope even though some shaft is being withdrawn.

    iv.    When the sigmoid is straight, advance the shaft while maintaining clockwise torque.

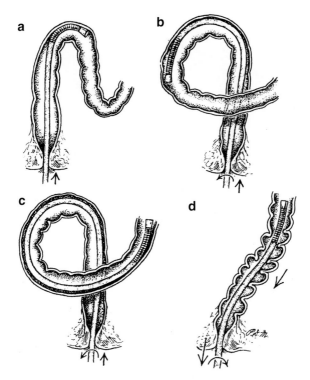

Fig. 44.2.  Intubation by looping. (**a**) The sigmoidoscope is advanced to the distal sigmoid. (**b**) Counterclockwise torquing during further advancement loops the proximal sigmoid in front of the distal sigmoid. (**c**) The looped sigmoid flattens the angle at the distal-descending colon. (**d**) Clockwise torquing and shaft withdrawal accordionizes the sigmoid.

c.  **Intubation by dither-torquing**: This method attempts to minimize stretching or deforming of the colon. If there are numerous adhesions in the pelvis or associated with the distal colon, then the rectosigmoid and sigmoid are likely to be characterized by several short angulated segments. There is insufficient redundancy to elongate or loop the sigmoid colon. Synchronous use of a back-and-forth movement with the shaft (dithering) while torquing left and right is very effective in showing the way to the lumen while encouraging the colon to accordionize, bit by bit, onto the scope (Fig. 44.3). This avoids the development of a large and often uncomfortable loop. When the sigmoid is tightly

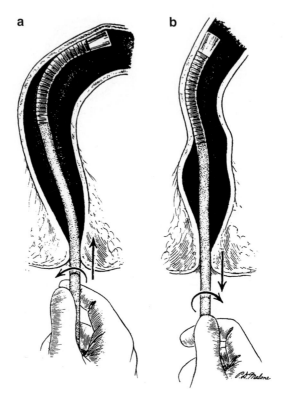

Fig. 44.3.   Intubation by dither-torquing. (**a**) The shaft is torqued counterclock-wise while advancing the shaft 10–15 cm. (**b**) The shaft is torqued clockwise while withdrawing the shaft 10–15 cm. Repetition of this cycle encourages the sigmoid to accordionize onto the sigmoidoscope.

nested in the pelvis, the dither-torquing method is usually the only way that intubation can be accomplished expeditiously.

i.   Move the right hand on the shaft in a repetitive fig-ure-of-eight motion. As one dithers forward for about 10 cm, torque in the clockwise direction. This is fol-lowed by dithering backwards while torquing coun-terclockwise. Performing this motion repeatedly, tends to accordionize the colon onto the scope, and usually reveals the direction of the lumen ahead.

ii.  Conceptually, the dither–torque approach tries to bring the colon back onto the scope shaft rather than just pushing the scope into the colon.

9.  Neither of the three approaches, described above, will work all of the time in all colons. One has to start the examination and be sufficiently fluid enough to change from one approach to another. A most helpful attitude to have during the examination is to spend as little time as possible with the lumen not in clear view. If one is moving the deflection tip all around unsuccessfully trying to get an idea of the lumen direction, time is being wasted. The shaft should be withdrawn until the lumen is visualized and then proceed forward. Not only is blind advancement counterproductive, it is more likely to be traumatic.

10.  During withdrawal, careful examination of the entire mucosal surface is obtained. At any point along the withdrawal, it may be necessary to torque first in one direction and then repeat the withdrawal with torquing in the other direction in order to see the entire mucosal surface. Because of the frequent presence of circular muscle hypertrophy and sharp angulation it may be necessary to vigorously use the deflection tip in order to see behind folds. As the distal rectum "cones-down" to the anal sphincter, withdrawal should proceed slowly so that a complete exam is accomplished. I am personally not in favor of routine retroflexion of the deflection tip unless there is a suspected lesion that cannot otherwise be explained. The rectum may have limited compliance and be at risk for injury from an unnecessary retroflexion maneuver.

# E.  Diagnostic Flexible Sigmoidoscopy

There are several potential applications of diagnostic flexible sigmoidoscopy.

## 1.  Screening for Colon Cancer

One of the major roles for flexible sigmoidoscopy is its place among screening strategies for the detection of neoplastic polyps and cancer. Although the instrument has a capacity to examine only one-third to one-half of the total surface area of the large bowel, it serves as an indicator for the entire colon and has an established role in the screening paradigm for colorectal cancer.

The American Cancer Society–the US Multi-Society Task Force (ACS-MSTF) suggests a flexible sigmoidoscopy every 5 years, starting at age 50 is an acceptable screening strategy for patients that have an average risk for colorectal cancer. In addition, the United States Preventative Services Task Force (USPSTF) accepts the same endoscopic parameter but adds the use of fecal occult blood testing, every 3 years. Another common strategy that is accepted by both task forces is the performance of a colonoscopy once every 10 years. The tradeoff appears to be examination of a shorter segment of colon more often or the entire colon less frequently. A large population study from the UK suggests that even a single lifetime flexible sigmoidoscopy examination can have a beneficial effect on colorectal mortality among nonhigh risk individuals. This randomized controlled study (2002) examined the effectiveness of flexible sigmoidoscopy in colorectal polyp and cancer screening; 170,038 asymptomatic individuals between the ages of 55 and 64 years were offered a first time screening by sigmoidoscopy; 112,939 subjects were placed in the control group and 57,099 were in the intervention group. Average follow-up interval was 11.2 years. The incidence of colorectal cancer was reduced by 33% and the mortality by 43% in the group subjected to the single flexible sigmoidoscopy screening.

Despite the presumptive superiority for colonoscopy versus flexible sigmoidoscopy in colorectal cancer screening, there is at this time a lack of compelling data that screening has to be colonoscopy and not flexible sigmoidoscopy. Ongoing prospective studies in this regard are not due to be completed for another 10–15 years.

## 2. Evaluation of Symptoms

There are multiple symptoms that occur relative to the anorectum: itching, pain, bleeding, and change in bowel habit. The requisite depth and type of endoscopic visualization will vary depending upon the patient's personal and family history and response to initial therapy. A 25-year-old female with anal pain and bright red rectal bleeding following a dieting effort to loose weight most likely will require only an anoscopy to document the presence of an anal fissure. On the other hand, a 62-year-old male, with similar symptoms, will require a full colonos-copy to insure that the source of bleeding is not a colon cancer.

When symptoms are highly suggestive of an anorectal source, then it is reasonable to limit visualization to the local anorectal area with anos-copy and the distal colorectum by flexible sigmoidoscopy. If a young patient has symptoms and findings compatible with internal hemor-rhoids, there is little rationale to automatically proceed with colonos-copy. If symptoms do not respond to appropriate therapy, then more aggressive investigation can be entertained.

## 3. Lower Gastrointestinal Hemorrhage

When symptoms are suggestive of a lower GI source of anemia or hemorrhage, a limited investigative approach is a compromise in the depth of care. The quality evaluation of presumed active lower GI hem-orrhage should generally default to a complete colon examination. Clearly, a history of iron deficiency anemia requires a full colonoscopy.

## F. Therapeutic Flexible Sigmoidoscopy

The flexible sigmoidoscope is basically a diagnostic instrument. Much of the therapy that is performed endoscopically of the colorectum requires the use of an energy source that has potential for igniting explosive gas mixtures, such as hydrogen and methane that may be resident within the colon. Bowel preparation for colonoscopy has a high likelihood of reducing the concentration of potentially explosive substances. In addition, the longer time required for colonoscopy results in considerable gas exchange that further lessens the likelihood of explosive gas mixtures. The same safety margin is usually not present for flexible sigmoidoscopy. Often, the only preparation is a single Fleet enema, shortly before the examination. If a neoplastic polyp is encoun-tered, the examination is no longer an asymptomatic screening proce-dure. With few exceptions, when a lesion has been found on flexible sigmoidoscopy that requires electrocoagulation treatment, the patient should be scheduled for complete colonoscopy and management of any neoplastic lesions. Consequently, the use of energy sources is not dis-cussed in this section.

## 1. Biopsy

When an abnormality is encountered, it is usually appropriate to perform a biopsy. This information helps direct further therapy. It is not infrequent to find one or more small, diminutive polyps in the rectosigmoid. It is reasonable to perform a cold biopsy in order to inform appropriate follow-up. If the tissue demonstrates normal or hyperplastic colon mucosa, there is not a mandate to proceed with full colonoscopy. However, if the gross appearance or histologic examination demonstrates a neoplastic lesion, e.g., tubular or villous adenoma, then the entire colon should be examined. In addition, if there is any residual tissue at the biopsy site, or additional polyps observed, they should be addressed with electrocoagulative removal. It should be born in mind that cold biopsy of a polyp that is not completely encompassed by the forceps has a high likelihood of leaving some residual neoplastic tissue. As a consequence, some endoscopists prefer to remove very small lesions by snare excision without the application of electrocautery. Although this approach offers a more complete removal of a diminutive polyp, it may not offer complete destruction. Snare removal, without electrocoagulation of small polyps is a rather common practice. Although there has not been a rigorous examination of the treatment of small neoplastic polyps without electrocoagulation, there has not been a plethora of adverse events, including subsequent malignant appearance associated with this treatment.

Although there are large bite forceps, the quantity of tissue in a single biopsy of a standard size forceps can be quite miniscule and poorly reflective of the tissue morphology. Rather than sniping at the mucosa, end on, it is often better to go at the mucosa tangentially, gathering a small strip of tissue into the jaws.

## 2. Management of Anastomotic Stricture

Distal colonic strictures can be treated at the time of flexible sigmoidoscopy. Those that are a result of a surgical anastomosis are able to be treated, preferably with a hydrostatic balloon dilator. If the stricture is very tight, e.g., 2–5 mm, it is safest to initially dilate with a balloon that achieves a 10 mm diameter. If symptoms persist, further dilatation to 20 mm diameter can be performed at a subsequent session. It is essential that the etiology of the stricture, anastomotic or idiopathic, be ascertained by biopsy and/or imaging before proceeding with endoluminal treatment. It should be noted that an anastomotic stricture associated with IPAA or coloanal anastomosis often involves very sensitive anorectal tissue. In general, dilatation without sedation is an intolerable circumstance, removing it from the average flexible sigmoidoscopy realm. In the case of a malignant distal colon stricture, temporary improvement may be obtained with the insertion of a stent. This can be used for palliative treatment or as means for permitting a bowel preparation prior to definitive surgery.

## 4. Foreign Body Removal

Foreign bodies of various shapes and intent are not infrequently encountered in the rectum and distal colon. In general, if a foreign body is suspected, it is appropriate to obtain at least a simple plain X-ray of the lower abdomen and upright of the chest before proceeding with endoscopic examination. The chest X-ray will help to determine if there is evidence of free air. The X-ray of the lower abdomen may inform the surgeon of the shape of the device. Some devices with appendages may be much less traumatic to insert than to remove. Very large diameter units may require the use of a nerve blocks or anesthesia to relax the sphincter unless it is already a patulous structure.

Frequently, the flexible sigmoidoscope can be a valuable tool in safe foreign body evaluation and extraction especially if the device is above the reach of an anoscope or rigid proctoscope. One of the most frequent categories of device is associated with sexual massage or dildos. These units are often of large diameter with a smooth surface providing no grasping features. Although history taking will usually inform the physician as what to expect, it is interesting how often individuals attempt to avoid details under embarrassing circumstances. If initial abdominal examination, blood studies, and imaging fail to suggest compromise of the visceral wall, then proceeding with endoscopic evaluation is appropriate. Assuming the device is not palpable on digital examination, proceed with flexible sigmoidoscopy. When the device is encountered, note whether or not there are any physical irregularities on the presenting surface that can be used to advantage to assist with retrieval. In the case of a mechanical massager, there might be a switch or dial that can be grasped with a snare. The snare and scope can then be slowly withdrawn. Unfortunately, large diameter devices, whether mechanical or biologic, as in the form of a cucumber, may occlude the lumen and resist removal due to suction on the proximal side. Under these circumstances, one can pass a Foley catheter alongside the device in order to introduce air above. Then, inflate the balloon to help pull the device distally. Alternatively, withdraw the video sigmoidoscope and replace it with a smaller diameter gastroscope to reach above the device to disrupt the negative pressure.

Special caution must be taken with body packers. These patients present with one or more condoms in the lower colon, filled with heroin or cocaine. It is imperative that the container not be damaged in order to avoid gross contamination and absorption of a fatal volume of narcotics. Unless the package is just above the anal sphincter, it may be better to approach under anesthesia where one or more packages can be gently massaged to the anus.

On occasion, a hollow tubular structure, such as a rectal tube or irrigation catheter will become displaced above the anal sphincter. If the edge of the tube cannot be firmly grasped with a biopsy forceps, a balloon catheter can be passed through the flexible sigmoidoscope and threaded into the catheter lumen. Distending the balloon can produce a firm grasp of the wayward catheter.

If the device is not retrieved with relative ease, using the techniques as described above, it is better to discontinue flexible sigmoidoscopy alone and consider the addition of anesthesia, laparoscopy, or hand-assisted bowel massage. It is poor judgment to continue a nonproductive endoscopic approach alone.

After the device has been removed by whatever means, a final endoscopic examination of the rectum and left colon is indicated to ascertain visceral integrity.

# G.  Complications

Intubation may be difficult in the presence of extensive diverticulosis or pelvic adhesions. A dense population of large-diameter diverticular orifices in association with circular muscular hypertrophy can confuse identification of the lumen. Do not proceed with shaft advancement in the absence of a clear view of the lumen. If the next proximal fold cannot be clearly identified through the prospective opening, one is more likely peering into a diverticulum rather than the lumen. My guiding measure is "If you only *think* that orifice is the lumen rather than *know* it is the lumen", then you are trying to intubate a diverticulum.

Pelvic adhesions may severely limit the degree of manipulation that one can apply to the sigmoid and descending colon. Prior gynecologic surgery, a history of peritoneal sepsis, and radiation injury are often responsible for severe adhesion formation. If the colon between the recto-sigmoid and the distal-descending colon is fixed into tightly nested loops, intubation may not be possible. Most likely, intubation without proper sedation, as with colonoscopy, will be unsuccessful. Some patients have a low pain threshold. This should be promptly recognized so that the examination can be appropriately terminated. It should be borne in mind that a patient who experiences undue discomfort during an initial examination will be reticent to seek prompt evaluation in the future when necessary.

Serious complications, e.g., perforation and bleeding, are extremely rare when the procedure is performed by qualified individuals. Inadequate scope cleaning procedures can result in chemical or infectious transmission of injury.

## Selected References

Atkin WS, Edwards R, Kralj-Hans I, Wooldrage K, Hart AR, Northover JM, Parkin DM, Wardle J, Duffy SW, Cuzick J, UK Flexible Sigmoidoscopy Trial Investigators. Once-only flexible sigmoidoscopy screening in prevention of colorectal cancer: a multicentre randomised controlled trial. Lancet. 2010;375(9726):1624–33.

Coller JA. Technique of flexible fiberoptic sigmoidoscopy. Surg Clin N Am. 1980;60: 465–97.

Harringotn L, Schub S. Complications of Fleet enema administration and suggested guidelines for use in the pediatric emergency department. Pediatr Emerg Care. 1997;13(3): 225–6.

Helikson MA, Parham WA, Tobias JD. Hypocalcemia and hyperphosphatemia after phosphate enema use in a child. J Pediatr Surg. 1997;32(8):1244–6.

Hoff G, Grotmol T, Skovlund E, Bretthauer M, Norwegian Colorectal Cancer Prevention Study Group. Risk of colorectal cancer seven years after flexible sigmoidoscopy screening: randomised controlled trial. Br Med J. 2009;338:b1846.

Levin TR, Conell C, Shapiro JA, Chazan SG, Nadel MR, Selby JV. Complications of screening flexible sigmoidoscopy. Gastroenterology. 2002;123(6):1786–92.

Neugut AI, Lebwohl B. Colonoscopy vs sigmoidoscopy screening: getting it right. JAMA. 2010;304(4):461–2.

Preston KL, Peluso FE, Goldner F. Optimal bowel preparation for flexible sigmoidoscopy-are two enemas better than one? Gastrointest Endosc. 1994;40(4):474–6.

West AB, Kuan SF, Bennick M, Largarde S. Glutaraldehyde colitis following endoscopy: clinical and pathological features and investigation of an outbreak. Gastroenterology. 1995;108:1250–5.

# 45. Diagnostic Colonoscopy

*Aman Banerjee, M.D.*
*Melissa S. Phillips, M.D.*
*Jeffrey M. Marks, M.D., F.A.C.S.*

## A. Indications

Not only is colonoscopy useful in diagnosing problems of the gastrointestinal tract, it is also the preferred method for colorectal cancer (CRC) screening by the American College of Gastroenterology and the American Cancer Society. As CRC is the second leading cause of cancer death, the importance of screening against this disease process may have significant impact on patient outcomes. Colonoscopy provides the ability to visualize the entire mucosal surface of the colon, to detect and identify both benign and malignant lesions, and to provide tissue removal of these areas, either for diagnosis or complete resection. Accepted indications for diagnostic colonoscopy are listed in Table 45.1 and include, in addition to detection of malignancy, the ability to evaluate and treat gastrointestinal hemorrhage, evaluate etiologies for changes in bowel habits, delineate extent of disease involvement in inflammatory bowel disease, and aid with intraoperative localization of lesions.

## 1. Indications for Colonoscopic Screening

The risk for developing CRC increases with age. The overall lifetime risk is approximately 5%, with 90% of cases occurring after the age of 50. Risk factors for the development of CRC include family or personal history of CRC or adenomatous polyps, history of inflammatory bowel disease, familial polyposis syndromes (FAP), and hereditary nonpolyposis colon cancer (HNPCC). These risk factors, as well as the number, type, and size of previously removed polyps are used to apply an algorithm for

N.J. Soper and C.E.H. Scott-Conner (eds.), *The SAGES Manual: Volume 1
Basic Laparoscopy and Endoscopy*, DOI 10.1007/978-1-4614-2344-7_45,
© Springer Science+Business Media, LLC 2012

Table 45.1.  Indications for diagnostic colonoscopy.

**Evaluation of gastrointestinal bleeding**
- Hemoccult positive stools
- Hematochezia when an anal or rectal source is not certain
- Melena after excluding an upper gastrointestinal tract source
- Unexplained iron deficiency anemia

**Surveillance for colon neoplasia**
- Following resection of carcinoma or neoplastic/adenomatous polyp
- When a cancer or neoplastic polyp has been found on screening sigmoidoscopy
- In patients at high risk for cancer
  First-degree relatives or multiple family members with colon cancer, Adenomatous polyps, or polyposis syndromes
  Cancer family syndrome
  Chronic ulcerative colitis or extensive Crohn's

**Inflammatory bowel disease**
- Determination of extent of disease
- Confirmation of diagnosis
- Cancer surveillance in chronic ulcerative colitis

**Evaluation of**
- Clinically significant abnormalities on barium enema
- Clinically significant diarrhea of unexplained etiology
- Suspected ischemic colitis
- Follow-up after acute diverticulitis
- Colonic anastomosis

**Intraoperative localization of lesions not apparent at surgery**

recommendations of screening colonoscopy, thus individualizing care for each patient. This chapter discusses the role of colonoscopy, which is the preferred method for screening. Alternatives available for colorectal screening include fecal occult blood test, sigmoidoscopy, and radiographic contrast enemas.

Recommendations for people of average risk include colonoscopy every 10 years starting at age 50. Patients with a family history of colon cancer, especially if a first degree relative, should undergo screening colonoscopy at an earlier age, either 40 years or at the age of 10 years less the age of diagnosis of the affected family member. Patients with personal history of CRC have an increased risk for both recurrence and new lesions, decreasing their recommended screening interval after initial surgical resection from 1 to 3 years depending on cancer location and stage.

Individuals with genetic cancer syndromes must be followed closely because of their elevated risk for developing a malignancy. For patients with HNPCC, current recommendations suggest colonoscopy every 1–2 years starting at age 25 or 10 years younger than the earliest age of CRC diagnosis in a family member. Annual colonoscopy is performed in these high risk patients after age 40. For patients with a family history of FAP and a positive genetic test, annual flexible colonoscopy is offered beginning at age 10 until age 40, after 40 the screening interval increases to every 3–5 years. Colectomy is performed when dysplastic polyps begin to develop.

## 2. Contraindications

a. Generally accepted contraindications to diagnostic colonoscopy included the presence of peritonitis or suspected colorectal perforation, severe acute diverticulitis, and fulminant colitis.

b. Patients who are unable to cooperate during the procedure or patients in whom adequate sedation cannot be achieved should have the procedure aborted.

c. Relative contraindications include large bowel obstruction, hemodynamic instability, symptomatic or large abdominal aortic aneurysms and recent myocardial infarction or pulmonary embolus.

d. Life expectancy less than 5 years is a relative contraindication for screening colonoscopy in patients without colonic symptoms, although the individual risks/benefits should be discussed with the patients.

# B. Patient Preparation

## 1. Anticoagulation Management

Anticoagulation management (including aspirin, nonsteroidal anti-inflammatory medications, clopidegrel, and warfarin) for elective diagnostic colonoscopy is a balance of three factors: the risk of bleeding on anticoagulation, the risk of bleeding related to the endoscopic procedure, and the risk to the patient in temporarily stopping the anticoagulation. For screening colonoscopy, current evidence supports that neither aspirin nor clopidrigrel increase the bleeding risk. There are scattered reports that therapeutic anticoagulation does not increase clinically significant bleeding for diagnostic procedures. In patients who may need to undergo a concomitant therapeutic procedure, the risk for bleeding is increased and specific considerations should be given. Please see Chap. 46 describing Therapeutic Colonoscopy and Complications for more specific details.

## 2. Bowel Preparation

Diagnostic accuracy and therapeutic safety depend upon the quality of bowel preparation. Inadequate preparation can result in missed lesions, increase procedure time, cause cancelation of procedure, and increase the risk for complications. To obtain a reliable examination, the entire bowel must be empty of fecal material to allow for visualization of all colonic mucosa. Ideally, the bowel preparation should cause minimal discomfort with appropriate evacuation of stool. It is also important to avoid large fluid shifts or electrolyte imbalances as these may lead to inadvertent cardiac or renal complications.

The day prior to the exam, patients should discontinue iron-containing medications and begin a clear liquid diet.

a. **Polyethylene glycol lavage** is the most common bowel preparation. The solution passes through the bowel without absorption, working as an osmotic laxative by drawing water into the bowel lumen. This regimen requires approximately 4 L of volume consumption, which can be in one- or divided-doses, over the 12 h before planned colonoscopy. This preparation is relatively safe in patients with renal failure, congestive heart failure, and advanced liver disease. It is also the preferred method for bowel preparation in infants and children. Addition of promotility agents to this regimen has not been shown to improve patient tolerance or quality of colonic preparation.

b. **Enemas** may be used in patients with poor distal preparation or in those with defunctionalized colons after surgical intervention.

c. **Alternative regimens** include varying combinations of low-volume polyethylene glycol lavage, bisacodyl, enemas, and magnesium citrate. These alternatives **should be avoided** in patients with cardiac failure, renal insufficiency, and ascites as these medications may aggravate preexisting conditions. **Mannitol** and other fermentable carbohydrates, including the addition of sugar to commercially available preparations, should be avoided as these may be fermented into explosive gases.

## 3. Antibiotic Prophylaxis

Endoscopic procedures carry a small risk of transient bacteremia which for diagnostic colonoscopy is around 4%. The risk, however, for clinically significant infections is rare. Antibiotic prophylaxis solely to prevent infective endocarditis is no longer recommended for patients before undergoing endoscopic procedures. Although routine antibiotic use is not recommended, special consideration must be given to patients with particularly high risks for adverse outcomes from infective endocarditis, such as those with prosthetic cardiac valve, prior endocarditis, cardiac transplant recipients, and patients with a repaired congenital heart defect incorporating prosthetic material or an implanted device. In such cases, prophylactic administration of amoxicillin or ampicillin may be considered.

## 4. Consent

The risks and benefits of the procedure are reviewed with the patient or the medical power of attorney, documentation of informed consent is placed in the patient's medical record. Any planned therapeutic interventions should also be clearly discussed. Complications of diagnostic colonoscopy are rare and increase when therapeutic procedures are performed concomitantly. These complications include bleeding, perforation, myocardial infarction, and cerebrovascular accidents and are detailed in Chap. 46. Knowledge of potential complications and their relative frequency aids in the informed consent process.

## C. Endoscopic Equipment

The flexible endoscope is available in multiple sizes and consists of a light source, camera, and instrument channels. The length of most colonoscopes is between 100 and 160 cm. The majority of endoscopes are videoscopes where light is transmitted to the tip of the instrument and reflected onto a charge-coupled device (CCD) chip. The CCD contain thousands of light sensitive points called pixels that then relay the image via wires electronically to the instrument head and onto a video monitor. Image resolution (the ability to distinguish two points that are close together) is directly related to the number of pixels. Standard resolution endoscopes produce an image of 480–576 scanning lines on screen. High-definition (HD) CCD can generate up to 1,080 scanning lines on screen. Several studies indicate that there may be increased detection of adenomas 1–5 mm in size with HD devices over standard resolution devices. The value of detecting and removing these adenomas remain unclear. The standard field of view is 180°.

**Chromoendoscopy** is a technique that employs the topical application of stains or pigments to the mucosal surface in order to improve localization, characterization, or diagnosis of a lesion. This can be done in an untargeted manner (panchromoendoscopy) or be targeted to specific lesions. Studies show that there is increased detection of adenomas and polyps with chromoendoscopy over that of standard colonoscopy. However, it is regarded as time intensive thus limiting its adoption into routine practice.

Digital chromoendoscopy consists of the use of newer filter technologies to narrow the red-green-blue wavelengths of light produced by conventional white light endoscopy to enhance microvessel architecture or pattern visualization. Narrow band imaging, or NBI, uses shorter wavelengths of light to enhance superficial mucosal vasculature and surface patterns. Hemoglobin absorbs a greater portion of the projected light thereby appearing darker on the image. This technology is available on most endoscopes and provides real-time information during colonoscopy.

# D.  Passing the Colonoscope: Normal Anatomy

## 1.  Monitoring and Sedation

Appropriate monitoring for patients undergoing conscious sedation includes telemetry with heart rate monitoring, pulse oximetry, and frequent blood pressure recordings. Capnography has been used for conscious sedation monitoring, especially in the setting of advanced endoscopic procedures, and is designed to detect carbon dioxide retention as a sign of over sedation before more dangerous events, such as desaturation, occur.

Conscious sedation is appropriate for most patients. Commonly used agents include a combination of a narcotic, such as fentanyl or demerol, and a benzodiazepine, such as midazolam. The dose is titrated in a stepwise manner until the desired level of sedation is accomplished. Reversal agents, including naloxone and flumenazil, should be immediately available. Propofol (2,6 diisopropyl phenol) is another medication option for conscious sedation and has a similar safety and efficacy profile to the narcotic/benzodiazepine combination mentioned above. All physicians and nurses involved in conscious sedation should be trained and certified with this procedure. For more details on sedation and monitoring, please refer to Chap. 39.

## 2. General Principles

Prior to the procedure, ensure that insufflation and suction are functioning properly. White balance the scope to obtain accurate color correction. Figure 45.1 shows the general set up of the endoscopy suite. The

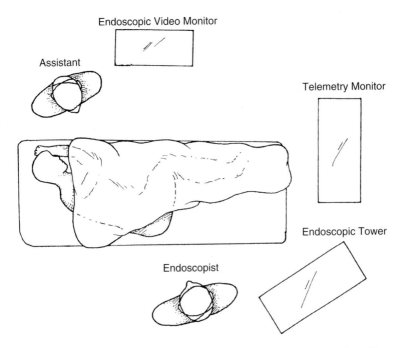

Fig. 45.1. **Endoscopy Suite Set Up**. A video monitor is placed in the direct line of sight of the endoscopist (who stands at the back of the patient) and the assistant (who stands in front of the patient). Monitoring equipment for EKG, blood pressure, and oxygen saturation are positioned at the foot of the bed.

patient should be positioned in the left lateral position. Anesthesia is induced and titrated to the desired level of sedation. A digital rectal exam is performed to lubricate the anus, relax the sphincter muscles, and evaluate for any distal mass lesions. In men, the prostate should also be evaluated.

## 3. Passing the Colonoscope

Lubricate the colonoscope to 10 cm and insert it into the anus while supporting the flexible tip with the index finger. Hold the shaft of the instrument between the thumb and fingers. A gauze sponge can aid in control of a lubricated instrument. Pass the scope into the proximal rectum while keeping the lumen in view. Rotating the shaft clockwise or counterclockwise and using the thumb to angulate up and down results in efficient passage of the scope. As compared to upper endoscopy which is dependent on the right-left controls, external rotation of the colonoscope to generate torque will aid in visualization of all aspects of the colonic mucosa. In general, care should be taken to insufflate as little air as possible for adequate visualization. If abdominal distension develops, the colon should be suctioned for decompression. Throughout the length of the colon, if the view of the lumen is lost, a 2–3 cm withdrawal of the scope with manipulation of the direction of the tip of the scope should bring the lumen back into view. During advancement of the scope, if resistance is encountered, the angulation controls should be checked as a fully angulated tip will not slide through the colon. Essential to the completion of the procedure is reduction of loop formation by the colonoscope. This is accomplished by pulling back and rotating the scope to straighten the redundancy before additional forward progress can be made.

### a. Rectum

Following insertion of the scope, the initial view is often obscured because the lens is pressed against the rectal mucosa. Air insufflation, pulling back on the scope and clockwise rotation of the scope will allow for visualization of the lumen. Suction out any residual fluid or residue to avoid leakage. Air leakage can be significant in patients with significant sphincter dysfunction, and an assistant may be required to push the perineal body against the colonoscope to minimize air leakage.

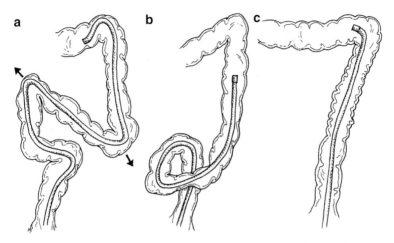

Fig. 45.2. **Loop Formation and Reduction**. (**a**) Formation of loops in the colon can cause patient discomfort, difficulty in advancing the scope, and may increase the risk of perforation. (**b**) Illustration of an alpha loop that has been formed in the sigmoid colon to allow passage into the descending colon. Clockwise torque is sometimes necessary to derotate the loop. (**c**) Reduction of the sigmoid loop can be accomplished by scope withdrawal and subsequent readvancement. Using a combination of push, pull, jiggle, and torque maneuvers, passage of the scope through the remainder of the colon can be accomplished.

## b. Sigmoid Colon

The sigmoid colon derives its name for its "S" shape in most individuals; it begins at the level of the iliac crest and ends at the third sacral vertebra. It is approximately 40–70 cm long when stretched and can collapse to 30–35 cm during the withdrawal phase. Because of the variable length of the sigmoid, it is important to document the location of identified lesions relative to endoscopic landmarks in addition to the location based on depth of the scope. The sigmoid colon has a mesentery of variable length and can be affected by prior surgery, radiation, or inflammation. Diverticuli are not uncommon. Their presence can cause luminal narrowing from chronic inflammation or, in the setting of multiple large diverticuli, may mislead an inexperienced endoscopist away from the true lumen. Instrument loops, detailed in Fig. 45.2, are common in the sigmoid and generally occur in an anterior–posterior formation creating a clockwise spiral loop. Outside pressure on the abdomen may oppose loop formation. Patients should be warned that they may feel a gas pain or stretching pain when pushing around a loop. Care must be taken to reduce these loops when possible to allow for forward progress through the remainder of the colon.

## c. Descending Colon

The descending colon is fixed to the retroperitoneum in the left paracolic gutter. The stretch created by advancing the colonoscope through the sigmoid colon can create an acute angle at the junction with the sigmoid colon. Should any difficulty be encountered, reduce this acute angle by pulling back on the scope; this should improve poor visibility. Deflation of the colon will also shorten the colon and decrease the acute angle. Take care to avoid pushing through any loop created in passage through the sigmoid colon. Pressing on the left lower quadrant or repositioning the patient to allow gravity to pull the colon into a better alignment may also allow for easier passage.

## d. Splenic Flexure

The splenic flexure is created by the extrinsic attachments of the splenocolic, pancreaticocolic, and phrenocolic ligaments to the colon. Visualization of the lumen may be lost when passing the flexure due to the acute angle. In such cases, the longitudinal bulge of the tenia coli serves as a consistent landmark that shows which axis to follow. Proceed carefully when traversing the splenic flexure as splenic avulsions or tears have been reported in the literature. Changing the patient to the right lateral position can pull the splenic flexure into a gentle curve. Finally, after passing the splenic flexure straighten the instrument and reduce all the loops to minimize problems navigating the proximal colon.

## e. Transverse Colon

The transverse colon is approximately 50 cm in length and is located between the hepatic and splenic flexures and may lay in a "U" shaped or "V" shaped curve. Once through the splenic flexure, the transverse colon can be clearly identified by its triangular lumen, created by extrinsic attachments to the gastrocolic ligament. Difficulty in navigating this area is usually due to loop formation in the sigmoid colon. Loop reduction by partial withdrawal and straightening of the scope can aid in passage through the transverse colon. Additionally, pressure applied to the left lower quadrant or mid-abdomen may help facilitate scope passage.

## f. Hepatic Flexure

The hepatic flexure is located at approximately the midaxillary line under the ninth and tenth costal cartilages. It has a characteristic purple-blue liver shadow, and there is usually a pool of liquid at the end of the transverse colon. Passage of the hepatic flexure can be accomplished by applying intermittent suction while withdrawing the scope. This technique is detailed in the next section and will often create paradoxical forward movement of the tip of the scope during reduction of a loop, allowing the hepatic flexure to be traversed.

## g. Ascending Colon and Cecum

The ascending colon is also triangular in appearance. The three colonic taeniae converge at the cecum, giving it its characteristic "Mercedes sign" or crow's foot where the appendiceal orifice can be found. The ileocecal valve can appear as a yellowish fold due to fatty infiltration, and occasionally may look flat. Liquid stool or gas bubbles sometimes can be seen emerging from it. Advancing the scope beyond the hepatic flexure will often lead to a paradoxical movement (i.e., tip of the scope moves backward with external advancement). If this occurs, pull back on the scope and apply intermittent suction. This will most often paradoxically push the tip of the scope forward toward the cecum. When performing this maneuver one must remember that the suction channel is located at the 6 o'clock position on the screen and can catch the mucosa. Mucosal trauma can be avoided by directing the tip the scope up as suction is applied. Having the patient turn, either into the supine or prone position, may also be helpful in allowing advancement the scope. It is important to ensure that one reaches the cecal pit and clearly identifies both the appendiceal orifice and the ileocecal valve. The only way to verify with 100% confidence that the ileocecal valve has been reached is to intubate the terminal ileum and visualize ileal mucosa. Ileal intubation should be performed in patients with concern of ileal disease, such as those with Crohn's disease.

## h. Scope Withdrawal

After reaching the cecum or terminal ileum, gradually withdraw the colonoscope, carefully inspecting the colonic mucosa circumferentially. A withdrawal time of at least 6 minutes is recommended to ensure adequate detection of adenomas, although this number may be higher during a teaching case with resident participation. If an area slips without adequate visualization of that area, readvance the colonoscope until a satisfactory exam is accomplished. After visualization of the anal verge, reinsert the colonoscope to the rectum and retroflex it. This allows for the evaluation of low rectal malignant disease as well as other benign processes, including internal hemorrhoids and fissures. After careful inspection, return the scope to the forward viewing direction and identify the lumen. Remove excess air using intermittent suction and withdraw the scope.

# E.  Passing the Colonoscope: Postsurgical Anatomy

After colon resections, the colon is generally shorter and colonoscopy is correspondingly easier and less time-consuming. If the sigmoid colon has been resected, the colon will appear straighter.

Anastomoses are recognized by visualizing either a suture or a staple line with its characteristic white scar. Occasionally, suture or staple material can be seen through the mucosa. Anastomoses may be created in many ways (end-to-end, side-to-side, or end-to-side) which may result in the creation of a blind pouch. It is very important to recognize the blind end and avoid forceful insertion, as this may lead to perforation. A sharp turn is frequently noted in stapled side-to-side, functional end-to-end anastomosis. Care should be taken to carefully examine all anastomotic sites after resection of previous malignancy to assure there is no local disease recurrence.

## 1.  Passing Scope Via Colostomy

Place the patient in the supine position. Both visual inspection and digital exam of the stoma to the level of the fascia is mandatory before introducing the scope. The remainder of the colonoscopy follows the above-mentioned principles. A problem particular to this situation is air leakage around the stoma, which could compromise insufflation. Applying mild pressure with a gauze sponge around the scope at the stoma level may be helpful.

# Selected References

[No authors listed] ASGE: The role of colonoscopy in management of patients with colonic neoplasia. Gastrointest Endosc 1999;50:921–4.

Banerjee S, Shen B, Baron TH, Nelson DB, Anderson MA, Cash BD, Dominitz JA, Gan SI, Harrison ME, Ikenberry SO, Jagannath SB, Lichtenstein D, Fanelli RD, Lee K, van Guilder T, Stewart LE. ASGE: antibiotic prophylaxis for GI endoscopy. Gastrointest Endosc. 2008;67:791–8.

Blacker DJ, Wijdicks EFM, McClelland RL. Stroke risk in anticoagulated patients with atrial fibrillation undergoing endoscopy. Neurology. 2003;61:964–8.

Cappell MS. Reducing the incidence and mortality of colon cancer: mass screening and colonoscopic polypectomy. Gastroenterol Clin North Am. 2008;37(1):129–60.

Davila RE, Rajan E, Baron TH, Adler DG, Egan JV, Faigel DO, Gan SI, Hirota WK, Leighton JA, Lichtenstein D, Qureshi WA, Shen B, Zuckerman MJ, VanGuilder T, Fanelli RD. ASGE: guidelines for colorectal cancer screening and surveillance. Gastrointest Endosc. 2006;63:546–57.

Dominitz JA, Eisen GM, Baron TH, Goldstein JL, Hirota WK, Jacobson BC, Johanson JF, Leighton JA, Mallery JS, Raddawi HM, Vargo 2nd JJ, Waring JP, Fanelli RD, Wheeler-Harbough J, Faigel DO. ASGE: complications of colonoscopy. Gastrointest Endosc. 2003;57:441–5.

Kim HN, Raju GS. Bowel preparation and colonoscopy technique: to detect non-polypoid colorectal neoplasms. Gastrointest Endosc Clin N Am. 2010;20:437–48.

Leighton JA, Shen B, Baron TH, Adler DG, Davila R, Egan JV, Faigel DO, Gan SI, Hirota WK, Lichtenstein D, Qureshi WA, Rajan E, Zuckerman MJ, VanGuilder T, Fanelli RD. ASGE: the role of endoscopy in the management of patients with inflammatory bowel disease. Gastrointest Endosc. 2006;63:558–65.

Lichtenstein DR, Jagannath S, Baron TH, Anderson MA, Banerjee S, Dominitz JA, Fanelli RD, Gan SI, Harrison ME, Ikenberry SO, Shen B, Stewart L, Khan K, Vargo JJ. ASGE: sedation and anesthesia in GI endoscopy. Gastrointest Endosc. 2008;68: 215–826.

Mandel JS, Bond JH, Church TS, Ederer F, Geisser MS, Mongin SJ, Snover DC, Schuman LM. Reducing mortality from colorectal cancer by screening for fecal occult blood. Minnesota colon cancer control study. N Engl J Med. 1993;328:1365–71.

Ponsky JL, editor. Atlas of surgical endoscopy. St. Louis, MO: CV Mosby-Year-Book; 1992.

Romano G, Belli G, Rotondano G. Colorectal cancer: diagnosis of recurrence. Gastrointest Endosc Clin North Am. 1995;5(4):831–41.

Rosch T, Lorenz R, Classen M. Endoscpic ultrasonography in the evaluation of colon and rectal disease. Gastrointest Endosc. 1990;36(2):S33–9.

Sauk J, Hoffman A, Anandasabapathy S, Kiesslich R. High-definition and filter-aided colonoscopy. Gastroenterol Clin North Am. 2010;39(4):859–81.

Senagore AJ. Intrarectal and intra-anal ultrasonography in the evaluation of colorectal pathology. Surg Clin North Am. 1994;74(6):1465–73.

Silverstein FE, Tytgat GNJ, Hunter J, editors. Atlas of gastrointestinal endoscopy. 2dth ed. New York, NY: Gower Medical; 1991.

Waye JD, Rex DK, Williams CB. Colonoscopy: principles and practice. 1st ed. Malden, MA: Wiley-Blackwell; c2003. p. 318–38. Chapter 29, Insertion Technique.

Wexner SD, Beck DE, Baron TH, Fanelli RD, Hyman N, Shen B, Wasco KE. ASGE: consensus document on bowel preparation before colonoscopy. Gastrointest Endosc. 2006;63:894–909.

Williams JE, Faigel DO. Colonoscopy reports and current state of performance measures. Gastrointest Endosc Clin N Am. 2010;20:685–97.

# 46. Therapeutic Colonoscopy and Its Complications*

*Aaron S. Fink, M.D.*

## A. Introduction

Polypectomy is the most common therapeutic maneuver performed during colonoscopy. This chapter discusses techniques for biopsy and polypectomy. It also discusses decompressive colonoscopy for Ogilvie's syndrome, volvulus reduction, endoscopic hemorrhoidal band ligation, and colonoscopic complications.

## B. Polypectomy

Polypectomy is an essential skill for all who perform colonoscopy. By breaking the adenoma → cancer sequence, this vital technique clearly reduces the incidence of colon cancer.

The risk of malignancy in a polyp depends on its histology and size (as many as 10% of polyps larger than 2 cm may be malignant). Given the inability to accurately predict histology based on appearance alone, most polyps—and certainly those over 0.5 cm—should be removed during colonoscopy. The site of any polyp concerning for malignancy should be marked with India ink to facilitate future localization at repeat colonoscopy or surgical exploration.

*C. Daniel Smith, M.D., Gregory Van Stiegmann, M.D., David W. Easter, M.D. made contributions to this chapter in the previous edition.

As described below, various techniques are used to remove polyps. The polyp's size and appearance (pedunculated, sessile, and flat) typically determine the optimal polypectomy technique.

1. *Cold Biopsy* is used to remove small polyps (1–3 mm); slightly larger polyps can be removed using jumbo forceps.
   a. Close the biopsy forceps on the polyp and gently pull, removing the grasped tissue from the mucosa.
   b. Following cold biopsy, carefully inspect the site for residual tissue requiring removal.

2. *Hot Forceps.* Due to the high incidence of residual tissue, this technique has fallen out of favor.
   a. Grab the tip of the polyp with the forceps and then gently pulled it into the lumen, "tenting" the mucosa.
   b. Apply electrocautery so as to destroy the polyp's base while preserving the entrapped tissue for histological examination.

3. *Snare Polypectomy* is the technique most frequently utilized for polypectomy and is preferred for polyps larger than 1 cm.
   a. Loop the snare over the polyp and tighten it around the polyp's base. If the polyp is pedunculated, position the snare so as to leave a small remnant of the stalk which can be grasped in the event of post-polypectomy bleeding. Sessile polyps are ensnared with a margin of normal mucosa adjacent to the polyp.
   b. If electrocautery is to be used, gently push the ensnared polyp away from the scope and pull it towards the lumen. Monopolar coagulation current is then applied, carefully moving the polyp back and forth so as to minimize contact with other portions of the colon wall. After several seconds, slowly tighten the snare until the polyp has been removed.

4. *Endoscopic Mucosal Resection* may allow endoscopic management of larger sessile polyps (>2 cm), possibly avoiding future surgical resection.
   a. Inject saline into the submucosa below the polyp, lifting it from the mucosa. Then, use the hot snare to resect the polyp either in an *en bloc* or piecemeal fashion.
   b. Residual polypoid tissue is commonly found following endoscopic mucosal resections. Thus, these resection sites should be reexamined colonoscopically in 2–6 months.

5.  *Polyp Retrieval.* Specimen retrieval following polypectomy can be challenging; 10–15% of specimens may be lost (see discussion regarding lost specimens under colonoscopic complications).

   a.  Retrieve small polyps by suctioning them through the suction channel into an in-line trap.

   b.  Slightly larger polyps can be transected with the snare to allow the resulting pieces to pass through the suction channel. Alternatively, use endoscopic grasping forceps to grab the specimen for removal with the colonoscope. In such situations, advance the forceps several centimeters to allow mucosal visualization as the colonoscope is withdrawn.

# C.  Decompressive Colonoscopy for Ogilvie's Syndrome

In acute colonic pseudo-obstruction (Ogilvie's syndrome), the colon becomes massively dilated without apparent mechanical obstruction. Conditions commonly associated with Ogilvie's syndrome are listed in Table 46.1. The cause is unknown but likely to be multifactorial.

The diagnosis is usually straightforward. The predominant clinical feature is abdominal distention which develops over 3–4 days. Bowel sounds are variably present and the abdomen is generally tense with

Table 46.1.  Conditions associated with Ogilvie's syndrome.

| | |
|---|---|
| **Nonabdominal surgery** | • Orthopedic surgery |
| **Blunt trauma** | |
| **Electrolyte abnormalities** | • Hypokalemia |
| | • Hypomagnesemia |
| | • Hypophosphatemia |
| **Chronic illness** | • Renal failure |
| | • Diabetes mellitus |
| | • Malignancy |
| | • Autoimmune disorders |
| | • Hypothyroidism |
| **Medications** | • Anticholinergic agents |
| | • Narcotics |
| | • Phenothiazines |
| | • Tricyclic antidepressants |

mild tenderness. Fever and leukocytosis are common. Plain abdominal X-rays frequently reveal massive dilatation of the proximal colon with relatively normal colonic diameter from the mid-transverse colon to rectum. Contrast enema is necessary to exclude mechanical obstruction. Radiographic demonstration of perforation mandates urgent laparotomy.

Initial therapy for this condition includes cessation of oral intake, nasogastric decompression, and correction of fluid and electrolyte abnormalities. All potentially exacerbating medications (such as narcotics) should be discontinued. Prokinetic agents, epidural anesthesia, frequent positional change, or ambulation may promote motility. Serial abdominal examinations and daily abdominal X-rays should be used to monitor response or progression. The cecum is at greatest risk of perforation owing to its thin wall and greater circumference. Colonoscopic decompression is indicated if cecal diameter exceeds 12 cm, or if there is persistence or progression of colonic dilatation despite conservative measures.

1. Set up the room and position the patient as for routine colonoscopy.
2. Minimize air insufflation during endoscope passage. The pathologic distention usually facilitates endoscope passage, which is often surprisingly easy.
3. Irrigate frequently with small volumes (50 mL) of saline through the endoscope's suction channel to help maintain channel patency and good visualization.
4. It is not necessary to reach the cecum with the colonoscope to effect decompression; the latter is especially true if the colon is distended beyond the hepatic flexure.
5. Carefully inspect the mucosa during insertion and withdrawal. Cyanotic or ischemic mucosa may indicate the need for operative intervention. Bloody drainage may be the only sign of proximal ischemia.
6. In this setting, use of an overtube must be done with care as its large size and stiff nature can complicate endoscope insertion and increase the risk of perforation or erosion.
7. After maximal insertion, begin to slowly remove the endoscope in 4–5 cm increments, applying intermittent suction until the colonic lumen collapses. Keep the tip of the endoscope in the middle of the bowel lumen. This position optimizes decompression of gas and liquid through the suction channel without trapping bowel mucosa.

8. Evaluate the success of the treatment with serial abdominal physical and radiographic examination.
9. A nasogastric tube or long intestinal tube may be passed with the colonoscope and left in place after scope removal.

# D. Decompressive Colonoscopy for Sigmoid Volvulus

Sigmoid volvulus occurs when the sigmoid abnormally twists or folds on its mesentery. Volvulus produces a closed-loop obstruction; the condition carries a high risk of mortality unless treated. The diagnosis may be suspected on the basis of clinical presentation and plain abdominal films (which may be diagnostic). Contrast studies may confirm the diagnosis if the typical" bird's beak deformity" is seen at the distal end of the twisted segment.

In the absence of signs of gangrene (elevated temperature, leukocytosis, abdominal tenderness with peritoneal signs), sigmoidoscopic reduction and decompression is the safest initial treatment for sigmoid volvulus. This intervention allows mucosal viability to be assessed; more importantly, the procedure may decompress the dilated loop and reduce the volvulus. Urgent laparotomy is mandated if necrotic mucosa is observed or if the volvulus cannot be reduced.

1. Begin preparing the patient for surgery so that operative intervention will not be delayed if endoscopic treatment fails.
2. Position the patient in the prone jackknife position. This position facilitates decompression by allowing the colon to fall away. The lateral decubitus position can also be used if the patient cannot tolerate the jackknife position.
3. Because the twist is low in the sigmoid, it can usually be reached with a **rigid sigmoidoscope**; use of this instrument may facilitate decompression.
   a. Minimize air insufflation during insertion.
   b. Carefully insert the rigid sigmoidoscope until the site of torsion is seen. Thoroughly inspect the mucosa at this point for signs of ischemia or necrosis.
   c. If the mucosa appears intact, gently advance the sigmoidoscope beyond the point of torsion. Entry into the volvulus results in a dramatic passage of gas and stool as the segment is decompressed.

    d.    After decompression, perform a limited examination of the bowel mucosa to ensure viability, then place a rectal tube well above the site of torsion, secure it to the perianal skin, and leave it in place for at least 48 h. This tube will maintain decompression and facilitate subsequent bowel preparation or further evaluation.

    e.    Alternatively, a soft, well-lubricated 40- to 60-cm rectal tube can be gently passed beyond the site of torsion under endoscopic vision to accomplish decompression. Obviously, this technique limits the ability to evaluate mucosal viability.

4.    Points of axial rotation and obstruction beyond the reach of a rigid scope require use of a flexible sigmoidoscope or a colonoscope.

    a.    Suction and an assistant are critical to safe completion of endoscopic evaluation and decompression.

    b.    Pass the colonoscope through the site of torsion, until the scope is passed beyond the site of obstruction. Gentle air insufflation may be used to facilitate endoscopic passage.

    c.    Decompression may be aided by attaching an external suction device to the colonoscope's biopsy channel. Alternatively, a long, soft, 14- to 16-French straight catheter can be attached to the colonoscope. After advancing past the torsion and into the proximal colon, this tube can be left in place for subsequent decompression.

5.    Endoscopic decompression and detorsion is successful in 85% of cases of sigmoid volvulus. Unfortunately, the condition frequently recurs; as such, an elective resection of the redundant segment may provide optimal benefit. Patients in whom endoscopic decompression fails, or in whom nonviable mucosa is seen on colonoscopy, require urgent surgery.

In contrast to sigmoid volvulus, endoscopic reduction and decompression is not effective for cecal volvulus. Although both colonoscopic and barium-assisted reduction of cecal volvulus have been described, successes have been limited and associated with high morbidity owing to delays in definitive management. Prompt laparotomy remains the mainstay of management for cecal volvulus, at which time the cecal volvulus is reduced or resected, depending on its viability.

# E.  Endoscopic Band Ligation Treatment of Internal Hemorrhoids

**Indications for treatment of internal hemorrhoids** include bleeding and prolapse. Hemorrhoids of grade 1, 2, or 3 are suitable for endoscopic treatment. Band ligation treatment is usually preceded with a Fleets enema. Thorough examination of the anorectum, including anoscopy and flexible sigmoidoscopy/colonoscopy is indicated for most patients with such symptoms.

1. Place the patient in the Sims position (left lateral decubitus with right knee flexed).
2. Sedation is usually not necessary.
3. Mount the ligating device on the endoscope and pass the endoscope just beyond the dentate line. When a "see-through" ligator is used, the dentate line is easily visualized as it is passed.
4. Perform ligations 1 cm or more above the dentate line to avoid patient discomfort.
5. The direct approach (Fig. 46.1) is simplest and best tolerated by most patients.
   a. Identify the largest hemorrhoid.
   b. Aspirate it into the ligating cylinder using endoscopic suction, and release the rubber band to produce ligation.
   c. Single-fire instruments require that the endoscope be removed and a second band loaded. Multi-fire devices do not require this maneuver.
   d. Repeat the ligation for additional hemorrhoids. Up to three ligations are done at one sitting.
   e. Patients with a short anal canal (often female patients) may be more easily approached with the endoscope retroflexed.
      i. Insert the endoscope with the attached ligating device into the rectum.
      ii. Retroflex the endoscope within the rectum to visualize the region above the dentate line.
      iii. The retroflexed view facilitates visualization and ligation when the anal canal is too short to permit a direct approach.
      iv. Use of the multi-fire device facilitates the retroflexed approach since removal and reloading are not required. From one to three ligations are done at one sitting as described in item 5.d.

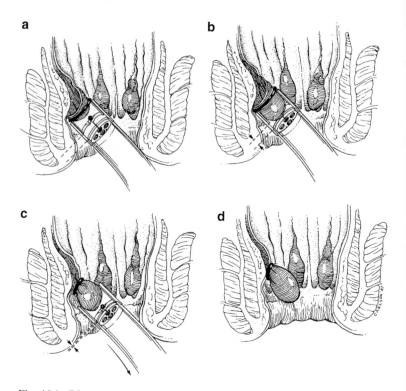

Fig. 46.1. Direct endoscopic ligation of internal hemorrhoids. (**a**) The endoscopist positions the ligator in contact with the hemorrhoid about 1 cm above the dentate line. (**b**) Endoscopic suction draws the hemorrhoid into the banding cylinder. (**c**) The elastic **O**-ring is released to ensnare the hemorrhoid. (**d**) The ligated hemorrhoid.

Patients with external hemorrhoids, some patients with large grade 3 hemorrhoids, and those with grade 4 hemorrhoids are **not suitable** for endoscopic therapy. Caution is indicated in patients who are neutropenic or have compromised immune function. These patients may have a higher risk of impaired healing or septic complications.

## F.  Complications of Colonoscopy

Complications are often worsened by delay in recognition and treatment. Inexperienced endoscopists are more likely to produce complications—including both technical and judgmental errors. At both the beginning and end of each procedure, review any risks and unusual events specific to the individual patient and procedure. For example, is the patient on antiplatelet medications? Was any undue difficulty experienced during the procedure?

Instruct the patient and/or guardian about the common presenting symptoms and signs of complications that can follow an "uneventful" colonoscopy. These generally include pain, bleeding, sensorium changes, nausea, and abdominal distention. Any worrisome event should prompt urgent physician contact and an appropriate evaluation.

## 1. Bleeding

a. **Cause and prevention**. Bleeding, the most common complication following colonoscopy, is usually a result of faulty hemostasis following biopsy. Resections of polyps exceeding 15 mm are at particular risk for continued or delayed bleeding.

Rarely, bleeding can occur from trauma to hemorrhoidal veins, from mucosal erosions caused by mechanical trauma, and very rarely from direct mechanical trauma resulting in splenic rupture. The best ways to prevent these injuries are to (1) anticipate potential problems, (2) correct coagulation disorders prior to and following any biopsy, (3) carefully inspect all biopsy sites minutes after manipulation, and (4) avoid overmedicating the patient (to the state of being unable to report undue pain).

b. **Recognition and management**. Do not aggressively pursue self-limited bleeding from biopsy sites, in order to avoid risk of perforation from the inappropriate use of excessive cautery. Less than half of biopsy sites will require additional cautery and/or the epinephrine injection.

After polypectomy, both immediate and delayed (>12 h) hemorrhage can occur. Following the removal of a pedunculated polyp, immediate bleeding can often be managed by capturing and then tightening the snare around the stalk remnant until bleeding ceases. If this maneuver fails or is not possible, the bleeding site can be injected with epinephrine, or secured with endoscopic clips or endoloops.

Delayed bleeding can occur from hours to as long as 30 days following colonoscopy. This complication requires immediate resuscitation, correction of any coagulating disorders, and usually repeat colonoscopy. If bleeding sites cannot be promptly controlled at colonoscopy, abdominal exploration is usually indicated; arterial embolization is probably contraindicated since the risk of perforation is already high. If the patient has clearly stopped bleeding after the replacement of fluids and correcting coagulation deficits, repeat colonoscopy may be deferred so as to minimize the risk of perforation at the biopsy site(s). Unaltered fresh blood per rectum should raise the suspicion of hemorrhoidal bleeding. Bleeding hemorrhoids require immediate banding or rarely open hemorrhoidectomy. Clinical fluid losses and/or shock without an obvious source should raise the concern of an occult splenic rupture. Emergency abdominal ultrasound (as for trauma patients) is indicated; any free fluid should prompt an immediate laparotomy.

## 2. Perforation

a.  **Causes and prevention**. Perforation following routine diagnostic colonoscopy occurs in approximately 0.8% of cases. This rate doubles following therapeutic procedures such as polypectomy. Prior surgery, diverticulitis, or any cause of preexisting intra-abdominal adhesions increase the procedure's difficulty and enhance the possibility of a colon perforation. Perforation is caused by barotrauma from excessive insufflation, direct mechanical trauma from the scope or inserted instruments, and compromised biopsy sites. Oversedation can increase the risk of this deadly complication since a reasonably alert patient can complain of overdistention and mechanical scope trauma. The rate of perforation increases with the size of any resected lesion and the amount of cautery used. Large lesions should prompt consideration of staged, partial resections. Miscellaneous causes of perforation include overzealous dilation of strictures, excessive laser ablation, and inappropriate use of biopsy instruments. Manipulations should occur under visual control at all times while using patience and caution.

b.  **Recognition and management**. Any departure from a smooth and uneventful colonoscopy should raise concern for a possible perforation. This complication is particularly of concern when the patient awakens with unexpected discomfort. Escalating pain is a very worrisome sign, and should prompt urgent evaluation, including abdominal radiographs. An elevated temperature, tachycardia, and/or a leukocytosis increase concerns. At the first suspicion of perforation, broad-spectrum antibiotics and fluid resuscitation should be considered. Upright chest X-ray and left lateral decubitis films are indicated to detect free intra-abdominal air. Computed tomography (CT) is more sensitive but also more costly and probably less rapidly available. The diagnostic modality selected [laparoscopy, CT, or other means of diagnosis (e.g., contrast enemas if CT is not available) should be tailored based on planned therapy for each finding. For example, if a "confined leak" will be treated expectantly, then CT scan may be indicated. Likewise, if the results of laparoscopic diagnosis or treatment are not trusted, one should not utilize laparoscopy for this situation. Intraperitoneal air is absent in about 12% of perforations. In selected patients, early suspicion and the absence of free air on plain radiographs may allow expectant management with broad-spectrum antibiotics. Delayed recognition and gross soilage requires a diverting colostomy and washout of the abdomen (note: consider laparoscopy). Of note, patients who are "poor surgical candidates" are those who are least likely to survive continued fecal soilage.

## 3. Infection

a.  **Causes and prevention**. While transmission of infectious material from one patient to another via colonoscopic equipment is possible, this event is fortunately quite rare. Proper attention to scope preparation, especially the mechanical scrubbing of all ports, channels, and instruments, is essential. Standard soaking protocols should be understood by all personnel and routinely used. Colonoscopy can and does produce a transient bacteremia; thus, antibiotic prophylaxis is indicated for patients with vascular prostheses or valvular abnormalities.

b.    **Recognition and management**. Delayed presentation of vague or confusing symptoms following colonoscopy should prompt a careful history, physical examination, and review of symptoms. Awareness of this possible iatrogenic complication will facilitate appropriate recognition and management.

## 4. Missed diagnosis

a.    **Causes and prevention**. Failure to diagnose an existing condition that warrants prompt treatment is a serious complication of colonoscopy. Inadequate bowel prep can certainly obscure significant colon and rectal neoplasia. This concern is particularly relevant in the three anatomic "silent areas" of the colon: the cecum, the most distal rectum, and the splenic flexure. A complete colonoscopic examination should always include examination of the cecum, which cannot be adequately visualized in up to 5–10% of cases. During colonoscopy, cecal intubation is usually assured when three of the following criteria are met: (1) transillumination of the cecum in the right lower abdomen, (2) convergence of the cecal haustra, (3) identification of the appendiceal lumen, (4) identification and/or cannulation of the terminal ileum, (5) clear recognition of the palpating hand in the right lower abdomen, or (6) the normal progression of intraluminal landmarks (e.g., hepatic flexure and capacious cecum). If doubt persists, fluoroscopy will confirm the colonoscope's exact location. Careful technique, including meticulous inspection of all potential blind spots as well as a retroflexed view of the anodermal junction, will minimize the chance of a missed lesion. If the preparation of the bowel is inadequate, thorough washing/irrigation of the retained feces should be attempted via the colonoscope. If the visual inspection remains incomplete, then a second exam with a more vigorous preparation is indicated at a later date.

b.    **Recognition and management**. Faulty judgment and pride can preclude recognition of an incomplete colonoscopy. Unless complications ensue, if a full diagnostic colonoscopy was initially indicated, then a full screening examination must be accomplished. If necessary, repeat colonoscopy and/or double-contrast barium enema should be scheduled. Alternatively, radiology colleagues should be approached to perform an "add-on" barium enema exam on the same day as the incomplete colonoscopy, thus sparing the patient a repeat bowel prep.

## 5. Lost specimens

a. **Causes and prevention**. Specimen retrieval may prove difficult at times, especially following snare polypectomy of small polyps. Careful cleansing of surrounding feces **prior** to polypectomy and optimal patient positioning (e.g., rolling the patient on their side, abdomen, or back) may prevent many frustrating situations.

b. **Recognition and management**. If a specimen is not initially retrieved, a series of maneuvers can be employed. Using an in-line suction trap, all debris and fecal material should be removed with suction when attempting to recover small lost specimens. Once the small polyp is found, it can often be immobilized at the suction port, allowing retrieval by removing the scope while applying constant suction. If the specimen is still not found upon scope removal, the suction trap should be carefully inspected and the endoscope's suction port should be probed. If the specimen remains lost, the diagnostic colonoscopy should be repeated. As a last resort, the patient should be instructed to use a collection "seat" on the home toilet and to screen all fecal matter over the next 2 days. Clearly, the best hope of retrieving a lost specimen rests with the diligent efforts of an experienced endoscopist.

## 6. Complications of endoscopic hemorrhoid ligation

a. **Pain**
   i. **Cause and prevention**. Pain is the most common complication of endoscopic hemorrhoidal ligation and usually indicates that the ligation site was too close to the dentate line.
   ii. **Recognition and management**. If severe pain occurs immediately following endoscopic ligation,

an anoscope may be inserted and the elastic band divided and removed with a pointed scissors. Repeat endoscopic ligation can then be performed at a more cephalad site if the patient is willing.

b. **Bleeding**. The patient should be advised to expect limited bleeding 3–6 days after endoscopic hemorrhoidal ligation treatment. Band breakage or dislodgment in the first 24–48 h can result in significant (>100 mL) bleeding; rarely, repeat banding or suture ligation via an anoscope may be required to control bleeding.

c. **Thrombosis of external hemorrhoids** occasionally follows band ligation of internal hemorrhoids. Most cases can be managed conservatively with sitz baths and analgesics.

d. **Pelvic sepsis**

   i. **Cause and prevention**. This **very** rare complication of hemorrhoidal band ligation has been reported most frequently in younger males and may be devastating. No specific preventive measures have been identified.

   ii. **Recognition and management**. The typical patient develops perineal pain, swelling, inability to urinate, and may be found to have cellulitis, perineal ulceration, or gangrene. These symptoms mandate hospital admission, urgent computed tomography of the pelvis (to rule out other pathology), intravenous antibiotics, examination under anesthesia, and possibly perineal debridement and colostomy. This complication has only been reported in a small number of cases. It may be wise to inform patients of both the symptoms associated with this complication as well as its rarity when obtaining informed consent.

## Selected References

Ballantyne GH. Review of sigmoid volvulus: history and results of treatment. Dis Colon Rectum. 1982;25:494–501.

Ballantyne GH, Brandner MD, Beart Jr RW, Ilstrup DM. Volvulus of the colon: incidence and mortality. Ann Surg. 1985;202:830–92.

Bat L, Melzer E, Koler M, Dreznick Z, Shemesh E. Complications of rubber band ligation of symptomatic internal hemorrhoids. Dis Colon Rectum. 1993;36:287–90.

Berkelhammer C, Moosvi SB. Retroflexed endoscopic band ligation of internal hemor-rhoids. Gastrointest Endosc. 2002;55(4):532–7.

Branum GB, Fink AS. Ogilvie's syndrome. In: Cameron JL, editor. Current surgical ther-apy. 6th ed. St Louis: CV Mosby-Year-Book; 1997.

Brothers TE, Strodel WE, Eckhauser FE. Endoscopy in colonic volvulus. Ann Surg. 1987;206:1–4.

Draganov PV. Colonoscopic polypectomy and associated techniques. World J Gastroenterol. 2010;16:3630–7.

Geller A, Petersen BT, Gostout CJ. Endoscopic decompression for acute colonic pseu-doobstruction. Gastrointest Endosc. 1996;44:144–50.

Jetmore AB, Timmcke AE, Gathright JB, et al. Ogilvie's syndrome: colonoscopic decom-pression and analysis of predisposing factors. Dis Colon Rectum. 1995;35:1135–42.

Komborozos VA, Skrekas GJ, Pissiotis CA. Rubber band ligation of symptomatic internal hemorrhoids: results of 500 cases. Dig Surg. 2000;17(1):1–6.

MacRae HM, McLeod RS. Comparison of hemorrhoidal treatment modalities. A meta-analysis. Dis Colon Rectum. 1995;38:687–94.

McCloud JM, Jameson JS, Scott AN. Life-threatening sepsis following treatment for hem-orrhoids: a systematic review. Colorectal Dis. 2006;8:748–55.

Rex DK. Colonoscopy and acute colonic pseudo-obstruction. Gastrointest Endosc Clin North Am. 1997;7(3):499–508.

Saunders MD. Acute colonic pseudo-obstruction. Gastrointest Endosc Clin North Am. 2007;17:341–60.

Smith CD, Fink AS. The management of colonic volvulus. In: Cameron JL, editor. Current surgical therapy. 6th ed. St Louis: CV Mosby-Year-Book; 1997.

Tolliver KA, Rex DK. Colonoscopic polypectomy. Gastroenterol Clin N Am. 2008;37:229–51.

# Appendix

SAGES issues and periodically revises *guidelines, position papers, patient information brochures*, and other materials on a variety of subjects related to endoscopy, laparoscopy, and education. Documents may be viewed or downloaded from the Internet at www.sages.org. Some videos are available free, others are available for purchase. This partial list includes materials available on October 27, 2011. Materials are constantly being added, so the reader is urged to bookmark the SAGES Web site and consult it frequently.

## A. Practice/Clinical Guidelines www.sages.org/publications/guidelines/guidelines.php

1. Guidelines for the Surgical Treatment of Esophageal Achalasia.
2. Guidelines for Diagnosis, Treatment, and Use of Laparoscopy for Surgical Problems during Pregnancy.
3. Guidelines for Surgical Treatment of Gastroesophageal Reflux Disease (GERD).
4. Guidelines for the Clinical Application of Laparoscopic Biliary Tract Surgery.
5. Guidelines for Laparoscopic Appendectomy.
6. Guidelines for Office Endoscopic Services.
7. Guidelines for Clinical Application of Laparoscopic Bariatric Surgery.
8. Guidelines for Diagnostic Laparoscopy.
9. Guidelines for Deppe Venous Thrombosis Prophylaxis During Laparoscopic Surgery.
10. Guidelines for Laparoscopic Resection of Curable Colon and Rectal Cancer.
11. Guidelines for the Surgical Practice of Telemedicine.

N.J. Soper and C.E.H. Scott-Conner (eds.), *The SAGES Manual: Volume 1 Basic Laparoscopy and Endoscopy*, DOI 10.1007/978-1-4614-2344-7, © Springer Science+Business Media, LLC 2012

# B.  Privileging Guidelines

1. Guidelines for Granting of Ultrasonography Privileges for Surgeons.
2. Guidelines for Institutions Granting Privileges Utilizing Laparoscopic and/or Thoracoscopic Techniques.
3. Guidelines for Institutions Granting Bariatric Privileges Utilizing Laparoscopic Techniques.
4. Granting of Privileges for Gastrointestinal Endoscopy.

# C.  Training Guidelines

1. Framework for Post-residency Surgical Education and Training.
2. Guidelines for Training in Diagnostic and Therapeutic Endoscopic Retrograde Cholangiopancreatography (ERCP).

# D.  Additional Materials

1. SAGES Laparoscopy Troubleshooting Chart.
2. SAGES/AORN MIS Checklist.
3. Position Papers/Statements.
4. Outlines for Education.
5. Implementation Manual for the World Health Organization Surgical Safety Checklist.

# E.  Patient Information Brochures (Selected Brochures Are Also Available in Spanish, French, Polish, and Vietnamese) www.sages.org/publications/patient_information/

1. Patient Information for Laparoscopic Anti-Reflux (GERD) Surgery from SAGES.
2. Patient Information for Upper Endoscopy from SAGES.

3. Patient Information for Laparoscopic Surgery for Severe Obesity from SAGES.

4. Patient Information for Laparoscopic Adrenal Gland Removal (Adrenalectomy) from SAGES.

5. Patient Information for Laparoscopic Spleen Removal (Splenectomy) from SAGES.

6. Patient Information for Laparoscopic Gall Bladder Removal (Cholecystectomy) from SAGES.

7. Patient Information for Laparoscopic Ventral Hernia Repair from SAGES.

8. Patient Information for Laparoscopic Colon Resection from SAGES.

9. Patient Information for Laparoscopic Appendectomy from SAGES.

10. Patient Information for Laparoscopic Spine Surgery from SAGES.

11. Patient Information for ERCP (Endoscopic Retrograde Cholangiopancreatography) from SAGES.

12. Patient Information for Laparoscopic Inguinal Hernia Repair from SAGES.

13. Patient Information for Flexible Sigmoidoscopy from SAGES.

# F. Other Educational Materials Listed at www. sages.org/education/index.php

1. The entire SAGES Educational Video Library is now freely accessible to any interested party at www.sages.org/video.

2. The Fundamentals of Laparoscopic Surgery is a comprehensive Web-based education module that includes hands-on basic skill training. Information is available at: www. flsprogram.org.

3. SAGES Grand Rounds provides a Grand Rounds style in-depth discussion of a selected topic by experts in the field.

4. SAGES Pearls breaks selected procedures down into core steps (video).

5. Top 21 Procedures Every Surgeon Should Know is a collection of videos.

# Index